Frailty in Children

Mario Lima • Maria Cristina Mondardini
Editors

Frailty in Children

From the Perioperative Management to the Multidisciplinary Approach

Springer

Editors
Mario Lima
Pediatric Surgery Unit
Sant'Orsola Hospital IRCCS
University of Bologna
Bologna, Italy

Maria Cristina Mondardini
Pediatric Intensive Care Unit
Sant'Orsola Hospital IRCCS
University of Bologna
Bologna, Italy

ISBN 978-3-031-24306-6 ISBN 978-3-031-24307-3 (eBook)
https://doi.org/10.1007/978-3-031-24307-3

This Springer imprint is published by the registered company Springer Nature Switzerland AG
The registered company address is: Gewerbestrasse 11, 6330 Cham, Switzerland

Foreword

The Oxford Dictionary defines the noun "frailty" as "weakness or poor health" and the adjective "frail" as "physically weak and thin" or "easily damaged or broken."

Surgeons deal every day with frail individuals either because the surgical disease itself is endangering their health status and/or (more often) because, in addition to the current disease, they may have comorbidities. An aging patient with intestinal obstruction has a serious problem, but if this happens in association with diabetes, coronary insufficiency, and emphysema, the problem becomes very serious. Except in emergency situations, elective surgery is delayed until the comorbidities are more or less under control, and this is why pre-operative tests and anesthetic consultations are mandatory.

Pediatric surgeons are not different from adult surgeons in this respect, and they have also to deal with similar situations although the age and the nature of comorbidities are usually different. In the core of the specialty the complexity of the situation may be extreme while performing surgery for newborns: A 900 g baby with respiratory distress syndrome, an open ductus, and stage 3 necrotizing enterocolitis is a very "frail" patient. The skin barrier is weak, immunity is developing, the g.i. tract is in the process of establishing a symbiotic flora, the lung is immature, and so are the clotting mechanisms and the brain. But prematurity is not the only dangerous comorbidity. A 3000 g term baby with left CDH, associated congenital heart disease, pulmonary insufficiency, and hypertension requiring ECMO may have more mature functions than a premature but shares the same extreme frailty. This could be extended to other surgical situations beyond the neonatal period. In addition, in a number of these clinical conditions there is no chance for "elective" surgery.

If I look back at my career as a pediatric surgeon extended along more than 50 years, I realize that these issues have become more and more complicated with the passage of time. When I was a trainee, almost half the patients with esophageal atresia died and so did the majority of babies with congenital diaphragmatic hernia or Wilms' tumor. Ventilation in newborns was at its beginnings, total parenteral nutrition was not yet available, and many of the supporting drugs currently used were not in the market. Survival of newborns below 1000 or even 1500 g was rare and our "frail" patients were the tip of the iceberg. Rapid progress made the iceberg emerge and it grew more and more until producing many of these cases that nowadays constitute a large share of our activity. We succeeded in improving survival and functional results but, frankly, at the expense of a much more complex specialty.

This is why this book on frailty is timely and appealing. Moreover, the editors, Mario Lima and Maria Cristina Mondardini, authors of a number of acknowledged books on various aspects of our specialty, planned a comprehensive coverage of the subject and recruited a set of first-class authors for different chapters.

The book is structured in five parts: After an introduction, the frailty of the newborn is covered extensively. The next parts analyze the multiple comorbidities that may cause additional frailty, the various actions pointed to improving therapeutic actions in this context, and the need for social support, continuity of care, and transition to adult care of these individuals that may require follow-up and support for life.

I predict that this volume will have great success and that many of us will be illuminated by this comprehensive view of the growing intricacies of our surgical activity.

Juan A. Tovar

Department of Pediatric Surgery,
Hospital Universitario La Paz
Madrid Spain

Emeritus Professor of Pediatrics,
Universidad Autonoma de Madrid
Madrid Spain

Contents

Part IV Operational Improvement Strategies

Part V Conclusions

Part I

Introductory Aspects

Frailty in Pediatrics: Definition and Care Needs

1

Franca Benini, Luca Maria Antoniello, and Miriam Duci

Abbreviations

AIDS	Acquired immune deficiency syndrome
CP	Cerebral palsy
ESPGHAN	European Society for Pediatric Gastroenterology Hepatology and Nutrition
GERD	Gastro-esophageal reflux disease
OS	Orthopedic surgery

1.1 Definition of Frailty in Pediatrics

The term "frailty" in the pediatric setting describes a state of increased health vulnerability with an increased risk of death, in particular with regard to children with life-threatening, life-limiting, or terminal conditions [1, 2]. In these patients, the condition of frailty is due to a multi-system physiological impairment, including neurological, endocrine, immune, and skeletal muscle failures. This leads to major and complex clinical needs, with great impairment of quality of life [3, 4].

In the last years, a novel conceptualization of frailty and complex care was provided. In the pediatric setting, complex care is now intended to comprise health and social needs in response to a recognized medical condition or for patients with undefined diagnosis [1].

This broader definition, which also considers the social sphere, implies that an adequate healthcare plan should be defined to promote physical growth and cognitive, emotional, and social development, especially if the intervention plan lasts for years. In this scenario, each clinical intervention must be decided taking into account the child's global well-being. In this perspective, the decision of "not doing," i.e., avoiding any intervention, should always be considered.

In particular, the importance of "not doing" concerns also a subgroup of frail children, namely, those requiring surgery. Examples vary and include children with congenital or acquired multiorgan disease, metabolic disorders, severe neurological conditions with marked functional impairment and patients with cancer/cancer survivors with residual disability. Awareness of frailty and associated risks for adverse health outcomes improves care and perioperative management for these vulnerable patients. Specific

F. Benini (✉)
Paediatric Palliative Care, Pain Service, Women's and Children's Health Department, University of Padua, Padua, Italy
e-mail: franca.benini@aopd.veneto.it

L. M. Antoniello · M. Duci
Paediatric Surgery Unit, Women's and Children's Health Department, University of Padua, Padua, Italy
e-mail: lucamaria.antoniello@aopd.veneto.it

M. Lima, M. C. Mondardini (eds.), *Frailty in Children*,
https://doi.org/10.1007/978-3-031-24307-3_1

guidelines should be defined and applied to ensure the best quality of care.

1.2 High Complexity of Frail Pediatric Patients: The Multidisciplinary Coordinated Approach as a Model of Care

Frail children require additional care and related services compared with children of the same age [2, 5].

The spectrum of illnesses that contribute to a frailty condition is wide and heterogeneous [6]. As mentioned above, these include neurological, muscular, oncological, respiratory, cardiological, and metabolic disorders, as well as syndromes, malformations, infections, and postanoxic conditions, with nononcological disease accounting for the wide majority of cases (cancer only accounts for 4.1%) [2, 6, 7].

Remarkably, children with human immunodeficiency virus (HIV)/acquired immunodeficiency syndrome (AIDS) living in low- to middle-income countries and those with congenital diseases living in high-income countries account for about half of the total number of frail children, followed by children with extreme prematurity and birth trauma and those with neurological conditions [7–9].

To further complicate this scenario, several frail children also lack a definite diagnosis: for them, it is important to define the extent of frailty and associated risks.

The variety in terms of age groups of frail children leads to a great heterogeneity of needs. Due to the discrepancy between chronological and biological age, they continue to have basic needs typical of early childhood (e.g., assistance in nutrition and daily hygiene) [10, 11].

Furthermore, the communication needs of both families and patients have to be considered when managing frail children. Parents or legal guardians must receive timely, detailed, and immediate information about the child's clinical condition and prognosis in an adequate and safe setting. They should also be informed about the benefits and limitations of the proposed interventions, and they should always be invited to participate in the decision-making process [12–14]. Especially when considering surgery, the intervention must be intended as a part of a shared healthcare plan, with goals beyond the immediate benefit of the surgery itself. Healthcare providers must investigate the family's actual level of understanding of the illness and prognosis and adapt communication accordingly. In addition, parents must be supported and guided to actively listen and respond to their child's concerns and feelings.

To face this great variety of care needs, a coordinated multidisciplinary approach represents the best model of care. Indeed, a multidisciplinary team possesses sufficient skills and abilities to support decision-making and respond to the variety of physical, psychological, emotional, and practical needs of the children and families [15, 16]. In addition, a competent multidisciplinary team should be able to coordinate the interventions of various players in the context of a comprehensive and mutually agreed plan of care [17].

Care at home is generally desired both by the child (as it allows him/her to live a normal daily life) and by the families (as it reduces physical and psychological discomfort and is economically advantageous). Home care ensures that the frail child is cared for in a family environment without the added distress of a less familiar and friendly environment, such as a hospital or hospice.

Frail children may require life-supporting devices. In this case, the multidisciplinary team should be able to support family members in training on their use, on the management of potential emergencies, and on how best to reorganize their house [18–20].

1.3 Surgical Interventions in Frail Children

Three main types of surgical interventions related to a condition of pediatric frailty can be identified: (1) surgery aimed at restoring a physiological function (e.g., gastrointestinal, orthopedic interventions), (2) surgery aimed at correcting malformations related to the underlying pathology, and (3) surgery aimed at symptom control (e.g., hip dislocation). Some examples are provided below.

One of the most common problems in frail children is feeding difficulties, which lead to growth failure and malnutrition. This impairment is due to neurological disorders and motor/mental impairments [21]. When dietary supplementation fails, gastrostomy placement needs to be considered to provide nutritional support and reduce hunger sensation. A noticeable improvement in the quality of life of caregivers in terms of time dedicated to medical maneuvers was also shown [22]. In neurologically impaired children, feeding difficulties are often associated with gastroesophageal reflux disease (GERD), with a prevalence between 14 and 7%, depending on the diagnostic criteria [23–25]. According to the European Society for Pediatric Gastroenterology Hepatology and Nutrition (ESPGHAN) guidelines, fundoplication should be considered in cases of failure of optimized medical therapy [26].

Some frail children with airway obstruction or neurological conditions might benefit from tracheostomy. Children with tracheostomy are among the most complicated patients, and they need multidisciplinary management by pulmonologists, pediatricians, otorhinolaryngologists, and pediatric surgeons for proper care and better outcome, given also the severe burden on families and caregivers [27].

Moreover, some patients presenting with dystonia/spasticity and/or chronic pain, which severely impact their quality of life, can benefit from an implantable baclofen pump [28]. Although the use of intrathecal pumps has been well described [29], the risk of device extrusion and infection needs to be considered. Therefore, the placement of pumps in the submuscular plane of the abdominal wall may provide a well vascularized and stable environment for this device, minimizing the risks related to displacement and infection [30].

In selected cases, such as patients with cerebral palsy (CP), orthopedic surgery (OS) plays an important role [31]. The main objectives of OS are to optimize function and prevent deformity. The most common procedures are the use of external fixators, orthopedic selective spasticity control surgery, and arm restoration, which lead to significant improvements in motor function. For instance, tenotomies of adductor longus and brevis are easy procedures and can improve the home caring of patients with spastic diplegia and hip and knee contractures. However, a less than optimal OS, performed without the support of the multidisciplinary medical and rehabilitation team, often leads to significant functional worsening of patients, including the loss of previous ambulatory capacity, as well as to increased burden for caregivers [32].

The biopsychosocial consequences of all the aforementioned procedures are profound. Therefore, in some cases, "not doing" is the best choice not only for patients but also for the caregivers. Indeed, carrying out medical procedures for the children as well as daily hygiene can become burdensome and stressful for parents. This burden can lead to fatigue, depression, and social isolation [33].

To provide a practical example that summarizes the above concepts, we report a description of a complex case in which multidisciplinary collaboration and effective and appropriate communication played an important role.

1.4 Multidisciplinary Collaboration for the Management of a Frail Child: A Case Report

A girl affected by neurological impairment due to perinatal asphyxia was admitted to our hospital for a 10-day history of abdominal pain and progressive feeding problems. Her mother was a single parent looking after her daughter. An abdominal X-ray revealed free air in the abdomen, and she therefore underwent exploratory laparotomy, and a colic perforation was found. Due to the extremely distended intestine, we decided to perform an ileostomy. During the postoperative course, we had to manage the enteral feeding problems that had already been present for around 1 year, associated with malnutrition signs.

We discussed with the family the need for gastrostomy (already rejected by the family) to allow the patient to gain weight and reduce hunger sensation. Initially, the mother disagreed with this medical decision as she wanted to continue to feed her per os, but after appropriate communication, we shared a common strategy, proper for that specific situation, in a multidisciplinary scenario in which the pediatric surgeon, pediatrician, dietician, anesthetist, and palliative physician were involved. We explained that gastrostomy was a good choice since this device did not exclude the possibility of continuing to feed her daughter per os. We performed a further percutaneous endoscopic gastrostomy.

The next step would be the closure of the ileostomy, but we decided not to perform that. Indeed, listening to the girl's family, we found out that ileostomy management was easier than continuous bowel irrigations for her constipation. Changing the bag and washing the stomy became quicker and less painful; therefore, we preferred not to perform another surgery. Furthermore, the risk of new episodes of subocclusion was less likely to happen with the stomy.

After 6 months, the mother was really satisfied with this shared therapeutical decision, and the girl was in good health.

This case shows that the management goals of these children are to improve the quality of life for both the child and their family, and sometimes, the better choice is "not doing."

1.5 Best Practice in the Field

Despite the fact that a broad conceptual definition of medical complexity exists, precise operational definitions are still critical and remain not fully defined [34]. Nevertheless, some best practices can be identified in the management of frail pediatric patients.

The first involves the analysis of the patient's needs based on a careful examination of the patient's history and his/her illness, family environment, thoughts, desires, and beliefs, when this is possible, according to age and situation. The collection of information related to his/her family, social role, culture, and religious belief is also crucial.

The interdisciplinary team plays a major role in sharing with the patient's family all the risk and benefit assessments of any possible therapeutic choice. This helps maintain the "right perspective." According to the situation, it allows healthcare providers to ensure tailored care for the child and his/her family in a correct balance between what science proposes and the actual viability of interventions. In this perspective, the term "health" is intended in its global meaning and not limited to the control of a symptom and/or the recovery of the organ/system function. This must influence all choices and decisions and must change the perspective of "doing everything technically possible" to "doing everything that the situation requires, maintaining a good quality of life."

It is important to leave the patient and family with the opportunity to evaluate the choices of the interdisciplinary team, giving them time to ask, express doubts, and propose, if useful, the willingness to seek a second opinion. The patient and family have the right to competent and honest communication to base their choices. The child's unalienable right is to express his/her opinion, which (according to age and degree of maturity) must always be taken into consideration and must guide choices and strategies in some situations. Parents must be listened to in their doubts and requests and must be accepted in their perplexities, beliefs, and anger, in a dynamic exchange, where competence, time, respect, and mediation skills are the most effective tools. However, involvement in selecting any specific medical treatment cannot be considered a complete decision-making responsibility, which remains, albeit in a continuous sharing, a medical choice. It is certainly not easy, but if supported and honestly informed, family members actively participate in the health choices for their child and can also accept the limit of "not doing," transforming this limit into a new "possibility."

These communications and choices become much easier and less burdensome when, in the course of the disease, clinicians have already faced the problem of the achievable goals of care and when a shared advanced care plan (ACP) is already defined with clear and honest goals. The preparation of an ACP is a key tool in the correct management of pediatric complexity [10]. The defined care program (intervention or nonintervention) must be implemented by providing the maximum competence, time, and willingness to communicate.

Home care must be arranged by sharing the clinical and/or psychological/organizational situation of the patient and family with the healthcare providers and the territorial team (PPC when available) and remaining open to discussing any new need.

Finally, shared monitoring of situations must be implemented, with the aim of preventing problems and managing needs.

The implementation of the aforementioned practices is not always easy; sometimes it clashes with a consolidated culture and practice, but training, information, and research supported by the increasingly available specific regulations and instruments, also for this category of patients, are the basis for dealing with these frequent and sometimes very tiring situations with greater competence.

References

1. Brenner M, Kidston C, Hilliard C, Coyne I, Eustace-Cook J, Doyle C, Begley T, Barrett MJ. Children's complex care needs: a systematic concept analysis of multidisciplinary language. Eur J Pediatr. 2018;177(11):1641–52.
2. Gallo M, Agostiniani R, Pintus R, Fanos V. The child with medical complexity. Ital J Pediatr. 2021;47(1):1–7.
3. Calcaterra V, Cena H, Ruggieri A, Zuccotti G, De Silvestri A, Bonalumi G, Pelizzo G. Metabolically unhealthy phenotype: a key factor in determining "pediatric" frailty. Pediatr Rep. 2021;13(3):340–6.
4. Feng Z, Lugtenberg M, Franse C, Fang X, Hu S, Jin C, Raat H. Risk factors and protective factors associated with incident or increase of frailty among community-dwelling older adults: a systematic review of longitudinal studies. PLoS One. 2017;12(6):e0178383.
5. Benini F, Pappadatou D, Bernadá M, Craig F, De Zen L, Downing J, Drake R, Freidrichsdorf S, Garros D, Giacomelli L, Lacerda A. International standards for pediatric palliative care: from IMPaCCT to GO-PPaCS. J Pain Symptom Manag. 2022;63:e529–43.
6. Jankovic M, De Zen L, Pellegatta F, Lazzarin P, Bertolotti M, Manfredini L, Aprea A, Memo L, Del Vecchio A, Agostiniani R, Benini F. A consensus conference report on defining the eligibility criteria for pediatric palliative care in Italy. Ital J Pediatr. 2019;45(1):1–5.
7. Connor JA, LaGrasta C, Porter C, Hurtig M, McHugh S, King E, Atkinson C, Hickey PA. The measurement of pediatric inpatient nursing using the complexity assessment and monitoring to ensure optimal outcomes (CAMEO©) tool. J Pediatr Nurs. 2020;51:42–8.
8. Connor SR, Downing J, Marston J. Estimating the global need for palliative care for children: a cross-sectional analysis. J Pain Symptom Manag. 2017;53(2):171–7.
9. Fraser LK, Bluebond-Langner M, Ling J. Advances and challenges in European paediatric palliative care. Med Sci. 2020;8(2):20.
10. DeCourcey DD, Silverman M, Oladunjoye A, Wolfe J. Advance care planning and parent-reported end-of-life outcomes in children, adolescents, and young adults with complex chronic conditions. Crit Care Med. 2019;47(1):101–8.
11. Noyes J, Pritchard S, Pritchard A, Bennett V, Rees S. Conflicting realities experienced by children with life-limiting and life-threatening conditions when transitioning to adult health services. J Adv Nurs. 2018;74(12):2871–81.
12. Verberne LM, Fahner JC, Sondaal SFV, Schouten-van Meeteren AYN, de Kruiff CC, van Delden JJM, Kars MC. Anticipating the future of the child and family in pediatric palliative care: a qualitative study into the perspectives of parents and healthcare professionals. Eur J Pediatr. 2021;180(3):949–57.
13. Bluebond-Langner M, Hargrave D, Henderson EM, Langner R. 'I have to live with the decisions I make': laying a foundation for decision making for children with life-limiting conditions and life-threatening illnesses. Arch Dis Child. 2017;102(5):468–71.
14. Papadatou D, Kalliani V, Karakosta E, Liakopoulou P, Bluebond-Langner M. Home or hospital as the place of end-of-life care and death: a grounded theory study of parents' decision-making. Palliat Med. 2021;35(1):219–30.
15. Weaver MS, Rosenberg AR, Tager J, Wichman CS, Wiener L. A summary of pediatric palliative care team structure and services as reported by centers caring for children with cancer. J Palliat Med. 2018;21(4):452–62.
16. Taylor J, Aldridge J. Exploring the rewards and challenges of paediatric palliative care work—a qualitative study of a multi-disciplinary children's hospice care team. BMC Palliat Care. 2017;16(1):73.

17. Friedrichsdorf SJ, Remke S, Hauser J, Foster L, Postier A, Kolste A, Wolfe J. Development of a pediatric palliative care curriculum and dissemination model: education in palliative and end-of-life care (EPEC) pediatrics. J Pain Symp Manag. 2019;58(4):707–720.e3.
18. Lazzarin P, Schiavon B, Brugnaro L, Benini F. Parents spend an average of nine hours a day providing palliative care for children at home and need to maintain an average of five life-saving devices. Acta Paediatr. 2018;107(2):289–93.
19. Kuhn E, Schalley S, Potthoff M, Weaver MS. The arc of generational care: a case series considering grandparent roles and care needs in pediatric palliative care. J Soc Work End Life Palliat Care. 2019;15(2–3):99–110.
20. Pandian V, Garg V, Antar R, Best S. Discharge education and caregiver coping of pediatric patients with a tracheostomy: systematic review. ORL Head Neck Nurs. 2016;34(1):17–8.
21. Vernon-Roberts A, Sullivan PB. Fundoplication versus post-operative medication for gastro-oesophageal reflux in children with neurological impairment undergoing gastrostomy. Cochrane Database Syst Rev. 2007;1:CD006151.
22. Sullivan PB, Juszczak E, Bachlet AM, Thomas AG, Lambert B, Vernon-Roberts A, Grant HW, Eltumi M, Alder N, Jenkinson C. Impact of gastrostomy tube feeding on the quality of life of carers of children with cerebral palsy. Dev Med Child Neurol. 2004;46(12):796–800.
23. Sullivan PB. Gastrostomy and the disabled child. Dev Med Child Neurol. 1992;34(6):552–5.
24. Reyes J, Tzakis AG, Todo S, Nour B, Starzl TE. Small bowel and liver/small bowel transplantation in children. Semin Pediatr Surg. 1993;2(4):289.
25. Gangil A, Patwari AK, Bajaj P, Kashyap R, Anand VK. Gastroesophageal reflux disease in children with cerebral palsy. Indian Pediatr. 2001;38(7):766–70.
26. Romano C, Van Wynckel M, Hulst J, Broekaert I, Bronsky J, Dall'Oglio L, Mis NF, Hojsak I, Orel R, Papadopoulou A, Schaeppi M. European Society for Paediatric Gastroenterology, Hepatology and Nutrition guidelines for the evaluation and treatment of gastrointestinal and nutritional complications in children with neurological impairment. J Pediatr Gastroenterol Nutr. 2017;65(2):242–64.
27. Chandran A, Sikka K, Thakar A, Lodha R, Irugu DV, Kumar R, Sharma SC. The impact of pediatric tracheostomy on the quality of life of caregivers. Int J Pediatr Otorhinolaryngol. 2021;149:110854.
28. Woolf SM, Baum CR. Baclofen pumps: uses and complications. Pediatr Emerg Care. 2017;33(4):271–5.
29. Lake W, Shah H. Intrathecal baclofen infusion for the treatment of movement disorders. Neurosurg Clin. 2019;30(2):203–9.
30. Bogue JT, Wald G, Iosim S, Greenfield JP, Otterburn DM. Submuscular placement of baclofen infusion pumps: case series and technique. Ann Plast Surg. 2020;85(S1):S8–11.
31. Nahm NJ, Graham HK, Gormley ME Jr, Georgiadis AG. Management of hypertonia in cerebral palsy. Curr Opin Pediatr. 2018;30(1):57–64.
32. Sharan D. Orthopedic surgery in cerebral palsy: instructional course lecture. Indian J Orthop. 2017;51(3):240–55.
33. Caicedo C. Families with special needs children: family health, functioning, and care burden. J Am Psychiatr Nurses Assoc. 2014;20(6):398–407.
34. Berry JG, Hall M, Cohen E, O'Neill M, Feudtner C. Ways to identify children with medical complexity and the importance of why. J Pediatr. 2015;167(2):229–37.

Part II

Frail Newborn Infants

Premature Infants

2

Silvia Martini and Luigi Corvaglia

Abbreviations

AGA	Adequate for gestational age
AREDF	Absent or reversed end-diastolic flow
BPD	Bronchopulmonary dysplasia
BSID	Bayley Scales of Infant Development
BW	Birth weight
CBF	Cerebral blood flow
CHDs	Congenital heart defects
COX	Cyclooxygenase
CP	Cerebral palsy
CPAP	Continuous positive airway pressure
CRP	C-Reactive protein
DA	Ductus arteriosus
ELBW	Extremely low birth weight
FiO_2	Fractional inspired oxygen
GA	Gestational age
IUGR	Intrauterine growth restriction
IVF	In vitro fertilization
IVH	Intraventricular hemorrhage
LBW	Low birth weight
LGA	Large for gestational age
LISA	Less invasive surfactant administration
NEC	Necrotizing enterocolitis
NICU	Neonatal intensive care unit
NSAIDs	Nonsteroidal anti-inflammatory drugs
PCA	Postconceptional age
PDA	Patent ductus arteriosus
PH	Pulmonary hemorrhage
PHI	Parenchymal hemorrhagic infarction
PHVD	Posthemorrhagic ventricular dilatation
PROM	Premature rupture of membranes
PVL	Periventricular leukomalacia
PVR	Pulmonary vascular resistance
RDS	Respiratory distress syndrome
ROP	Retinopathy of prematurity
SGA	Small for gestational age
VEGF	Vascular endothelial growth factor
VLBW	Very low birth weight

S. Martini (✉) · L. Corvaglia
Neonatal Intensive Care Unit, IRCCS Azienda Ospedaliero-Universitaria di Bologna, Bologna, Italy
e-mail: silvia.martini9@unibo.it; luigi.corvaglia@unibo.it

2.1 Preterm Birth

2.1.1 Epidemiology

Preterm birth is defined as a delivery occurring before 37 completed weeks' gestation and represents a leading cause of neonatal and childhood mortality worldwide, accounting for 965,000 deaths in the neonatal period and an additional 125,000 deaths in the first 5 years of life.

Each year, approximately 15 million neonates are born preterm, indicating a global preterm birth rate of about 11%; of these births, nearly

M. Lima, M. C. Mondardini (eds.), *Frailty in Children*,
https://doi.org/10.1007/978-3-031-24307-3_2

85% occur between 32 and 36 weeks' gestation, 10% between 28 and 31 weeks' gestation, and the remaining 5% prior to the achievement of 28 weeks [1, 2].

The percentage of preterm deliveries has steadily risen over the last couple of decades. Advances in medical technologies and therapeutic perinatal and neonatal care have substantially improved the rates of survival among preterm infants, even at the lowest gestational ages. However, compared to full-term-born infants, the survival of preterm neonates is burdened by increased rates of short- and long-term morbidities and, in particular, neurologic and developmental impairment, which can range from major disabilities such as cerebral palsy, mental retardation, and sensory impairments to more subtle disorders like language and learning problems, attention-deficit/hyperactivity disorder, and behavioral difficulties. Hence, preterm birth is a critical global problem because of its implications for morbidity and mortality, as well as its socioeconomic liability [3].

The burden of prematurity, however, is influenced not only by the gestational age (GA), which determines the extent of the immaturity of organs and systems, but also by available health resources. As such, preterm birth rates vary significantly among different geographical regions according to their income levels, with approximately 90% of all premature births occurring in low- and middle-income settings. Except for the United States, which, with an estimated rate of 12%, is the principal contributor among developing countries, the global burden of prematurity predominantly falls on countries with fewer resources to manage the medical, social, and economic complexities of caring for preterm infants. Consistently, the survival rate of infants born before 28 weeks of GA is nearly 90% in high-income settings but falls to 10% in low-income ones [2].

2.1.2 Etiology and Risk Factors

Although the etiologic pathways underlying a preterm delivery still need to be completely clarified, a large series of well-known risk factors has been identified. These risk factors have long been distinguished between factors that cause a spontaneous onset of labor or a premature rupture of amniotic membranes and maternal or fetal conditions that represent a clinical indication for iatrogenic preterm delivery. Some clinical conditions could be considered risk factors for both spontaneous and iatrogenic preterm births. According to Stout et al. there is a substantial, but imperfect, agreement between reviewers for the classification of preterm birth into spontaneous and indicated subtypes; incorrect classification may occur 5–15% of the time, even with experienced research personnel [4]. Hence, these limitations have led to the proposal of a new classification system that considers the following maternal, fetal, and obstetrical conditions.

Maternal risk factors

- Acute and chronic diseases: these include hypertension, preeclampsia, eclampsia, diabetes, acute or chronic kidney disease, heart failure, hyperthyroidism, and infections (both bacterial and viral).
- Age: pregnancy onset prior to 16 years and after 35 years has been related to an increased risk of premature delivery.
- Body weight: both low and excessive body weight prior to pregnancy as well as inappropriate variation of weight during pregnancy are associated with an increased risk of premature labor.
- Socioeconomic and educational status: there is a tight relationship between a low maternal socioeconomic status and/or education level and preterm delivery. As an example, the rate of preterm birth in Norway was 9.7% in women with a low level of education and 5.9% in women with a high level.
- Ethnicity: beyond any predictable etiological cause of preterm birth and with the same range of risk factors, varying rates have been noticed among different ethnic groups. The relatively heterogeneous population of the United States provides a good example for this observation: in 2013, the preterm birth rate was 16.3% in non-Hispanic black women, 11.3% in Hispanic women, and only 10.2%

in non-Hispanic white women. Additionally, when considering deliveries <32 weeks, this rate was twofold higher in non-Hispanic black women compared to non-Hispanic white women. Although the reason for the significant differences in preterm birth rates between racial groups is not fully understood, a possible hypothesis is that it is related to underlying social and economic inequalities [5].

- Maternal smoking during pregnancy: this habit is a major determinant of poor pregnancy and neonatal outcomes, including preterm birth and low birth weight (LBW); in particular, more than 20% of LBW cases are related to this habit. The mechanisms through which maternal smoking leads to these adverse outcomes are related to the effects of carbon monoxide, which binds to fetal hemoglobin, causing a state of chronic fetal hypoxia, and of nicotine, which increases placental and fetal vascular resistances. Such abnormalities of placental morphology, including microscopic infarction, obstructive endarteritis as well as decidual necrosis, have been associated with cigarette smoke [6].

Fetal risk factors

- Fetal erythroblastosis: this condition, which is associated with an increased risk of preterm birth, is caused by the transplacental passage of maternal immunoglobulin G (IgG) antibodies targeting red blood cell antigens in the fetal circulation; based on the fetal blood phenotype group, these antibodies can destroy red blood cells, leading to fetal reticulocytosis, anemia, and, in the most severe cases, hydrops with subsequent circulatory failure. The various alloantigen types that can be involved include AB0, anti-RhD, anti-RhE, anti-Rhc, anti-Rhe, anti-RhC, anti-Kell, and multiantigen combinations, with anti-RhD type being the most common cause of fetal hemolysis [7].
- Intrauterine growth restriction (IUGR, also known as fetal growth restriction): this is a complex and multifactorial condition that is often associated with iatrogenic preterm delivery. Fetal growth may be restricted due to constitutional reasons (i.e., small parental build) or because of genetic abnormalities or congenital infections. However, the leading cause of IUGR is uteroplacental insufficiency, characterized by altered placental vascularization with increased resistance of the placental vessels [8]. This condition alters gas and nutrient exchanges at the placental interface, and the ensuing chronic fetal hypoxia and undernutrition are responsible for the declining growth rates. Premature delivery of IUGR fetuses may be required in the presence of hemodynamic fetal impairment secondary to the effects of persistently increased placental vascular resistances, which can be diagnosed by evidence of absent or reversed end-diastolic flow (AREDF) in the umbilical arteries of the fetus or, in the most severe cases, impaired Doppler flowmetry in the ductus venosus. In order to compensate for the reduced perfusion ensuing from uteroplacental insufficiency, a vascular redistribution of fetal blood flow often occurs in AREDF cases, aiming to preserve the perfusion and, subsequently, the development of vital organs (e.g., brain, heart, adrenal glands) at the expense of peripheral and splanchnic circulation. This adaptive response is known as the "brain-sparing reflex" and is characterized by Doppler evidence of a decreased pulsatility index of the middle cerebral artery [9]. Consequently, body growth significantly declines, whereas the cranial circumference is less impaired. In addition to this relative preservation of brain growth, some data suggest that fetuses make other adaptations to adverse intrauterine conditions, such as the acceleration of lung and brain maturation [10].
- Fetal abnormalities: congenital heart defects (CHDs), and especially right ventricular outflow tract obstructions, are associated with an increased risk of spontaneous preterm birth [11].

Obstetrical risk factors

- Multiple pregnancies: it is not only associated with delivery at lower gestational ages, but it is also an important risk factor for intrauterine growth restriction.
- In vitro fertilization (IVF): compared to naturally conceived pregnancies, IVF is associated

with a 1.78-fold increase in spontaneous preterm birth risk [12].

- Placental abruption: this rare yet serious complication occurs acutely when the placenta partly or completely detaches from the inner uterine wall before delivery, causing heavy maternal bleeding and concomitant disruption of fetal perfusion and of the subsequent oxygen and nutrient supply.
- Placental implantation abnormalities: according to a recent metanalysis, the preterm delivery rates for low-lying/marginal placenta, placenta previa, placenta accreta, vasa previa, and velamentous cord insertion are 26.9%, 43.5%, 57.7%, 81.9%, and 37.5%, respectively [13].
- Uterine malformations (e.g., bicornuate uterus, septate uterus, etc.) or other pathological conditions (e.g., uterine fibromas) that hinder intrauterine fetal growth and development.
- Cervical insufficiency: this condition occurs when weak cervical tissue dilates in the earlier phases of pregnancy and usually in the absence of contractions, causing either premature birth or the loss of an otherwise healthy pregnancy.
- Premature rupture of membranes (PROM): this condition, characterized by the early rupture of the amniotic membranes with subsequent loss of amniotic fluid and oligohydramnios, occurs in 2–4% of all pregnancies and is known to represent a primary cause of nearly 50% of preterm deliveries. PROM is usually associated with an underlying infection of the placental tissue and the amniotic layers, defined as chorioamnionitis (see below).
- Chorioamnionitis: genital tract infection is associated with 25–40% of preterm births based on microbiological studies [14]. This range may be an underestimation limited by poor strategies suitable for the detection of infections. Microorganisms can reach the amniotic cavity and fetus by ascent from the lower genital tract or, more rarely, by hematogenous distribution or after invasive medical procedures. Bacterial vaginosis is a leading cause of chorioamnionitis and is associated with a two- to fourfold increase in the risk of preterm birth [15]. As a consequence of the infection, chemokines and cytokines enhance neutrophil activity and the synthesis and release of matrix metalloproteinases, which lead to a remodeling of the extracellular matrix within the cervix and the placental interface, favoring the rupture of membranes. Moreover, the enhanced prostaglandin production associated with the infection represents a strong stimulus to uterine contractility [16]. Altogether, these events comprehensively contribute to a preterm onset of labor.

2.1.3 The Preterm Newborn

2.1.3.1 Classification

According to the GA at which preterm birth occurs, premature infants can be classified into the following categories

- Moderate to late preterm infants: 32–36^{+6} weeks
- Very preterm infants: 28–31^{+6} weeks
- Extremely preterm infants: <28 weeks

In addition to gestational age, preterm infants can be defined also according to their birth weight (BW)

- Low birth weight (LBW): <2500 g
- Very low birth weight (VLBW): <1500 g
- Extremely low birth weight (ELBW): <1000 g

The neonatal weight is influenced not only by the gestational age but also by the fetal conditions during pregnancy; therefore, according to the adequacy of BW for GA, preterm neonates can be also classified as follows:

- Appropriate for gestational age (AGA) if BW is between the 10th and 90th percentile for GA, i.e., within the normal range.
- Small for gestational age (SGA) if BW is below the 10th percentile, indicating that intrauterine growth was below the normal range for GA. This condition is particularly frequent after pregnancies complicated by IUGR. SGA babies can be also classified as symmetric or asymmetric based on the ratio

between the head and abdominal circumference. In asymmetrical SGA, which is most common and often results from late IUGR resulting from placental insufficiency, this ratio is increased, whereas symmetrical SGA presents with an overall growth restriction (both circumferences are reduced compared to standard) and usually results from an earlier IUGR condition.

- Large for gestational age (LGA) if BW is above the 90th percentile, indicating that intrauterine growth exceeded the normal range for GA. This condition is less frequent among preterm infants and can be constitutional or underlie pathological conditions, (e.g., maternal diabetes or genetic abnormalities).

2.1.3.2 Clinical Features

Preterm infants show specific phenotypical features, listed below, that are more evident at lower GAs

- The size is small, with a disproportionately large head, while the thoracic diameter is reduced. The cranial fontanels, and in particular the anterior one, are ampler than in term infants. The limbs are thin, with tapered fingers.
- The skin is reddish and thin, prone to breakdown injuries, and covered by a fine lanugo. Superficial capillaries and veins are evident. Subcutaneous fat layers are scarcely represented, giving preterm babies a sharper and less rounded looking.
- Ear cartilage is commonly not yet well defined, while recoils are mostly absent. At GAs <26 weeks, eyelids can be still fused together or only partially open. The eyes seldom present a wide movement range or intense light reactions.
- The abdomen is prominent and distended, with an evident venous reticulum. Abdominal rectus diastasis and umbilical and inguinal hernias are common findings.
- The heart rate is set at higher ranges compared to term infants (e.g., 150–190 bpm); bradycardic spells are frequent, secondary to the periodic breathing pattern or to apneic episodes. Blood pressure is correlated to GAs: normal values of mean arterial blood pressure should be equal to or greater than the corresponding GA or postconceptional age (PCA).
- The tone is decreased due to the scarce and immature muscle tissue and to neural immaturity; hence, antigravity movements are often hindered, and limb posture may appear extended rather than flexed.
- Due to neural immaturity, the sucking–swallowing coordination may be poor or lacking at lower GAs, leading to feeding difficulties requiring tube feeding. Moreover, gastric emptying gastrointestinal transit is often delayed, contributing to the development of feeding intolerance and constipation.
- In female preterm infants, hypertrophy of the clitoris is a common finding, while in males, testicles are often not palpable in the scrotum because their descent in the inguinal canal usually occurs after 29 weeks' gestation.

2.2 Complications of Preterm Birth

2.2.1 Thermoregulation Impairment

The maintenance of body temperature, defined as thermoregulation, is a complex process that involves gluconeogenesis and lipolysis. The following clinical characteristics place preterm infants at extremely high risk of heat loss, with subsequent hypothermia:

- High surface/volume body ratio
- Permeable epidermal layer of the skin
- Thin subcutaneous fat layer
- Reduced brown adipose tissue
- Underdeveloped autonomic control of the skin vasculature [17]

The loss of heat through evaporation from the skin and the lungs is predominant within the first days of life, and in some cases, it might exceed urinary output. The clinical consequences of hypothermia are severe and include metabolic acidosis due to peripheral vasoconstriction, raised pulmonary pressures, hypoglycemia, dehydration, and bleeding tendency due to the inhibition of the coagulation cascade. As such, reduced body temperature at admission in the neonatal intensive care unit (NICU) has been largely associated with an increased burden of neonatal morbidity and mortality in preterm neonates [18, 19]. Moreover, the more energy is needed to maintain body temperature, the less is available for growth and brain development. Hence, maintaining preterm infants' body temperature within normal ranges, i.e., 36–37.5 °C for skin measurements, is fundamental to improving their outcomes, and for this reason, servo-controlled incubators and heating radiators have been developed to prevent excessive heating losses in the delivery room and during NICU stay.

2.2.2 Respiratory Distress

Neonatal respiratory distress syndrome (RDS) is the most common respiratory complication occurring in preterm infants, with an increasing incidence of decreasing GA. The most important risk factors are prematurity and low birth weight; among others, male gender, maternal diabetes, perinatal asphyxia, and delivery in the absence of labor are encountered.

RDS results from a deficiency of surfactant due to either inadequate production or surfactant inactivation in the context of immature lungs. Surfactant is a lipid mixture comprising 70–80% phospholipids, 10% protein, and 10% neutral lipids. In around 20 weeks of gestation, lamellar bodies begin to form in the cytoplasm of the cuboidal epithelium of the bronchioles, and these cells differentiate into type 2 cells, which are responsible for surfactant production. Surfactant-specific lipoproteins, namely SP-A, SP-B, SP-C, and SP-D, form inside lamellar bodies at the apical surface of type 2 cells and are subsequently released into the alveoli by exocytosis. Among these proteins, SP-B and SP-C contribute to lowering the surface tension of air-fluid interfaces in both the small airways and alveoli, preventing their collapse and the entering of interstitial fluid into the airspace [20].

Due to the immaturity of their lungs, preterm infants have a lower quantity and decreased activity of surfactant, which results in increased surface tension in the alveoli and an enhanced risk of atelectasis. Widespread and repeated atelectasis damages the respiratory epithelium, causing a cytokine-mediated inflammatory response that increases the leakage of protein-rich fluid from the vascular space into the alveoli, thus triggering surfactant inactivation [21]. Many infants with RDS may require mechanical ventilation support to achieve the pressure amounts needed to avoid alveolar collapse; in turn, mechanical ventilation causes further damage as well as inflammation in the developing lung due to the overdistension of the alveoli [22] and to the oxidative stress generated by high fractional inspired oxygen (FiO_2), which additionally contributes to the inactivation of the surfactant through protein and lipid peroxidation processes [23].

RDS signs and symptoms typically occur within a few minutes after birth and consist of nonspecific respiratory symptoms, such as decreased breath sounds, cyanosis, tachypnea, expiratory grunting, nasal flaring, and subcostal, intercostal, or suprasternal retractions. Auscultation reveals uniformly decreased air entry. Prompt diagnosis and treatment require an overall assessment of perinatal risk factors, clinical presentation, radiographic findings, and evidence of hypoxemia on blood gas analysis. The partial pressure of arterial oxygen (PaO_2) on an arterial blood gas should lie within the 50–80 mmHg range, while partial pressure of arterial carbon dioxide ($PaCO_2$) should be between 40 and 55 mmHg, with the pH >7.25 [24].

The pathognomonic radiological features of RDS include diffuse atelectasis, described as a ground-glass reticulogranular appearance, reduced lung volumes, and with air bronchograms due to the air-tissue interface formed between alveolar collapse in the background, with the air-filled larger airways in the foreground. Chest X-rays may be useful for the differential diagnosis between RDS and other lung conditions with a similar clinical presentation, such as pulmonary air leak disorders, pneumonia, meconium aspiration, or CHD. A cardiac ultrasound assessment may add useful information for identifying persistent pulmonary hypertension or an underlying cyanotic CHD. A workup for infectious etiologies, including complete blood counts and C-reactive protein (CRP), may be useful for ruling out RDS as a possible presentation of bacterial sepsis or viral congenital infection [24].

RDS prevention starts antenatally with the maternal administration of corticosteroids in case of possible preterm delivery in the next 7 days between 23 and 34 weeks' GA [25]. This treatment has been shown to effectively decrease not only RDS incidence and severity but also the rates of mortality and periventricular leukomalacia (PVL) in the face of any increase in maternal mortality [26].

The therapeutic management of neonates with RDS is based on the monitoring of oxygenation and ventilation, with pulse oximetry and serial blood gas evaluations, exogenous surfactant therapy, assisted ventilatory support, and supporting care (e.g., fluid and electrolyte management, antibiotic therapy, nutritional support, etc.) [25].

The targeted treatment for surfactant deficiency is endotracheal surfactant replacement. Surfactant administration decreases the risk of pneumothorax, interstitial emphysema, intraventricular hemorrhage (IVH), and bronchopulmonary dysplasia (BPD) and reduces neonatal mortality. According to European consensus guidelines, surfactant is administered to immature babies with FiO_2 >0.3 [25]. To date, different natural surfactants prepared from minced bovine, porcine, or calf lung extracts are available with similar efficacy [27], while clinical trials on synthetic surfactants are ongoing. Surfactants can be administered either by standard endotracheal intubation, which represents the standard technique, or through less invasive surfactant administration (LISA) techniques using thin intratracheal catheters or, alternatively, laryngeal masks [28]; nevertheless, further investigations are required to determine whether the LISA technique is preferred over endotracheal intubation for surfactant administration.

If neonates maintain an adequate respiratory drive, with FiO_2 <0.3, after surfactant administration, it is possible to switch them to noninvasive modalities of respiratory support, which are usually preferred as they decrease the risk of mortality and BPD compared to invasive ventilation. A widely used first-line strategy is the early initiation of continuous positive airway pressure (CPAP) to provide a constant distending airway pressure, associated with surfactant administration. RDS neonates that do not respond to CPAP, develop respiratory acidosis or hypoxemia, or have severe apneas require endotracheal intubation and mechanical ventilation. The goal of mechanical ventilation includes the provision of adequate respiratory support while balancing the risks of volutrauma, barotrauma, and oxygen toxicity. Time-cycled pressure-limited ventilation is the currently preferred initial mode of ventilation in preterm infants with RDS. High-frequency oscillatory ventilation is often used as a rescue modality if high conventional ventilator support is required or if there are concerns for pulmonary air leaks or, empirically, in extremely preterm infants to minimize lung injury [25].

The prognosis of infants managed with antenatal steroids, exogenous surfactants, and respiratory support is excellent, showing survival rates of up to 95% with advanced care in developed countries, whereas RDS-related mortality rates are still significantly higher in preterm infants born in low-income countries, where the mortality rate for premature infants with RDS is significantly higher, at times close to 100% [29]. However, while surfactant replacement has decreased the morbidity associated with RDS, many neonates continue to experience such acute complications as air-leak syndromes, and short- and long-term sequelae, such as BPD, discussed in the following paragraph, and neurodevelopmental delay and cerebral palsy, whose incidence is higher in infants at lower GA ranges who received prolonged mechanical ventilation [30].

2.2.3 Bronchopulmonary Dysplasia

BPD is defined as a multifactorial, chronic pulmonary disease typically observed in preterm infants who developed RDS and required prolonged respiratory support. Despite the significant advances in RDS management occurring over the past decades, such as surfactant replacement and less invasive ventilation modalities, the burden of BPD is still remarkably high at lower GAs and BW, with an estimated incidence ranging between 40 and 68% in VLBW infants, depending on the definition of BPD used. Other antenatal and postnatal risk factors associated with BPD development include a lack of antenatal steroid administration, maternal smoking, maternal hypertension, chorioamnionitis, family history of asthma, male sex, white race, SGA, inadequate nutrition, prolonged mechanical ventilation, and neonatal infections [31].

While before the introduction of surfactant replacement and noninvasive respiratory supports lung injury associated with BPD mainly resulted from the detrimental effects of mechanical ventilation, such as barotrauma and oxygen injury, these new strategies have led to a significant change in the characteristics of BPD. Compared to "old BPD," this "new BPD" is associated with diminished airway damage and alveolar septal fibrosis, but its pathological hallmarks are dysmorphic microvasculature and alveolar simplification [32]. This is consistent with the underlying pathophysiological mechanisms, according to which lung injury is mainly driven by an enhanced inflammatory response that triggers the release of proinflammatory cytokines (e.g., interleukins 6 and 8, tumor necrosis factor alpha, etc.) and angiogenic factors [vascular endothelial growth factor (VEGF), angiopoietin 2], which ultimately results in aberrant tissue repair, dysregulated angiogenesis, and arrested alveolar development [33].

The diagnosis of BPD is made clinically, based on oxygen requirements at 36 weeks PCA or at discharge home, whichever came first, in infants born at ≤32 weeks' gestation. In 2001, the National Institute of Child Health and Human Development (NICHD) workshop proposed the current definition, in which infants get diagnosed with mild, moderate, or severe BPD at 36 weeks PCA based on their respiratory support at that time [34]. This definition, however, still has many deficiencies and does not adequately predict respiratory outcomes; hence in 2016, the NICHD workshop on BPD further revised this definition, including the newer modes of noninvasive ventilation for BPD severity stratification [35].

In addition to persistent oxygen dependence, infants with BPD may present with peripheral edema, chronic hypoxemia, and other signs of right heart failure and are more prone to recurrent respiratory infections. Important secretions may obstruct the trachea or main bronchus, and it is not rare to observe concomitant tracheomalacia or bronchomalacia. These neonates may also present feeding difficulties and require prolonged parenteral nutrition [36].

Chest radiographs in BPD infants show decreased lung volumes, hyperinflation, areas of atelectasis, pulmonary edema, and interstitial emphysema. Infants with moderate or severe BPD also need to be screened for pulmonary hypertension at 36 weeks PCA using echocardiography since the estimated prevalence of this condition in severe BPD ranges between 20 and 40% and significantly worsens BPD-related morbidity and mortality [37].

The main aim in the management of preterm neonates with BPD is to limit further injury to their lungs, optimize lung function, detect associated complications, and support their growth.

Whenever feasible, noninvasive ventilation should be preferred to mechanical ventilation; if this is not possible, care should be taken to limit barotrauma and volutrauma. Exposure to hyperoxia is also critical in the pathogenesis of BPD and should be limited by keeping SpO_2 target ranges within the recommended thresholds (90–94%) [25].

Systemic corticosteroids, such as dexamethasone or hydrocortisone, are frequently used in BPD to reduce inflammation and facilitate extubation or scale the respiratory support down. However, due to concerns about long-term neurodevelopment, their use should be limited to infants with severe BPD who remain ventilator dependent with high oxygen requirements [37]. Although inhaled corticosteroids may reduce the neurodevelopmental burden associated with steroid treatment, current literature does not demonstrate support for their routine use in BPD prevention [38].

Based on the severity of their lung disease, total fluid volumes may be restricted to less than 150 mL/kg/day to prevent pulmonary edema and improve gas exchange. Thiazides and loop diuretics are commonly used over 3 weeks after birth in ventilator-dependent infants with an increasing requirement of positive end-expiratory pressure despite fluid restriction to improve short-term pulmonary mechanics. However, a systemic review of the available literature does not show any improvement in long-term clinical outcomes [39]. Eventually, due to the increased work of breathing and to concomitant feeding difficulties, infants with BPD need an increased amount of energy (e.g., up to 150 kcal/kg/day) and proteins to promote lung growth and repair. Milk fortifiers can be used to enrich maternal or donor breast milk and increase its caloric contents.

Unfortunately, the structural alveolar and vascular abnormalities associated with BPD persist into adulthood and are responsible for several long-term sequelae, such as significantly increased rates of hospital readmission during their first year of life; increased risk of developing reactive airway disease, asthma, and emphysema; and worse outcomes following viral bronchiolitis. Moreover, BPD also affects the neurodevelopmental outcome and is associated with a higher prevalence of delays in motor and language skills [40]. Hence, infants with BPD require a multidisciplinary follow-up that includes a neonatologist, a pediatric pulmonologist, a respiratory therapist, a nutritionist, physical and occupational therapists, and child life specialists.

2.2.4 Patent Ductus Arteriosus

The ductus arteriosus (DA), or ductus botalli, is an arterial vessel interposed between the pulmonary artery and the descending aorta. During antenatal life, oxygenated blood enters the fetal circulation from the placental interface through the umbilical vein, and via the inferior vena cava, it reaches the right atrium. Here, a tissue flap known as the Eustachian valve directs the great majority of this blood across the foramen ovale into the left atrium, from which it enters the left ventricle and is ejected into the systemic circulation. The venous return collected by the superior vena cava, inferior vena cava, and coronary sinus is collected in the right atrium, directed into the right ventricle across the tricuspid valve, and then ejected into the pulmonary artery. However, due to the high pulmonary vascular resistance (PVR) that characterizes the antenatal circulation, only a small proportion of blood reaches the pulmonary circuit, while 80–90% of this flow is shunted across the DA into the descending aorta toward the lower half of the body [41]. Hence, the DA plays a key role in maintaining fetal circulation; however, the transition from fetal to neonatal circulation, which occurs after birth, entails the closure of intra- and extracardiac shunts, such as DA, as their hemodynamic role becomes obsolete. Under physiological conditions, postnatal DA closure is regulated by exposure to oxygen and vasodilators. Oxygen induces the release of the potent vasoconstrictor endothelin-1 at the ductal level, whereas vasodilator substances such as prostaglandin E_2, prostacyclin, and nitric oxide contribute to DA patency [42]. In preterm infants, however, several factors may contribute to the disruption of the physiological DA closure. First, the immature DA is characterized by a thinner muscular wall compared to the term duct, with smooth muscle cells that are less sensitive to oxygen-related vasoconstriction and more sensitive to prostaglandin E_2- and prostacyclin-related vasodilative effects. The increased circulating levels of systemic inflammatory mediators and prostaglandins, which are observed in the preterm population, further contribute to the failure of spontaneous DA closure in this population [43]. Moreover, it has been observed that platelets are recruited into the DA lumen during closure, probably promoting a thrombotic sealing of the constricted DA [42]; therefore, thrombocytopenia [44] or an impaired platelet function [45] may contribute to persistent ductal patency. Consistently, the prevalence of a patent ductus arteriosus (PDA) increases with decreasing GA, and even the achievement of spontaneous closure may take up to several days to occur: in a large retrospective study on preterm infants who did not receive active medical or surgical treatment for PDA closure, the median closing time ranged from 6 days in infants ≥30 weeks of gestation to 71 days in those <26 weeks [46]. Hence, in the absence of targeted interventions, a significant proportion of extremely preterm neonates may be exposed to prolonged transductal shunting with potential pathophysiological implications [47].

PDA can be either symptomatic or asymptomatic, depending upon the transductal shunt volume and direction: a small left-to-right shunt is usually asymptomatic, especially among late preterm infants, whereas a higher flow across the patent duct may have different hemodynamic effects depending on PVR, as illustrated in Fig. 2.1.

Following preterm birth, the decrease in PVR may be slower than in term neonates due to the immaturity of the lung parenchyma, respiratory distress, and metabolic acidosis frequently seen in the early postnatal phases. The persistence of high PVR (Fig. 2.1a) prolongs the right-to-left or bidirectional shunting across the PDA, with subsequent reduction of pulmonary perfusion, low oxygen saturation levels, and increased need for supplemental oxygen and invasive respiratory support. If pulmonary blood flow decreases, the venous return to the left atrium is also decreased, and so are the left ventricle preload and cardiac output, leading to decreased perfusion and oxygenation in end-target organs. As a consequence, a raise in lactate and acidosis, which contribute to increasing PVR, may occur, feeding a detrimental vicious cycle that eventually leads to the development of pulmonary hypertension [48]. Persistently elevated PVR increases the afterload of the right ventricle, which gradually becomes hypertrophic and/or dilated. The resulting bowing of the interventricular septum toward the left ventricle further compromises left ventricular output, leading to biventricular dysfunction. Systemic hypotension requiring cardiovascular support often coexists during these phases.

Conversely, if PVR gradually decreases during the transitional period (Fig. 2.1b), a left-to-right shunt across the PDA may progressively become hemodynamically significant. Pulmonary hyperperfusion increases pulmonary venous

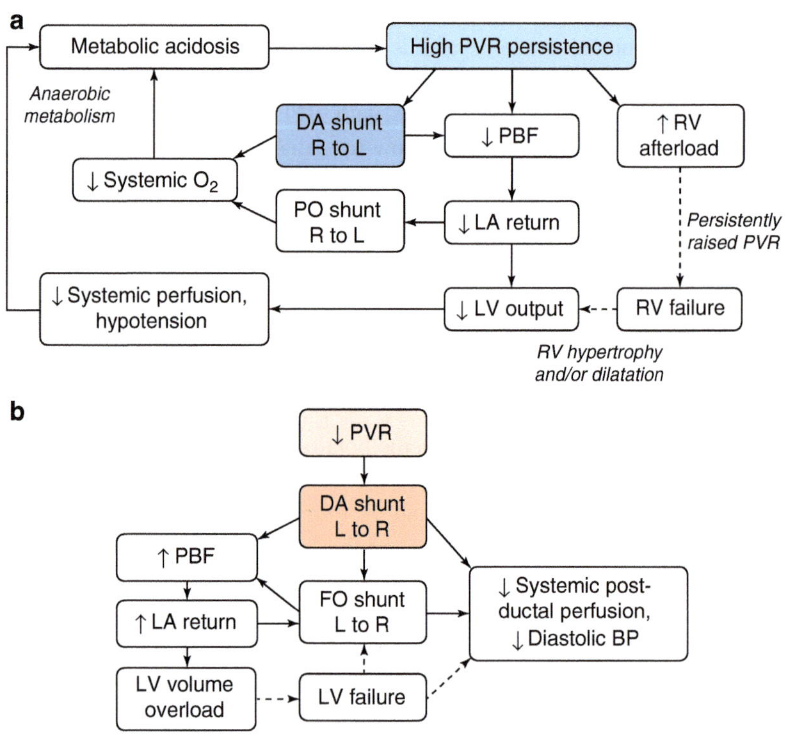

Fig. 2.1 Events associated with different directions of transductal shunt (scenarios **a** and **b**), depending on pulmonary vascular resistance (PVR). *BP* blood pressure, *DA* ductus arteriosus, *LV* left ventricle, *L* left, *PBF* pulmonary blood flow, *R* right, *RV* right ventricle

return with volume overload of the left ventricle and systemic hypoperfusion below the ductal level. Increased venous return to the left atrium may raise left atrial pressure and reverse the direction of shunting through the foramen ovale, thus further worsening pulmonary hyperperfusion and low systemic blood flow. Moreover, due to the diastolic dysfunction that characterizes the preterm myocardium [49], the left ventricle may struggle to adapt to the increased stroke volume, eventually progressing to left ventricular failure in the case of wide or prolonged left-to-right transductal shunting.

The signs and symptoms of PDA depend not only on the characteristics, magnitude, and duration of the transductal shunt but also on the individual adaptive ability of the immature myocardium as well as additional concomitant factors (e.g., fluid intakes, metabolic and ventilatory status). A continuous heart murmur on the parasternal line in proximity to the second intercostal space is a common finding in the presence of PDA. In the presence of a hemodynamically significant left-to-right transductal shunt, tachycardia, low diastolic blood pressure, tachypnea, and costal retractions are often evident, whereas if the shunt across the PDA is predominantly right to left, hypoxemia, hypotension, and signs of systemic venous congestion may prevail. Several of these signs, however, are not specific and may overlie a concomitant RDS, which can be further worsened by a hemodynamically significant PDA.

PDA persistence in preterm neonates has been associated with increased mortality and several major complications [50–54]; among these, the most relevant that typically occur during the transitional period are IVH and pulmonary hemorrhage (PH). Deshpande et al. [47] have proposed two potential pathophysiological models in which the interaction between the immature preterm myocardium and the exposure to an unrestrictive transductal shunt during postnatal transition are important contributors to the development of both PH and IVH in preterm neonates with a PDA. In particular, a delayed adaptation of the myocardial function to the volume overload resulting from transductal shunting left to right may increase left atrial pressure and pulmonary venous hypertension, placing the infant at risk of PH. The temporal association between this functional disturbance and the typical timing of PH onset (usually 48 h after birth) is noteworthy [53]. On the other hand, myocardial adaptation to the loading changes, which usually occurs within the first 48 h of life, may result in a sudden increase in cerebral blood flow (CBF), predisposing to IVH, whose incidence is highest during the first 72 h after preterm birth [55].

On the above basis, a thorough and integrated clinical and echocardiographic assessment in preterm neonates presenting with a PDA is essential, and subsequent hemodynamic management should be adopted according to the underlying cardiovascular physiology, aiming to prevent unfavorable outcomes [56].

Conservative management of PDA includes fluid restriction (110–130 mL/kg/day, associated with urine output monitoring) and increasing end-expiratory pressure to treat the pulmonary edema resulting from pulmonary overflow. The use of diuretics is not infrequent, although raises controversy of not being supported by evidence of improved outcomes and being possibly associated with electrolyte derangements, which are difficult to manage in extremely preterm neonates [57].

Pharmacologic treatment with nonsteroidal anti-inflammatory drugs (NSAIDs) such as indomethacin and ibuprofen or paracetamol, which hinder prostaglandin synthesis, should be considered in preterm neonates with a hemodynamically significant PDA with left-to-right shunt and is likely required in ELBW infants whose PDA persists despite conservative management. Indomethacin is a nonselective cyclooxygenase (COX)-1 and COX-2 inhibitor introduced for pharmacological PDA treatment in the mid-1970s; since then and for a long time, it had been the treatment of choice despite its association with renal impairment and gastrointestinal complications such as necrotizing enterocolitis (NEC) and spontaneous intestinal perforation secondary to its vasoconstrictor effects on splanchnic circulation [58]. Ibuprofen causes a nonselective competitive inhibition of COX-1 and COX-2 and, since the mid-1990s, has emerged as a valid alternative to indomethacin, demonstrating equal efficacy on PDA closure but lower risks of NEC and renal insufficiency [59]. Paracetamol inhibits the peroxidase site of prostaglandin H2 synthase and has also been associated with selective COX-2 inhibition. Over the past decade, multiple small studies have supported the efficacy of paracetamol for PDA closure; therefore, its use has progressively increased, although data from large randomized-controlled trials are expected. Due to its different mechanism of action, paracetamol is associated with poorer antiplatelet activity compared to nonselective NSAIDs, which inhibit COX-1-mediated platelet aggregation [60].

If a hemodynamically significant PDA persists despite pharmacologic therapy and is associated with increased respiratory support or renal impairment or if pharmacologic closure is contraindicated (e.g., in the case of acute renal failure), surgical ligation can be performed [61]. Surgical complications of PDA include injury to the recurrent laryngeal nerve with subsequent vocal cord palsy, occlusion of the descending aorta, injury to the pulmonary artery and phrenic nerve, and postligation left ventricular dysfunction [57].

2.2.5 Intraventricular Hemorrhage

IVH is a major complication of prematurity, with an incidence that is inversely proportional to GA. IVH etiology is multifactorial but primarily lies in the intrinsic fragility of the germinal matrix vasculature and in CBF disturbances resulting from the impairment of the physiological mechanisms of cerebral autoregulation. The prevalence of IVH is highest during the first 72 h after preterm birth, suggesting that brain circulation is especially vulnerable in this period [62].

The germinal matrix lies on the upper part of the caudate lobe and among the periventricular area, and it is abundantly represented before 34 weeks' gestation, and after this period, it progressively reduces its size. The microvasculature of the germinal matrix is characterized by an abundance of angiogenic blood vessels with an immature basal lamina, decreased pericytes, and deficient glial fibrillary acidic protein in the ensheathing astrocyte endfeet [63].

Due to the inefficiency of autoregulatory mechanisms, preterm neonates often present a passive CBF, which fluctuates as systemic blood flow varies. Several conditions affecting systemic blood pressure, such as hypovolemia, acidosis, PDA, or RDS requiring mechanical ventilation, may lead to CBF fluctuations, which are translated into repeated episodes of cerebral ischemia and reperfusion. The occurrence of these CBF fluctuations in the early postnatal period likely contributes to the rupture of fragile germinal matrix vessels, which represents the trigger event for IVH development. Consistently with this mechanism, CBF fluctuations characterized by a transient phase of hyperperfusion [55, 64] and a greater burden of impaired autoregulation have been detected using different techniques in preterm infants developing IVH during the transitional period [65–67]. Moreover, it has also been observed that, in mechanically ventilated neonates, severe IVH was preceded by a global abolishment of CBF reactivity to both $PaCO_2$ and blood pressure, whereas milder IVH did not [68]. As such, the maintenance of a stable CBF since the early postnatal period and the prevention of hypoxic and hypotensive states represent fundamental neuroprotective strategies in the preterm population.

Germinal matrix bleeding may disrupt the ependymal lining and extend into the ventricles, causing progressing degrees of IVH, detailed in Table 2.1. Serial cranial ultrasound scans through the anterior fontanel are fundamental for IVH diagnosis and grading. Although the Papile criteria [69] are still largely used in clinical and research settings, a more descriptive and precise nomenclature has been proposed by Volpe [70].

Based on its extension, IVH may have different clinical presentations [71]

- Silent presentation: this presentation accounts for 25–50% of all IVH cases and, in particular, for IVH grade I or II, which does not tend to

Table 2.1 IVH grading according to Papile and Volpe [70]

Papile's grading	Volpe's grading
Grade 1: Subependymal hemorrhage	Grade 1: IVH confined to the germinal matrix region
Grade 2: IVH without ventricular dilatation	Grade 2: IVH filling ≤50% of the lateral ventricle and/or without ventricular dilatation
Grade 3: IVH causing ventricular distension and dilatation	Grade 3: IVH filling >50% of the lateral ventricle and/or resulting in ventricular dilatation
Grade 4: IVH with parenchymal hemorrhage	IVH with periventricular hemorrhagic infarction (PHI) in the surrounding parenchyma

evolve and is detected at routine cranial ultrasound assessments.

- Stuttering course: this is the most frequent in IVH grades III–IV and evolves over a few hours to several days. It is characterized by nonspecific findings, such as hypotonia, hyporeactivity, decreased or abnormal spontaneous movements, and evidence of abnormal electrical brain activity.
- Catastrophic deterioration: this presentation, which rapidly evolves over minutes to hours, is least common and is usually associated with the most severe IVH grades. Clinical signs include stupor or coma, hypoventilation or apnea, decerebrate posture, generalized tonic seizures, and cranial nerve abnormalities, such as fixed mydriasis. Other features of this presentation include a bulging anterior fontanelle, severe hypotension, bradycardia, metabolic acidosis, and inappropriate antidiuretic hormone secretion.

Depending on its severity, IVH can lead to important neurological and neurodevelopmental sequelae. The destruction of the germinal matrix resulting from IVH and the damage to the glial precursors located in this area may be associated with poor neurodevelopmental outcomes. Moreover, severe IVH may be complicated by the development of a parenchymal hemorrhagic infarction (PHI) in the periventricular white matter. PHI was formerly believed to represent a parenchymal extension of the IVH; however, evidence from microscopic studies has revealed that perivascular hemorrhage follows the distribution of the medullary veins in the periventricular white matter and tends to be concentrated near the ventricular angle, where these veins become confluent, leading to venous infarction. PHI frequently results in a large porencephalic cyst, which can be isolated or accompanied by smaller cysts [70].

An additional common complication of severe IVH is posthemorrhagic ventricular dilatation (PHVD), occurring in 30–50% of infants with an IVH grade III/IV. PHVD is a consequence of the obstruction of the cerebrospinal fluid flow caused by the formation of a clot at any level among basilar cisterns in the posterior fossa, the cerebral aqueduct, or the arachnoid villi. Serial cranial ultrasound scans are useful not only to diagnose PHVD and quantify ventricular dilatation with specific measures, such as the ventricular index and anterior horn width, but also to follow up on its progression. Head circumference should be also measured sequentially in any baby with PHVD. Neurosurgical intervention is required in nearly 40–60% of preterm infants with PHVD, aiming to mitigate secondary brain injury and, in particular, damage to the white matter. There is significant variability in the timing of and approach to intervention; early interventions include initial lumbar puncture and the surgical insertion of a ventricular access device, whereas ventriculoperitoneal shunts are used in the case of progressive PHVD after early intervention. Symptoms of increased intracranial pressure, including bulging fontanels, rapid increase in head circumference, vomiting, bradycardia, or sunsetting appearance of the eyes, require urgent intervention. PHVD has been associated with cognitive and motor deficits, particularly in progressive cases requiring ventriculoperitoneal shunts [72].

2.2.6 White Matter Injury

The typical patterns of white matter injury observed in preterm infants mainly consist in PVL and diffuse white matter gliosis.

PVL is a form of white matter injury characterized by the loss of premyelinating oligodendrocytes and determines a high risk of neurodevelopmental impairment. The principal initiating pathogenetic factors in PVL appear to be repeated cycles of cerebral ischemia-reperfusion and systemic inflammation, which, by activating excitotoxicity and free radical damage, lead to the death of the vulnerable premyelinating oligodendrocytes. The cerebrovascular anatomy and physiology of premature infants, namely, the presence of arterial border and end zones and impaired CBF regulation, underly the peculiar sensitivity of white matter to ischemic insults, resulting in PVL. This type of injury typically involves the periventricular white matter and can be characterized by macroscopic or microscopic lesions.

The focal white matter damage observed in PVL is caused by deep necrosis of the periventricular white matter with a loss of all cellular elements. The typical areas involved are the arterial watershed zones, which lie between the penetrating branches of the middle, anterior, and posterior cerebral arteries. The resulting focal necrotic lesions may be either macroscopic or microscopic. While macroscopic lesions tend to evolve to form confluent cystic cavities, which are visible on cranial ultrasounds, microscopic necrosis alternatively evolves in white matter scars characterized by marked astrogliosis and microgliosis. It has been estimated that the latter form accounts for the majority of PVL cases; however, it is not easily diagnosed by cranial ultrasound and requires to be visualized with brain magnetic resonance imaging, it being therefore underdiagnosed [70].

Diffuse white matter injury is characterized by diffuse gliosis of preoligodendrocytes without focal necroses. The first step leading to this type of injury is a decrease in premyelinating oligodendrocytes, which is counteracted by an increase in oligodendroglial progenitors. The latter cells, however, are unable to undergo appropriate maturation and are particularly vulnerable to hypoxic-ischemic insults. Although it has not yet been conclusively established, it is likely that diffuse white matter gliosis represents the mildest form of injury in a spectrum that includes cystic PVL as the most severe form [73].

Neurological and neurodevelopmental outcomes following white matter injury depend on the patterns of injury. In the presence of white matter cystic lesions, the cysts' location is relevant for determining these outcomes: if the cysts are limited to the frontal or anterior parietal lobes, even though large or extensive, they are normally not associated with cerebral palsy (CP), whereas the risk of spastic diplegia or quadriplegia is particularly high with bilateral parieto-occipital cysts. In the latter case, cerebral visual impairment is also possible due to the involvement of optic radiation. On the other hand, diffuse white matter injury is associated with lower neurodevelopmental scores, with major impairments of cognitive and motor outcomes. An altered white matter structure has a long-term impact on neural connectivity and may underlie the behavioral and social-emotional problems growingly observed in children born very preterm, especially at prescholar and scholar ages [74].

2.2.7 Necrotizing Enterocolitis

NEC is a life-threatening gastrointestinal complication of prematurity and has an estimated incidence of 7% among hospitalized VLBW infants, which increases with decreasing BW and GA [75]. NEC represents a major cause of morbidity and mortality in the preterm population; the related mortality rates can reach up to 50% in surgical cases and have remained mainly unchanged over the past decades.

The pathophysiology of NEC is multifactorial and involves several different risk factors. First, the anatomical and functional immaturity of the preterm gut determines reduced intestinal motility, which affects the clearance of the intestinal lumen, increases the permeability of the intestinal mucosa, and alters the physiological mucosal defense mechanisms. In particular, the expression of Toll-like receptor 4 (TLR-4), which modulates intestinal development during pregnancy, is still enhanced in preterm neonates and can be abnormally activated by otherwise physiological intraluminal stimuli, such as feeds or the gut microbiota [76]. The crucial role of intestinal dysbiosis in NEC pathogenesis has also been largely established. The large use of wide-spectrum antibiotics in early life phases, as well as other medications, such as H_2-blockers or proton pump inhibitors, delayed the initiation of enteral feeds, and the use of formula feeding rather than maternal or donor milk favors a dysbiotic shift of the gut microbiome, characterized by low diversity and an increase in Proteobacteria and a decrease in Bacteroidetes and Firmicutes [77, 78]. This less physiological gut microbiome stimulates the immature immune system and activates TLR-4, initiating an inflammatory cascade that disrupts mucosal integrity and triggers necrotic modifications in the immature gut. An additional contributor to NEC development is ischemia, which can result from postnatal hemodynamic disturbances ensuing from hypotension, hemodynamically significant PDA, etc. or from vascular remodeling ensuing from antenatal IUGR with evidence of brain sparing. In this case, ischemic intestinal perforation may represent the predominant feature. Gut ischemia may also be secondary to local inflammatory processes triggered by the TLR-4 and associated with an increased expression of endothelin-1, which determine an imbalance between vasodilators and vasoconstrictor factors in the intestinal microcirculation [79].

The initial mucosal damage ensuing from the abovementioned mechanisms further alters the integrity of the gut mucosa, and as a consequence, gut bacteria can translocate within the inner layers of the intestinal wall, releasing inflammatory toxins that further contribute to necrotic damage [80].

NEC clinical presentation is highly variable, nonspecific, and subtle. Gastrointestinal signs included abdominal distension, abundant bilious or bloody gastric residuals, bilious vomiting, hematochezia, evidence of abdominal dyschromic, or erythematous areas. At physical examination, decreased bowel sounds, visible intestinal loops, and erythema of the abdominal wall, abdominal tenderness to palpation, or a palpable abdominal mass are typical findings. As the diseases progress, a progressive systemic deterioration characterized by recurrent apneas, respiratory failure, lethargy, decreased peripheral perfusion, hypotension, and decreased urine output often occurs. Electrolytic and glucose imbalance; blood cell count abnormalities, such as leukopenia, anemia, and thrombocytopenia; and increased CRP are also common findings.

The most important test required to make NEC diagnosis is an abdominal radiograph, including anterior–posterior and lateral decubitus views; evidence of dilated bowel loops with transmural edema and pneumatosis intestinalis, characterized by the visualization of small amounts of air within the bowel wall, is pathognomonic. Portal venous air is not always present but is a poor prognostic sign when found as it indicates an incipient bowel perforation at early stages; free air in the abdomen may be seen when perforation has occurred. In borderline cases, X-rays should be repeated serially until a definitive diagnosis and treatment can be established. Abdominal ultrasounds performed by trained personnel can be useful for identifying signs of intestinal pneumatosis and free air in the portal system or within the peritoneum and ascites and for the early detection of intestinal wall ischemia [80].

The combination of clinical and radiological findings allows classifying NEC cases according to the modified Bell staging criteria [81, 82] based on systemic, intestinal, and radiological signs, detailed in Table 2.2.

The first intervention in the case of suspected NEC is to stop all enteral feedings and all undertaken total parenteral nutrition, putting the intestine at rest. A nasogastric tube should be placed to evaluate gastric residuals and to decompress the dilated bowels. Intravenous broad-spectrum antibiotics (e.g., vancomycin, piperacillin and tazobactam, metronidazole) should be commenced, and correction of electrical disorders should be performed. In the case of systemic deterioration, breathing and circulation must be supported based on the infant's vital signs. Fluid resuscitation and inotropes are indicated for hypotension, while endotracheal intubation and mechanical ventilation may be

Table 2.2 Bell's staging criteria for NEC classification

Stage	Classification	Systemic signs	Gastrointestinal signs	Radiological findings
IA	Suspected NEC	Temperature instability, apnea, bradycardia, lethargy	Increased pregavage residuals, mild abdominal distention, emesis, guaiac-positive stool	Normal or intestinal dilation, mild ileus
IB			Bright red blood from the rectum	
IIA	Proven NEC—mild		Same as above + absent bowel sounds ± abdominal tenderness	Intestinal dilation, ileus, pneumatosis intestinalis
IIB	Proven NEC—moderate	Same as above + mild metabolic acidosis and thrombocytopenia	Same as above + abdominal tenderness ± palpable mass	Same as above + portal venous gas ± ascites
IIIA	Advanced NEC	Same as above + hypotension, severe apnea, respiratory and metabolic acidosis, disseminated intravascular coagulation, neutropenia	Same as above + signs of generalized peritonitis, marked tenderness, marked abdominal distention, skin dyschromia	Same as above + ascites
IIIB	Advanced NEC with bowel perforation			Same as above + pneumoperitoneum

required in the case of respiratory failure. If this conservative therapy is effective, infants may resume enteral feedings within several days or 1–2 weeks once NEC signs have resolved. The presence of normal bowel movements and the gradual improvement of radiological findings determine the restoration of bowel function.

In infants who have worsening conditions or signs of bowel perforation or who do not respond to medical therapy, surgical intervention is indicated. The abdomen is usually approached by laparotomy; only unquestionably necrotic or perforated intestinal portions are removed, trying to spare the maximum bowel length. Due to the risk of local ischemia, primary anastomosis is generally contraindicated, and a diverting ostomy is usually utilized, especially in severe cases or if there is evidence of peritonitis; the stoma can be reversed following recovery [83]. In extremely preterm and unstable neonates, laparotomy may be not tolerated; in these cases, if bowel perforation occurs, the bedside insertion of a peritoneal drain may be considered an alternative treatment [84].

NEC prognosis depends on its severity and the promptness of establishing treatment. The adoption of preventive strategies such as more targeted use of proton pump inhibitors or antibiotics and increased use of maternal or donor milk [85] and probiotics [86] has allowed achieving a slight decrease in overall NEC rates. However, the related mortality rates remain high, ranging from 20% in Bell's stages ≥2 to 50% or higher in ELBW neonates, or in severe cases, it requires surgical treatment [87]. Complications include postoperative adhesions and scarring, which may lead to stricture and obstruction. In the case of extensive bowel resections, other complications include short bowel syndrome, intestinal failure, nutritional deficiencies, and subsequent poor growth. Neonates requiring prolonged total parenteral nutrition may develop liver failure [88]. Eventually, a significant proportion of newborns with NEC, particularly those with the most severe Bell's stages resulting in intestinal failure, may develop moderate to severe neurodevelopmental delay; the inflammatory status and hemodynamic instability that accompany NEC onset, together with the resulting nutritional deficiencies, are the main contributors to adverse neurodevelopmental outcomes [89].

2.2.8 Retinopathy of Prematurity

Retinopathy of prematurity (ROP) is a condition characterized by retinal vascular proliferation, which typically affects premature infants undergoing prolonged oxygen therapy. The estimated incidence of any ROP stage is nearly 70% among infants with BW ≤1250 g [90].

Physiological hypoxia during antenatal life increases the levels of the vascular endothelial growth factor (VEGF), thus facilitating retinal angiogenesis, which starts from the 22nd week and continues after term, until its complete achievement.

The vascularization of nasal and temporal retinal portions is not completed until 32 and 40 weeks' GA, respectively; hence, following preterm birth, the vascularization of these areas is completed in the extrauterine environment. Due to the concomitant pulmonary immaturity, which often requires supplemental oxygen, the physiologic intrauterine hypoxia that was previously driving retinal vascularization is replaced by a state of hyperoxia, which inhibits VEGF transcription; as a result, retinal vascularization is delayed, and the developing capillaries undergo significant vasoconstriction. Subsequently, the increasingly metabolically active yet poorly vascularized retina becomes hypoxic and stimulates a secondary increase in VEGF, which replaces normal angiogenesis with a predominantly pathological vascular overgrowth in the developing retinal portions [91].

The most important risk factors for ROP are GA, BW, and supplemental oxygen need; in particular, increasing concentrations of O_2 are directly correlated with the risk of ROP development, and the duration of oxygen therapy is a significant risk factor for severe ROP. Hence, oxygen therapy regulation, by maintaining SpO_2 within the 90–94% range, is fundamental for ROP prevention [92].

ROP screening consists in fundus oculi evaluation following pupil dilation with phenylephrine and is of crucial importance for premature infants born ≤32 weeks GA or with BW ≤1500 g. Fundus examinations should begin at 4 weeks postnatal age or >30 weeks' PCA [93].

Based on the findings observed at the border of the vascular and avascular retina, ROP can be classified according to the following stages.

- Stage 1: evidence of a thin but clear demarcation separating the avascular retina anteriorly from the vascularized retina posteriorly, with the abnormal branching of vessels leading up to it
- Stage 2: evidence of a high crest along the demarcation line that extends above the retinal plane
- Stage 3: extraretinal fibrovascular proliferation or neovascularization extending from the ridge into the vitreous
- Stage 4: evidence of a partial retinal detachment, which can be extrafoveal (stage 4A) or foveal (stage 4B).
- Stage 5: tractional total retinal detachment

"Plus" disease is characterized by an increased venous dilation and arteriolar tortuosity of the retinal vessels in the posterior pole. Although plus disease can be present at any stage, it indicates vascular shunting and is a marker of severe ROP. The retinal zones involved by ROP are three: zone I refers to a concentric area centered on the optic disc with a diameter twice the distance between the center of the optic nerve and the fovea, zone II is a circle centered on the optic disc ending at the ora serrata, and zone III includes the temporal retina [94].

The decision to treat depends on the type of ROP. While a follow-up observation is recommended for zone I stage 1 or 2 without plus disease or zone II stage 3 without plus disease, treatment is indicated in any stage zone I ROP with plus disease, zone I stage 3 with or without plus disease, or zone II stage 2 or 3 with plus disease. The current standard treatment for ROP is argon and diode laser photocoagulation treatment to the avascular retina. The use of anti-VEGF agents, such as intravitreal bevacizumab, has also been proposed as a possible therapeutic strategy, but it requires further validation, especially for safety concerns [94].

Retinal detachment, which occurs in ROP stages 4 and 5, is the most frequent complication of ROP and is associated with a significantly high risk of poor visual outcomes, including visual acuity reduction to light perception or total blindness, and may require vitrectomy. Threats to visual acuity persist through childhood: the most common sequelae are myopia, whereas other late complications include glaucoma, amblyopia, cataract, and strabismus. Children with the greatest visual impairment (e.g., vision limited to light perception or no light perception) have significantly higher rates of developmental disability, epilepsy, and special education needs [95].

2.2.9 Neurodevelopmental Sequelae

Delicate extrauterine development, together with multiple prematurity-related complications and other factors that accompany their hospital stay, such as repeated painful stimulations and parental separation, is a major challenge for the neurodevelopment of children born preterm. In particular, the main factors that have been found to correlate with adverse neurodevelopmental outcomes include the following [96]:

- BW <750 g or GA <25 weeks
- Male sex
- Chorioamnionitis
- Low pH on umbilical arterial cord blood
- Periventricular hemorrhage grades III and IV and related complications (PVHI, PHVD)
- Periventricular leukomalacia or white matter abnormalities
- Neonatal seizures
- Prolonged mechanical ventilation
- Bronchopulmonary dysplasia
- Neonatal meningitis
- Subnormal head circumference at hospital discharge
- Coexisting congenital malformation
- Low parental education and parental deprivation

For this reason, a neurodevelopmental follow-up is routinely established after hospital discharge in order to evaluate the neurodevelopmental milestones and the development of motor, cognitive, and language functions following preterm birth. The Bayley Scales of Infant Development (BSID) is a widely used scoring tool for developmental assessment over the first 42 months of age. BSID consists of three components investigating cognitive, language, and motor skills; two parent-report subtests reflecting adaptive and social-emotional behaviors are also included in the evaluation [97].

To date, a large amount of literature on preterm infants' neurodevelopmental up to scholar age is available. At 2 years of corrected age, the rates of moderate to severe neurodevelopmental impairment are striking at the lowest GAs, being as high as 80% in infants born before 25 weeks' gestation. Adverse neurodevelopmental outcomes after extremely preterm birth include intellectual disability (5–36%), CP (9–18%), blindness (0.7–9%), and deafness (2–4%) [98]. On the other hand, moderate to late preterm infants are not exempt from neurodevelopmental sequelae, although usually less severe; however, due to the high prevalence of preterm births >32 weeks' gestation, even minor neurodevelopmental deficits may have a significant impact [99].

In recent years, it appears that specific neurological and developmental sequelae, such as severe CP, are occurring at lower rates compared to former data; it is likely that advances in neonatal medical intensive care may have contributed to this improvement. However, milder impairments, including attention-deficit/hyperactivity disorder, executive function deficits, visuomotor problems, learning disabilities, and behavior problems, are remarkably high among preterm-born children, occurring in 50–70% of VLBW infants. Moreover, it should be considered that many developmental deficits in cognition, behavioral development, and social adaptive functioning may emerge at older ages even in the absence of established neurodevelopmental impairment in prescholar ages, and this demonstrates the need for a longer follow-up of the preterm-born population.

References

1. Harrison MS, Goldenberg RL. Global burden of prematurity. Semin Fetal Neonatal Med. 2016;21:74–9.
2. Walani SR. Global burden of preterm birth. Int J Gynaecol Obstet. 2020;150:31–3. https://doi.org/10.1002/IJGO.13195.
3. Frey HA, Klebanoff MA. The epidemiology, etiology, and costs of preterm birth. Semin Fetal Neonatal Med. 2016;21:68–73.
4. Stout MJ, Busam R, Macones GA, Tuuli MG. Spontaneous and indicated preterm birth subtypes: interobserver agreement and accuracy of classification. Am J Obstet Gynecol. 2014;211:530.e1–4. https://doi.org/10.1016/J.AJOG.2014.05.023.
5. Manuck TA. Racial and ethnic differences in preterm birth: a complex, multifactorial problem. Semin Perinatol. 2017;41:511–8.
6. Ion R, Bernal AL. Smoking and preterm birth. Reprod Sci. 2015;22:918–26. https://doi.org/10.1177/1933719114556486.
7. Fan J, Lee BK, Wikman AT, Johansson S, Reilly M. Associations of rhesus and non-rhesus maternal red blood cell alloimmunization with stillbirth and preterm birth. Int J Epidemiol. 2014;43:1123–31. https://doi.org/10.1093/IJE/DYU079.
8. Zur RL, Kingdom JC, Parks WT, Hobson SR. The placental basis of fetal growth restriction. Obstet Gynecol Clin N Am. 2020;47:81–98. https://doi.org/10.1016/J.OGC.2019.10.008.
9. Ferrazzi E, Bozzo M, Rigano S, Bellotti M, Morabito A, Pardi G, Battaglia FC, Galan HL. Temporal sequence of abnormal Doppler changes in the peripheral and central circulatory systems of the severely growth-restricted fetus. Ultrasound Obstet Gynecol. 2002;19:140–6. https://doi.org/10.1046/J.0960-7692.2002.00627.X.
10. Amiel-Tison C, Cabrol D, Denver R, Jarreau PH, Papiernik E, Piazza PV. Fetal adaptation to stress. Part I: acceleration of fetal maturation and earlier birth triggered by placental insufficiency in humans. Early Hum Dev. 2004;78:15–27. https://doi.org/10.1016/J.EARLHUMDEV.2004.03.002.
11. Matthiesen NB, Østergaard JR, Hjortdal VE, Henriksen TB. Congenital heart defects and the risk of spontaneous preterm birth. J Pediatr. 2021;229:168–174.e5. https://doi.org/10.1016/J.JPEDS.2020.09.059.
12. Cavoretto P, Candiani M, Giorgione V, Inversetti A, Abu-Saba MM, Tiberio F, Sigismondi C, Farina A. Risk of spontaneous preterm birth in singleton pregnancies conceived after IVF/ICSI treatment: meta-analysis of cohort studies. Ultrasound Obstet Gynecol. 2018;51:43–53. https://doi.org/10.1002/UOG.18930.
13. Vahanian SA, Lavery JA, Ananth CV, Vintzileos A. Placental implantation abnormalities and risk of preterm delivery: a systematic review and meta-analysis. Am J Obstet Gynecol. 2015;213:S78–90. https://doi.org/10.1016/J.AJOG.2015.05.058.
14. Nadeau HCG, Subramaniam A, Andrews WW. Infection and preterm birth. Semin Fetal Neonatal Med. 2016;21:100–5. https://doi.org/10.1016/J.SINY.2015.12.008.
15. Leitich H, Bodner-Adler B, Brunbauer M, Kaider A, Egarter C, Husslein P. Bacterial vaginosis as a risk factor for preterm delivery: a meta-analysis. Am J Obstet Gynecol. 2003;189:139–47. https://doi.org/10.1067/mob.2003.339.
16. Goldenberg RL, Hauth JC, Andrews WW. Intrauterine infection and preterm delivery. N Engl J Med. 2000;342:1500–7. https://doi.org/10.1056/NEJM200005183422007.
17. Knobel RB, Guenther BD, Rice HE. Thermoregulation and thermography in neonatal physiology and disease. Biol Res Nurs. 2011;13:274–82. https://doi.org/10.1177/1099800411403467.
18. De Almeida MFB, Guinsburg R, Sancho GA, Rosa IRM, Lamy ZC, Martinez FE, Da Silva RPGVC, Ferrari LSL, De Souza Rugolo LMS, Abdallah VOS, Silveira RDC. Hypothermia and early neonatal mortality in preterm infants. J Pediatr. 2014;164:271–5. https://doi.org/10.1016/j.jpeds.2013.09.049.
19. de Siqueira Caldas JP, Ferri WAG, Marba STM, Aragon DC, Guinsburg R, de Almeida MFB, Diniz EMA, Silveira RCS, Alves Junior JMS, Pavanelli MB, Bentlin MR, Ferreira DMLM, Vale MS, Fiori HH, Duarte JLMB, Meneses JA, Cwajg S, Carvalho WB, Ferrari LSL, Silva NMM, da Silva RPGVC, Anchieta LM, Santos JPF, Kawakami MD. Admission hypothermia, neonatal morbidity, and mortality: evaluation of a multicenter cohort of very low birth weight preterm infants according to relative performance of the center. Eur J Pediatr. 2019;178:1023–32. https://doi.org/10.1007/s00431-019-03386-9.
20. Whitsett JA, Weaver TE. Hydrophobic surfactant proteins in lung function and disease. N Engl J Med. 2002;347:2141–8. https://doi.org/10.1056/NEJMRA022387.
21. Nitta K, Kobayashi T. Impairment of surfactant activity and ventilation by proteins in lung edema fluid. Respir Physiol. 1994;95:43–51. https://doi.org/10.1016/0034-5687(94)90046-9.
22. Donn SM, Sinha SK. Minimising ventilator induced lung injury in preterm infants. Arch Dis Child Fetal Neonatal Ed. 2006;91:226–30.
23. Marseglia L, D'Angelo G, Granese R, Falsaperla R, Reiter RJ, Corsello G, Gitto E. Role of oxidative stress in neonatal respiratory distress syndrome. Free Radic Biol Med. 2019;142:132–7.
24. Yadav S, Lee B, Kamity R. Neonatal respiratory distress syndrome. Treasure Island (FL): StatPearls Publishing; 2021.
25. Sweet DG, Carnielli V, Greisen G, Hallman M, Ozek E, Te Pas A, Plavka R, Roehr CC, Saugstad OD, Simeoni U, Speer CP, Vento M, Visser GHA, Halliday HL. European consensus guidelines on the management of respiratory distress syndrome—2019 update. Neonatology. 2019;115:432–50.

26. Roberts D, Brown J, Medley N, Dalziel SR. Antenatal corticosteroids for accelerating fetal lung maturation for women at risk of preterm birth. Cochrane Database Syst Rev. 2017;3(3):CD004454.
27. Ardell S, Pfister RH, Soll R. Animal derived surfactant extract versus protein free synthetic surfactant for the prevention and treatment of respiratory distress syndrome. Cochrane Database Syst Rev. 2015;8(8):CD000144.
28. Herting E, Härtel C, Göpel W. Less invasive surfactant administration (LISA): chances and limitations. Arch Dis Child Fetal Neonatal Ed. 2019;104:F655–9.
29. Kamath BD, MacGuire ER, McClure EM, Goldenberg RL, Jobe AH. Neonatal mortality from respiratory distress syndrome: lessons for low-resource countries. Pediatrics. 2011;127:1139–46. https://doi.org/10.1542/PEDS.2010-3212.
30. Sun H, Zhou Y, Xiong H, Kang W, Xu B, Liu D, Zhang X, Li H, Zhou C, Zhang Y, Zhou M, Meng Q. Prognosis of very preterm infants with severe respiratory distress syndrome receiving mechanical ventilation. Lung. 2015;193:249–54. https://doi.org/10.1007/S00408-014-9683-5.
31. Jensen EA, Schmidt B. Epidemiology of bronchopulmonary dysplasia. Birth Defects Res A Clin Mol Teratol. 2014;100:145–57. https://doi.org/10.1002/BDRA.23235.
32. Bancalari E, Jain D. Bronchopulmonary dysplasia: 50 years after the original description. Neonatology. 2019;115:384–91. https://doi.org/10.1159/000497422.
33. Morty RE. Recent advances in the pathogenesis of BPD. Semin Perinatol. 2018;42:404–12. https://doi.org/10.1053/J.SEMPERI.2018.09.001.
34. Ehrenkranz RA. Validation of the National Institutes of Health consensus definition of bronchopulmonary dysplasia. Pediatrics. 2005;116:1353–60. https://doi.org/10.1542/peds.2005-0249.
35. Higgins RD, Jobe AH, Koso-Thomas M, Bancalari E, Viscardi RM, Hartert TV, Ryan RM, Kallapur SG, Steinhorn RH, Konduri GG, Davis SD, Thebaud B, Clyman RI, Collaco JM, Martin CR, Woods JC, Finer NN, Raju TNK. Bronchopulmonary dysplasia: executive summary of a workshop. J Pediatr. 2018;197:300–8.
36. Sahni M, Mowes AK. Bronchopulmonary dysplasia. Treasure Island (FL): StatPearls Publishing; 2021.
37. Wu KY, Jensen EA, White AM, Wang Y, Biko DM, Nilan K, Fraga MV, Mercer-Rosa L, Zhang H, Kirpalani H. Characterization of disease phenotype in very preterm infants with severe bronchopulmonary dysplasia. Am J Respir Crit Care Med. 2020;201:1398–406. https://doi.org/10.1164/rccm.201907-1342OC.
38. Shah VS, Ohlsson A, Halliday HL, Dunn M. Early administration of inhaled corticosteroids for preventing chronic lung disease in very low birth weight preterm neonates. Cochrane Database Syst Rev. 2017;1:CD001969. https://doi.org/10.1002/14651858.CD001969.PUB4.
39. Stewart A, Brion LP, Ambrosio-Perez I. Diuretics acting on the distal renal tubule for preterm infants with (or developing) chronic lung disease. Cochrane Database Syst Rev. 2011;2011:CD001817. https://doi.org/10.1002/14651858.cd001817.pub2.
40. Anderson PJ, Doyle LW. Neurodevelopmental outcome of bronchopulmonary dysplasia. Semin Perinatol. 2006;30:227–32. https://doi.org/10.1053/j.semperi.2006.05.010.
41. Kiserud T. Physiology of the fetal circulation. Semin Fetal Neonatal Med. 2005;10:493–503. https://doi.org/10.1016/j.siny.2005.08.007.
42. Hamrick SEG, Hansmann G. Patent ductus arteriosus of the preterm infant. Pediatrics. 2010;125:1020–30.
43. Gonzalez A, Sosenko IRS, Chandar J, Hummler H, Claure N, Bancalari E. Influence of infection on patent ductus arteriosus and chronic lung disease in premature infants weighing 1000 g or less. J Pediatr. 1996;128:470–8. https://doi.org/10.1016/S0022-3476(96)70356-6.
44. Alyamac Dizdar E, Ozdemir R, Nur Sari F, Yurttutan S, Gokmen T, Erdeve O, Emre Canpolat F, Uras N, Suna Oguz S, Dilmen U. Low platelet count is associated with ductus arteriosus patency in preterm newborns. Early Hum Dev. 2012;88:813–6. https://doi.org/10.1016/j.earlhumdev.2012.05.007.
45. Sallmon H, Weber SC, Hüning B, Stein A, Horn PA, Metze BC, Dame C, Bührer C, Felderhoff-Müser U, Hansmann G, Koehne P. Thrombocytopenia in the first 24 h after birth and incidence of patent ductus arteriosus. Pediatrics. 2012;130:e623–30. https://doi.org/10.1542/peds.2012-0499.
46. Semberova J, Sirc J, Miletin J, Kucera J, Berka I, Sebkova S, O'Sullivan S, Franklin O, Stranak Z. Spontaneous closure of patent ductus arteriosus in infants ≤1500 g. Pediatrics. 2017;140:4258. https://doi.org/10.1542/peds.2016-4258.
47. Deshpande P, Baczynski M, McNamara PJ, Jain A. Patent ductus arteriosus: the physiology of transition. Semin Fetal Neonatal Med. 2018;23:225–31. https://doi.org/10.1016/j.siny.2018.05.001.
48. Singh Y, Tissot C. Echocardiographic evaluation of transitional circulation for the neonatologists. Front Pediatr. 2018;6:140. https://doi.org/10.3389/fped.2018.00140.
49. Finnemore A, Groves A. Physiology of the fetal and transitional circulation. Semin Fetal Neonatal Med. 2015;20:210–6. https://doi.org/10.1016/j.siny.2015.04.003.
50. Sellmer A, Bjerre JV, Schmidt MR, McNamara PJ, Hjortdal VE, Høst B, Bech BH, Henriksen TB. Morbidity and mortality in preterm neonates with patent ductus arteriosus on day 3. Arch Dis Child Fetal Neonatal Ed. 2013;98:F505–10. https://doi.org/10.1136/archdischild-2013-303816.
51. Noori S, McCoy M, Friedlich P, Bright B, Gottipati V, Seri I, Sekar K. Failure of ductus arteriosus closure is associated with increased mortality in preterm infants. Pediatrics. 2009;123:e138–44. https://doi.org/10.1542/peds.2008-2418.

52. Schena F, Francescato G, Cappelleri A, Picciolli I, Mayer A, Mosca F, Fumagalli M. Association between hemodynamically significant patent ductus arteriosus and bronchopulmonary dysplasia. J Pediatr. 2015;166:1488–92. https://doi.org/10.1016/j.jpeds.2015.03.012.
53. Kluckow M, Evans N. Ductal shunting, high pulmonary blood flow, and pulmonary hemorrhage. J Pediatr. 2000;137:68–72. https://doi.org/10.1067/mpd.2000.106569.
54. Evans N, Kluckow M. Early ductal shunting and intra ventricular haemorrhage in ventilated preterm infants. Arch Dis Child Fetal Neonatal Ed. 1996;75:F183–6.
55. Noori S, McCoy M, Anderson MP, Ramji F, Seri I. Changes in cardiac function and cerebral blood flow in relation to peri/intraventricular hemorrhage in extremely preterm infants. J Pediatr. 2014;164:264–70. https://doi.org/10.1016/j.jpeds.2013.09.045.
56. de Boode WP. Individualized hemodynamic management in newborns. Front Pediatr. 2020;8:580470. https://doi.org/10.3389/fped.2020.580470.
57. Ungerleider GD, Williams DA, Ungerleider RM. Patent ductus arteriosus. In: Critical heart disease in infants and children. Amsterdam: Elsevier; 2021. p. 536–43. https://doi.org/10.1016/B978-1-4557-0760-7.00043-7.
58. Shelton EL, Singh GK, Nichols CG. Novel drug targets for ductus arteriosus manipulation: looking beyond prostaglandins. Semin Perinatol. 2018;42:221–7. https://doi.org/10.1053/j.semperi.2018.05.004.
59. Ohlsson A, Walia R, Shah SS. Ibuprofen for the treatment of patent ductus arteriosus in preterm or low birth weight (or both) infants. Cochrane Database Syst Rev. 2013;2013(4):CD003481.
60. Graham GG, Davies MJ, Day RO, Mohamudally A, Scott KF. The modern pharmacology of paracetamol: therapeutic actions, mechanism of action, metabolism, toxicity and recent pharmacological findings. Inflammopharmacology. 2013;21:201–32.
61. Martini S, Galletti S, Kelsall W, Angeli E, Agulli M, Gargiulo GD, Chen SE, Corvaglia L, Singh Y. Ductal ligation timing and neonatal outcomes: a 12-year bicentric comparison. Eur J Pediatr. 2021;180:2261–70. https://doi.org/10.1007/s00431-021-04004-3.
62. Volpe JJ. Intraventricular hemorrhage in the premature infant—current concepts. Part II. Ann Neurol. 1989;25:109–16. https://doi.org/10.1002/ana.410250202.
63. Ballabh P. Intraventricular hemorrhage in premature infants: mechanism of disease. Pediatr Res. 2010;67:1–8.
64. Cimatti AG, Martini S, Galletti S, Vitali F, Aceti A, Frabboni G, Faldella G, Corvaglia L. Cerebral oxygenation and autoregulation in very preterm infants developing IVH during the transitional period: a pilot study. Front Pediatr. 2020;8:381. https://doi.org/10.3389/fped.2020.00381.
65. O'Leary H, Gregas MC, Limperopoulos C, Zaretskaya I, Bassan H, Soul JS, Di Salvo DN, Du Plessis AJ. Elevated cerebral pressure passivity is associated with prematurity-related intracranial hemorrhage. Pediatrics. 2009;124:302–9. https://doi.org/10.1542/peds.2008-2004.
66. Sortica da Costa C, Cardim D, Molnar Z, Kelsall W, Ng I, Czosnyka M, Smielewski P, Austin T. Changes in hemodynamics, cerebral oxygenation and cerebrovascular reactivity during the early transitional circulation in preterm infants. Pediatr Res. 2019;86:247–53. https://doi.org/10.1038/s41390-019-0410-z.
67. Hoffman SB, Cheng YJ, Magder LS, Shet N, Viscardi RM. Cerebral autoregulation in premature infants during the first 96 hours of life and relationship to adverse outcomes. Arch Dis Child Fetal Neonatal Ed. 2019;104:F473–9. https://doi.org/10.1136/archdischild-2018-315725.
68. Pryds O, Greisen G, Lou H, Frils-Hansen B, Friis-Hansen B. Heterogeneity of cerebral vasoreactivity in preterm infants supported by mechanical ventilation. J Pediatr. 1989;115:638–45. https://doi.org/10.1016/s0022-3476(89)80301-4.
69. Papile LA, Burstein J, Burstein R, Koffler H. Incidence and evolution of subependymal and intraventricular hemorrhage: a study of infants with birth weights less than 1500 g. J Pediatr. 1978;92:529–34. https://doi.org/10.1016/S0022-3476(78)80282-0.
70. Volpe JJ. Brain injury in premature infants: a complex amalgam of destructive and developmental disturbances. Lancet Neurol. 2009;8:110–24.
71. Inder TE, Perlman JM, Volpe JJ. Preterm intraventricular hemorrhage/posthemorrhagic hydrocephalus. In: Volpe's neurology of the newborn. Amsterdam: Elsevier; 2018. p. 637–98. https://doi.org/10.1016/B978-0-323-42876-7.00024-7.
72. Valdez Sandoval P, Hernández Rosales P, Quiñones Hernández DG, Chavana Naranjo EA, García Navarro V. Intraventricular hemorrhage and posthemorrhagic hydrocephalus in preterm infants: diagnosis, classification, and treatment options. Childs Nerv Syst. 2019;35:917–27. https://doi.org/10.1007/S00381-019-04127-X.
73. Khwaja O, Volpe JJ. Pathogenesis of cerebral white matter injury of prematurity. Arch Dis Child Fetal Neonatal Ed. 2008;93:F153–61. https://doi.org/10.1136/adc.2006.108837.
74. Agut T, Alarcon A, Cabañas F, Bartocci M, Martinez-Biarge M, Horsch S, Agut T, Alarcon A, Arena R, Bartocci M, Bravo M, Cabañas F, Carreras N, Claris O, Dudink J, Fumagalli M, Govaert P, Horsch S, Parodi A, Pellicer A, Ramenghi L, Roehr CC, Steggerda S, Valverde E. Preterm white matter injury: ultrasound diagnosis and classification. Pediatr Res. 2020;87:37–49.
75. Alsaied A, Islam N, Thalib L. Global incidence of necrotizing enterocolitis: a systematic review and meta-analysis. BMC Pediatr. 2020;20:344. https://doi.org/10.1186/s12887-020-02231-5.
76. Isani MA, Delaplain PT, Grishin A, Ford HR. Evolving understanding of neonatal necrotizing enterocolitis. Curr Opin Pediatr. 2018;30:417–23. https://doi.org/10.1097/MOP.0000000000000629.

77. Rose AT, Patel RM. A critical analysis of risk factors for necrotizing enterocolitis. Semin Fetal Neonatal Med. 2018;23(6):374–9. https://doi.org/10.1016/j.siny.2018.07.005.
78. Mshvildadze M, Neu J, Shuster J, Theriaque D, Li N, Mai V. Intestinal microbial ecology in premature infants assessed with non-culture-based techniques. J Pediatr. 2010;156:20–5. https://doi.org/10.1016/j.jpeds.2009.06.063.
79. Watkins DJ, Besner GE. The role of the intestinal microcirculation in necrotizing enterocolitis. Semin Pediatr Surg. 2013;22:83–7. https://doi.org/10.1053/j.sempedsurg.2013.01.004.
80. Epelman M, Daneman A, Navarro OM, Morag I, Moore AM, Kim JH, Faingold R, Taylor G, Gerstle JT. Necrotizing enterocolitis: review of state-of-the-art imaging findings with pathologic correlation. Radiographics. 2007;27:285–305. https://doi.org/10.1148/rg.272055098.
81. Bell MJ, Ternberg JL, Feigin RD, Keating JP, Marshall R, Barton L, Brotherton T. Neonatal necrotizing enterocolitis. Therapeutic decisions based upon clinical staging. Ann Surg. 1978;187:1–7.
82. Kliegman RM, Walsh MC. Neonatal necrotizing enterocolitis: pathogenesis, classification, and spectrum of illness. Curr Probl Pediatr. 1987;17:213–88.
83. Papillon SC, Short SS, Ford HR. Necrotizing enterocolitis. In: Newborn surgery. 4th ed. Cham: Springer; 2021. p. 653–9. https://doi.org/10.4324/9781315113968.
84. Henry MCW, Moss RL. Neonatal necrotizing enterocolitis. Semin Pediatr Surg. 2008;17:98–109. https://doi.org/10.1053/j.sempedsurg.2008.02.005.
85. Patel AL, Kim JH. Human milk and necrotizing enterocolitis. Semin Pediatr Surg. 2018;27:34–8. https://doi.org/10.1053/j.sempedsurg.2017.11.007.
86. Sharif S, Meader N, Oddie SJ, Rojas-Reyes MX, McGuire W. Probiotics to prevent necrotising enterocolitis in very preterm or very low birth weight infants. Cochrane Database Syst Rev. 2020;10:CD005496. https://doi.org/10.1002/14651858.CD005496.pub5.
87. Jones IH, Hall NJ. Contemporary outcomes for infants with necrotizing enterocolitis-a systematic review. J Pediatr. 2020;220:86–92.e3. https://doi.org/10.1016/j.jpeds.2019.11.011.
88. Ou J, Courtney CM, Steinberger AE, Tecos ME, Warner BW. Nutrition in necrotizing enterocolitis and following intestinal resection. Nutrients. 2020;12:520. https://doi.org/10.3390/nu12020520.
89. Hickey M, Georgieff M, Ramel S. Neurodevelopmental outcomes following necrotizing enterocolitis. Semin Fetal Neonatal Med. 2018;23:426–32.
90. Blencowe H, Lawn JE, Vazquez T, Fielder A, Gilbert C. Preterm-associated visual impairment and estimates of retinopathy of prematurity at regional and global levels for 2010. Pediatr Res. 2013;74:35–49. https://doi.org/10.1038/pr.2013.205.
91. Hellström A, Smith LEH, Dammann O. Retinopathy of prematurity. Lancet (London, England). 2013;382:1445–57. https://doi.org/10.1016/S0140-6736(13)60178-6.
92. Higgins RD. Oxygen saturation and retinopathy of prematurity. Clin Perinatol. 2019;46:593–9.
93. Fierson WM. Screening examination of premature infants for retinopathy of prematurity. Pediatrics. 2018;142:e20183061. https://doi.org/10.1542/peds.2018-3061.
94. Brown AC, Nwanyanwu K. Retinopathy of prematurity. Treasure Island (FL): StatPearls Publishing; 2021.
95. Norman M, Hellström A, Hallberg B, Wallin A, Gustafson P, Tornqvist K, Håkansson S, Holmström G. Prevalence of severe visual disability among preterm children with retinopathy of prematurity and association with adherence to best practice guidelines. JAMA Netw Open. 2019;2:e186801. https://doi.org/10.1001/jamanetworkopen.2018.6801.
96. Duncan AF, Matthews MA. Neurodevelopmental outcomes in early childhood. Clin Perinatol. 2018;45:377–92.
97. Balasundaram P, Avulakunta ID. Bayley scales of infant and toddler development. Treasure Island (FL): StatPearls Publishing; 2020.
98. Jarjour IT. Neurodevelopmental outcome after extreme prematurity: a review of the literature. Pediatr Neurol. 2015;52:143–52.
99. Woythaler M. Neurodevelopmental outcomes of the late preterm infant. Semin Fetal Neonatal Med. 2019;24:54–9. https://doi.org/10.1016/J.SINY.2018.10.002.

3 Newborns with Congenital Malformations

Guido Cocchi and Vincenzo Davide Catania

Abbreviations

AD	Autosomal dominant
AR	Autosomal recessive
CM	Congenital malformation
MRI	Magnetic resonance imaging
NIPT	Noninvasive prenatal testing
NS	Noonan syndrome

3.1 Introduction

Congenital malformations (CMs) are one of the main causes of the global burden of disease. CM may result in disabilities that may be physical, intellectual, or developmental. The disabilities can range from mild to severe. It is quite difficult to define CM in one sentence only. CMs are defined as structural or irreversible functional anomalies of prenatal origin that can affect almost one or more parts of the body, regardless of their cause. CMs may be diagnosed during pregnancy, at birth, during life, or postmortem. It is generally accepted that 3–4% of children are affected by congenital malformations [1–4].

Some CMs can be treated with surgical or nonsurgical options, such as cleft lip and/or palate, clubfoot, and atresia or stenosis. Others, including heart defects, neural tube defects, and Down syndrome (DS), can cause lifelong impacts. Different degrees of CMs require different surgical approaches: from cosmetic (exeresis of a postaxial polydactyly) to high surgical treatment (heart transplant in severe hypoplastic left heart syndrome and similar extreme forms of congenital heart disease) or with the use of therapeutic treatment for all the person's life (i.e., congenital hypothyroidism) [5–8].

The impact of CMs on clinical and social approaches is high. Almost all birth defect syndromes are rare, and a practicing physician would be expected to see only a limited number of such cases in his professional life. Because of the rarity of some disorders, even a specialist in this field will never gain experience in all of them. The recognition and analysis of various component anomalies are fundamental to reaching a correct diagnosis, with implications on the best way to treat and approach the defects [2, 9, 10].

G. Cocchi (✉)
Paediatric Unit, Department of Pediatrics, Sant'Orsola Hospital, IRCSS, University of Bologna, Bologna, BO, Italy
e-mail: guido.cocchi@unibo.it

V. D. Catania
Pediatric Surgery, Sant'Orsola Hospital, IRCSS, University of Bologna, Bologna, BO, Italy
e-mail: vincenzodavide.catania@aosp.bo.it

M. Lima, M. C. Mondardini (eds.), *Frailty in Children*,
https://doi.org/10.1007/978-3-031-24307-3_3

3.2 Pathogenetic Mechanism

Four different pathogenetic mechanisms of structural anomalies are indicated by the terms deformation, disruption, dysplasia, and malformation [7]

1. *Deformation*: this is caused by an abnormal external force acting on the fetus during its development. It results in the abnormal growth and formation of fetal structures. Fetuses that grow in a uterine environment where not enough amniotic fluid is present (oligohydramnios) may have a flattened face (Fig. 3.1) due to the compression of the head against the uterine wall, with no room for movement. Similar considerations could be made for positional foot abnormalities, such as calcaneovalgus foot or metatarsus adduct (Fig. 3.2) [4].
2. *Disruption*: this results from destructive processes that alter the fetal structure during organogenesis, i.e., in amniotic bands. The mechanism causing this injury is still unclear, but the resulting lesions range from shallow constricting rings with modifications of the lymphatic and hematological circulation to determine amputation or cutaneous rings, above all, in the distal parts of the fetal body, i.e., hands or feet.
3. *Dysplasia*: it is due to an abnormal cellular organization or function within a specific tissue, resulting in clinically evident structural and anatomical changes. It is a histologic diagnosis and refers to focal diffuse or segmentally arranged primitive structures. An important aspect of most dysplastic conditions is their continued course. Since the tissue itself is abnormal, clinical effects may persist or worsen as long as the tissue contin-

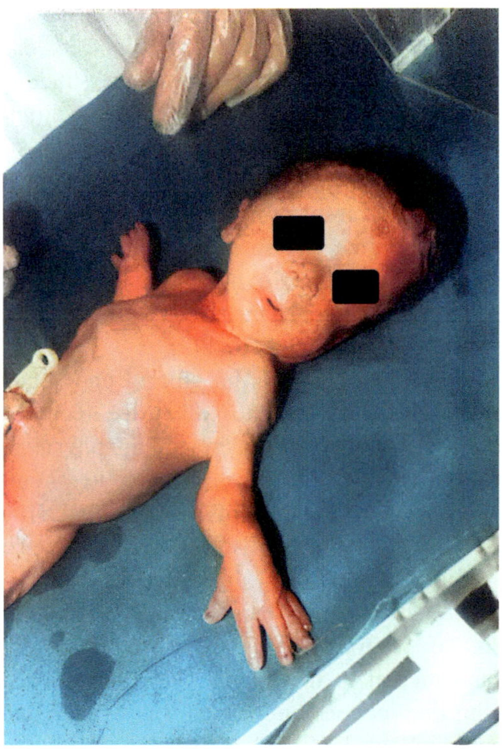

Fig. 3.1 Newborn with a flattened face. Pregnancy was complicated by polyhydramnios, with subsequent compression of the head against the uterine wall with no room for movement

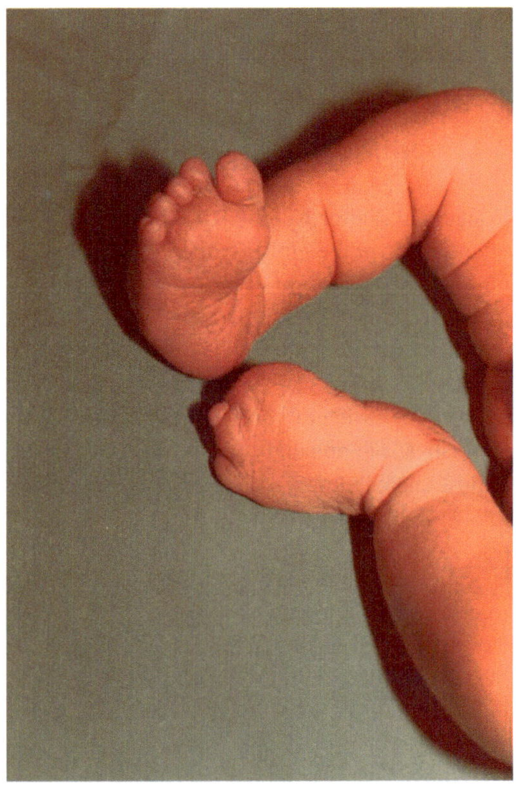

Fig. 3.2 Left finger-foot amputation and right metatarsus adductus foot

ues to grow or function. Almost all the dysplasia forms seem to be caused by a major mutant gene. Examples include metabolic disorders such as storage diseases, i.e., skeletal (achondroplasia) and ectodermal dysplasia (hypohidrotic ectodermal dysplasia XL-R) or renal dysplasia. Dysplasia can continue to produce dysmorphic changes throughout life.

4. *Malformation*: malformations are structural defects in the body due to abnormal embryonic development. They could be consequences of the failure or inadequate completion of embryological processes. As the earliest developmental alteration happens, more important is the damage to the tissue or organ involved. Alterations in the cellular and/or molecular interactions within any particular organ can cause abnormal development, which leads to defective organogenesis till the death of the embryo. The anomaly does not imply any specific etiology but is related to an early error in embryonic development. The result of damage in the fetal period is above all related to the growth and complexity of already differentiated organs, and true malformations arising in this period are quite rare.

3.3 Clinical Classification of Congenital Malformations

The best way to approach the complexity of CMs is to consider the relationship of one defect to another. An anomaly that occurred as isolated has a different significance if the same defect occurs in connection with others [11–15].

(a) Single defects

Malformation occurs only in one single organ or part of the body. In this group are included the majority of birth defects: congenital heart defects, esophageal and gastrointestinal atresia, anorectal atresia, cleft lip/palate, or atresia auris (Figs. 3.3 and 3.4). Most of these conditions are thought to have a multifactorial origin. These may result as a consequence of the impact of environmental factors with multiple genes not able to determine the effect by themselves. In a few other cases, a genetic cause is recognized not always based on Mendelian inheritance patterns, which leads one to think of the role of minor genes. Rarely do the single-system defects, however, show a high degree of concordance in monozygotic twins, which supports the hypothesis of nongenetic factors in their origin.

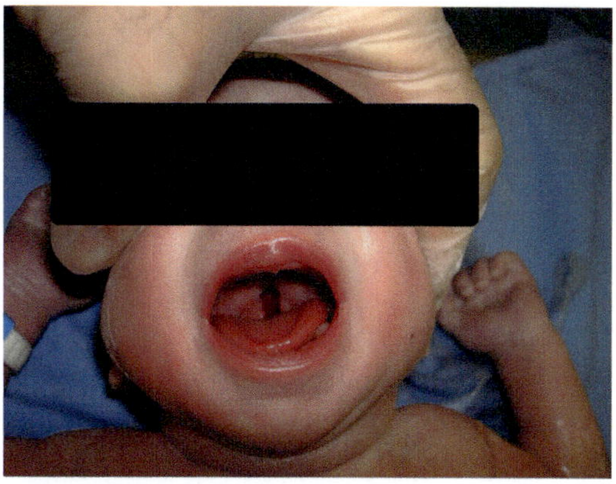

Fig. 3.3 Hard and soft cleft palate

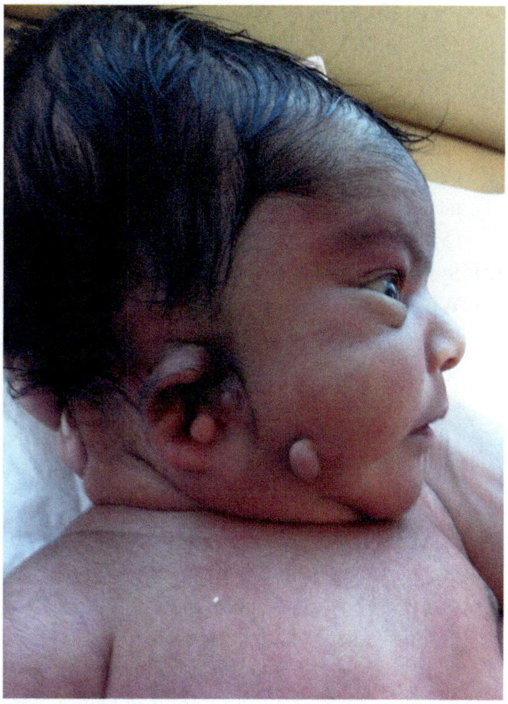

Fig. 3.4 Right mandibular hypoplasia, microtia and accessory prearicular tags. (Hemifacial Microsomia)

(b) Sequences
A sequence is a group of related anomalies that generally originate from a single initial major anomaly that alters the development of other surrounding or related tissues or structures [4]. Malformation sequences may be caused by genetic as well as environmental factors. The primary anomaly interferes with regular embryologic developmental processes, and at birth, the neonate seems to show multiple defects. The oligohydramnios sequence (Potter sequence) is a well-known example where agenesis of the kidneys or other urinary tract anomalies leads to pulmonary hypoplasia and deformations on the fetus, like a dysmorphic face. Spina bifida, for example, is frequently associated with clubfoot, which is closely related to spinal cord injury. The Pierre-Robin sequence, too, is an example in which a set of abnormalities affecting the head and face, consisting of hypoplasia of the mandibular area (micrognathia), glossoptosis (an incorrect placement or displacement of the tongue), that can result in an obstruction of the airways. Early mandibular retrognathia is the primary anomaly that can explain the cascade of events. Most neonates affected by the Pierre-Robin sequence show cleft palate, even though it is not generally considered necessary for the diagnosis of the condition [5, 11, 14, 16].

(c) Syndromes
When multiple congenital anomalies, which are not part of one sequence but may involve several sequences, are thought to be due to a single cause, this is called a syndrome (from Greek "syn" and "drome," in other words, "running together") [4]. When the etiology of a syndrome is detected, the initial designation, known as eponymous, should be abandoned in favor of the specific etiological origin. For chromosomal anomalies, the definitive name should arise from the altered chromosome: for example, Down syndrome, by the eponymous John Langdon Down, who in 1866 described for the first time the condition, should be better defined as trisomy 21 (T-21) for the presence of chromosome 21 triplicate. In the same way, DiGeorge syndrome, reported by DiGeorge in 1965 (also known as conotruncal anomaly face syndrome, described by Takao in 1976, and velocardiofacial syndrome, described by Shprintzen in 1978), should be better described as CATCH 22 syndrome due to the variable deletion of genetic materials by the long arm of chromosome 22. In the case of monogenic disorders, which are caused predominantly by a lesion of a single gene, the phenotypic manifestation may depend, to various extents, on additional genetic variants in the same or other genes, on epigenetic changes, and on environmental factors. In the Noonan syndrome (NS), the most frequent monogenic disorder occurring approximately in 1000–2500 children, the first most common genetic cause is still PTPN11 mutations, observed in 42.5% of NS patients, but many other mutations are described to be associated with NS. All these related disorders are defined as a group of rare conditions caused by mutations in the genes of the Ras-MAPK pathways, better known as RASopathies [14]. Mutations in the alpha-L-iduronidase lead to a deficiency in the glycosidase alpha-L-iduronidase; known as Hurler syndrome, it should be defined as mucopolysaccharidosis type 1 (MPS-1). In some other cases of multiple congenital anomalies, the pattern should be recognized while the etiology and pathogenesis are unknown. In this case, we should speak of association.

(d) Associations
Associations are usually sporadic conditions with a very low risk of recurrence. They are related to each other as a group of anomalies whose occurrence is explained by chance. These conditions emphasize the lack of uniformity in clinical presentation from case to case. VACTERL association comprises varied anomalies that are used as an acronym of the conditions shown at birth as anomalies of vertebrae (V), anal atresia (A), cardiac defects (C), tracheoesophageal atresia (TE),

renal anomalies (R), and limb defects (L). Most children with this condition, however, do not present all these anomalies at the same time but rather show a varying combination of these from this list. The condition is often sporadic with a low risk of recurrence. Until now, it is not possible to identify a common etiology, and a great deal is to be learned about this type of congenital abnormality. Another method that is useful in the presence of one of these malformations is to try and exclude the presence of some other defects. In presence of anal atresia or limb defects, it is necessary to exclude cardiac, renal, spine, and esophageal malformations. The prognosis is related to the severity of the malformation that the newborn presents and the possibility of surgical treatment [2, 17, 18].

3.4 Etiology of Congenital Malformations

For many CMs, the cause is unknown. Most of them are caused by multiple factors, yet at the same time, they are related to each other. Kalter and Warkany (1983) reviewed the knowledge of the etiology of major congenital malformations [11]. CMs are divided into five categories, and the relative contribution of each causal category was estimated:

1. Genetics: one or more genes might undergo a change or mutation that can lead to genetic disorders or illnesses. Some genetic conditions are caused by mutations in a single gene. These conditions are usually inherited in one of several patterns of Mendelian inheritance, depending by the gene involved. Different patterns of Mendelian inheritance—autosomal dominant (AD), autosomal recessive (AR), X-linked dominant (X-LD), and X-linked recessive (X-LR)—are principal examples of genetic patterns of inheritance. In other conditions, a gene or a part of a gene might be missing.
2. Chromosomal abnormalities: in some cases, a chromosome (Turner syndrome: 45, X0) or a part of a chromosome (CATCH 22 syndrome) might be missing. In other cases, such as with Down syndrome, chromosome 21 is triplicate (trisomy 21).
3. Environmental causes: exposure to drugs, chemicals, or toxic substances, i.e., alcohol exposure, can cause fetal alcohol spectrum disorders; exposure to antiepileptic drugs (valproic acid, hydantoin) can determine specific features, i.e., fetal valproate syndrome or fetal hydantoin syndrome. Exposure to maternal infections can produce infectious embryo-fetopathy too: maternal infection early in pregnancy, i.e., the *rubella virus*, can cause a miscarriage or serious birth defects [congenital rubella syndrome (CRS)]. *Toxoplasma gondii* and, Zika virus can determine teratogenic effects as eye-related manifestations of disease, other organ-related manifestation of disease as microcephaly.
4. Multifactorial disorders: these are due to a combination of the effects of multiple genes or the interactions between hereditary tendencies and nongenetic, usually undefined, factors, like the environment. This group of disorders includes a broad range of congenital birth defects, including cardiac malformations, neural tube defects, and cleft lip and/or palate. The underlying mechanisms by which the genes and the environment interact to cause these conditions are largely unknown.
5. Unknown causes: the dividing line between the categories multifactorial malformations and malformations of unknown etiology is not clear-cut. For multifactorial disorders, the genes and the environmental factors involved are often unknown. On the other hand, for malformations of unknown etiology, it is often assumed that genetic as well as environmental factors might be involved. The attribution of the 70% of malformations of multifactorial or unknown etiology to either one of these two categories is more or less a matter of subjective estimation. Family and twin studies have shown that these diseases have a genetic component, however. It is also clear that there are environmental contributors.

Knowledge of the etiology of congenital malformations is increasing gradually through the continued research of geneticists, embryologists, teratologists, pathologists, epidemiologists, and several other professionals. The estimate, however, that 70% of congenital anomalies are of unknown or multifactorial etiology still seems to be true [6, 7, 19].

3.4.1 Patterns of Inheritance

The diagnosis of a genetic disorder is based on a particular clinical pattern of symptoms and/or signs characteristic of the condition or by laboratory confirmation of the altered gene or gene products associated with the disorders [6]. It is important to distinguish between diseases that are genetic and those that are familial. A genetic disorder is determined completely or partially by altered genetic material. A familial disorder is one that is more common in the relatives of an affected individual than in the general population: some familial disorders are genetic, and others are caused by environmental exposure. The recognition of the pattern of inheritance not only assists in clinical diagnosis but also provides essential information for counseling family members about a recurrence risk in future pregnancies [4, 7].

3.4.2 Autosomal Dominant Inheritance

In an AD disorder, the mutated gene is a dominant gene located in one of the autosomes. Only one mutated gene is necessary to determine this type of disorder. AD disorders present some peculiarities in most circumstances: (1) any child of an affected parent has a 50% chance of inheriting the disorder, (2) phenotypically normal family members do not transmit the condition to their offspring, (3) there is no difference in impact between males and females, and (4) a significant proportion of cases involves new fresh mutation. An example of AD is Marfan syndrome.

3.4.3 Autosomal Recessive Inheritance

AR disorders are those in which two copies of the mutant gene in a homozygous state are necessary to cause the condition. The affected child inherits one copy of the mutated gene from each parent. The parents of a child with an AR condition usually do not have the condition. Unaffected parents are called carriers because they carry one copy of the mutant gene and can pass it to their children. An example of an AR condition is cystic fibrosis.

3.4.4 X-Linked Inheritance

The X chromosome has many genes that are important for growth and development. The Y chromosome is much smaller and has fewer genes. Females have two X chromosomes (XX); therefore, if one of the genes on an X chromosome has a change, the normal gene on the other X chromosome can compensate for the changed copy. If this happens, the female is usually a healthy carrier of the X-linked condition. In some cases, females show mild signs of the condition. Males have X and Y chromosomes (XY); therefore if one of the genes on the male's X chromosome has a mutation, he will be affected by the condition. Conditions that are inherited in this way are called X-linked recessive conditions [18].

(a) X-Linked Dominant Inheritance

Even though the most X-linked conditions are recessive, X-linked conditions can rarely be passed on in a dominant way. X-linked dominant disorders are seen more commonly in females than in males or, in the case of some diseases, affect only females. This means that even though a female inherits one changed copy of the gene, the changed gene will be enough to cause the condition. In males, it is thought that the hemizygous are so severely affected that they likely do not survive. This may be reflected in the familial pedigree of multiple miscarriages or male infant deaths. An affected female has a 50% chance of having affected children (sons and daughters). An affected male will have all daughters affected, but all sons will be unaffected. Examples of X-linked dominant disorders include X-linked lissencephaly, oral-facial-digital syndrome type I, and Rett syndrome [8, 17, 20].

(b) X-Linked Recessive Inheritance
If a female carrier has a son, she will pass on either the X chromosome with the normal gene or the X chromosome with the changed gene. Each son, therefore, has a 50% chance of inheriting the changed gene and being affected by the condition. There is also a 50% chance that the son will inherit the X chromosome with the normal gene, and for this, he will not be affected by the condition. This chance remains the same for every son. If a female carrier has a daughter, she will pass on either the X chromosome with the normal gene or the X chromosome with the changed gene. Each daughter therefore has a 50% chance of inheriting the changed gene. If this happens, the daughter will be a carrier, like her mother. There is also a 50% chance that the daughter will inherit the normal gene. If this happens, she will not be a carrier and will be totally unaffected by the condition. This chance remains the same for every daughter. If a male who has an X-linked condition has a daughter, he will always pass on the changed gene to her. All his daughters will therefore be carriers; they will usually not have the condition, but they are at risk of having affected sons. If a male who has an X-linked condition has a son, his son will never inherit the condition. Some examples of X-LR include hemophilia, Duchenne muscular dystrophy, and Fabry disease [17].

3.5 Prevention of Congenital Anomalies

Primary prevention represents the protection of the health of every person and of the community by activities that limit risk exposure or increase the immunity of individuals at risk. This could be achieved by preserving a good nutritional state, immunizing against infectious diseases of all community members, and making the environment as safe as possible. Those measures prevent the onset of illness or injury before the disease process begins [1, 16, 21]. Primary prevention is aimed at reducing the occurrence of new cases of the disease. Examples of successful primary prevention programs in the field of congenital malformations are the reduction of the prevalence of congenital rubella syndrome by vaccination and decreased prevalence of neural tube defects, both primary and recurrent, by the use of folic acid supplementation. Often, primary prevention is possible if the etiology of the defect is known. For most congenital malformations, this is impossible. One relevant aspect is the precocious detection, through the different techniques of prenatal diagnosis, of malformation and trying to identify and detect the severity and possibility of some kind of pharmacological or surgical treatment to find the best solution.

3.6 Prenatal Diagnosis

Until the early 1970s, the prenatal diagnosis of congenital anomalies focused on detecting chromosomal abnormalities by amniocentesis. Over the last two decades, prenatal diagnosis has benefited from advances in ultrasound technology. Now, fetal and postnatal ultrasound is a well-established technique for the early detection of abnormalities, and a precocious diagnosis may have important implications for the following:

(a) Obstetric and neonatal management: women carrying fetuses with identified or suspected malformations move to tertiary centers for further evaluation, counseling, and management. The task is to differentiate between lesions that could be incompatible with postnatal life, lesions that will necessitate a supporting person for the life of the patients, and lesions that are correctable through surgery or not.

(b) Morphologic anomalies detected by ultrasound could be associated with other defects and sometimes are components of syndromes that are difficult to identify in prenatal life. For these cases, genetic counseling is crucial. It is possible to associate specific genetic analysis to detect microscopic and submicroscopic chromosome abnormalities, like single-gene disorders, leading to relevant improvements in detection, such as congenital anomalies.

Invasive prenatal diagnosis continues to be the gold standard for pregnancies at increased risk for chromosomal and other genetic diseases. Chorionic villus sampling is the procedure of choice for the first trimester, whereas amniocentesis is the most common procedure during the mid-trimester. Prenatal diagnostic testing is available for an ever-increasing number of disorders. At first, prenatal tests focused on Down syndrome, while, actually, prenatal genetic testing can now detect a far broader array of conditions. Advances in genetic and genomic medicine have led to a dramatic increase in the availability of genetic testing, including in the prenatal period. At the same time, prenatal screening has also seen improvements, with the development of cell-free deoxyribonucleic acid (DNA) screening, like expanded carrier screening for a broad array of inherited conditions. This technique has extended fetal screening despite maternal age.

Patients should have pretest counseling that explains the benefits and limitations of invasive prenatal diagnostic testing, the conditions that will and will not be detected, and the risks of the procedures. Prenatal genetic testing has many benefits, like providing reassurance when there are no anomalies or identifying cases that will benefit from proper in utero or neonatal management. One of the goals is to guarantee the appropriate location and staffing for the delivery of affected infants and to provide the option of pregnancy termination for individual families that make that choice.

A new methodology for determining the risk of a fetus being affected by chromosomal and genetic disorders is noninvasive prenatal testing (NIPT). This testing analyzes small fragments of DNA that are circulating in pregnant blood. DNA fragments are free-floating, and they are called cell-free DNA (cfDNA). These small fragments usually contain fewer than 200 DNA building blocks (base pairs) and arise when cells die off and get broken down, and their contents, including DNA, are released into the bloodstream. These fragments originate from placenta cells that have the same fetus DNA. NIPT is used to check chromosomal disorders, such as aneuploidy (presence of an extra or a missing chromosome). Examples of extra chromosomes for autosomes are Down syndrome (T-21), Edward syndrome (T-18), and Patau syndrome (T-13), while for gonosomes, one well-known condition is Klinefelter syndrome (47, XXY). Another example of a missing copy for gonosomes is Turner syndrome (45, X0). All autosomes' monosomy is incompatible with life. The accuracy of the NIPT test varies for each disorder. NIPT can include screening for additional chromosomal anomalies, such as deletion (i.e., del 22q11) or duplication (i.e., mosaic tetrasomy 12p or Pallister–Killian syndrome).

NIPT is beginning to be used to test for genetic disorders caused by variants (changes in single genes). As technology improves and the cost of testing decreases, researchers expect that NIPT will become available for many more genetic conditions. In the low-risk population, prenatal diagnosis generally consists of screening procedures using ultrasound and maternal serum biochemistry.

Ultrasound technology continues to advance. Three-dimensional ultrasound imaging and the development of new markers should help improve diagnostic accuracy. Routine ultrasound screening does appear to reduce adverse outcomes in fetuses diagnosed with congenital anomalies.

However, limitations include operator variability, fetal position, gestational age effects (poor visualization, skull ossification), and tissue definition. Early studies using magnetic resonance imaging (MRI) in the evaluation of fetal morphology were hindered by fetal motion. Current software and hardware for MRI now allow the performance of MR examinations with high-quality images, permitting fetal imaging without maternal or fetal sedation. Although fast MRI techniques are widely available, few practitioners have knowledge of fetal anatomy and pathology with this technique.

Preliminary studies suggest that MRI may improve diagnostic accuracy and change counseling for many fetal central nervous system lesions and not as fetal abdominal, lung, and pelvic masses or congenital diaphragmatic hernia [22–24].

3.7 Communicating Diagnosis

Nowadays, fetal medicine provides reliable medical data about congenital abnormalities, and intrauterine diagnostic techniques are increasingly safe. The diagnosis that was not feasible a few decades ago can be elaborated with safety and certainty, generating ethical and legal responsibilities for the doctor who recognizes a malformation and communicates a specific diagnosis or the suspect of a diagnosis. When the mother and the couple are informed that the child is affected by a condition with a high risk of a congenital defect, fear and anxiety are increased. The "idealized child," after the communication of bad news, will be replaced by the "real child," who may be affected by some abnormalities as well as some defects that can require postnatal surgical or long-term pharmacological treatment, as well as the association to some degree of cognitive disability. The reactions go through shock, disbelief, denial, frustration, anger, and even irritation directed at the doctor who is to relay the bad news. The sudden change in the expectations of the desired pregnancy and the replacement with this news generates an emotional reaction in the mother above all and the couple too, which can range from the total protection of their baby to the rejection of the pregnancy and asking the for termination of the pregnancy. The communication becomes critical and can worsen by a low or incomplete preparation of the doctor who is in charge of communicating the clinical conditions of the child. Frequently, the parents have negative memories of the moment they receive them, not only because of their content but also because of the way they were informed—with inability, little empathy, and insensitivity [4, 5]. However, the way to report bad news must be learned and improved to understand how it can interfere with the physician-patient relationship. The communicating doctor must clarify, as much as possible, the aspects of the condition and, consequently, keep confidential the information obtained in the medical practice. Therefore, communication is one of the main critical aspects of this phase as it is a fundamental condition of human relations. In the same context, parents should be informed about all possible care attitudes and outcomes, such as the possibility of treatment and taking care of assistance after the birth of the baby by a team of doctors who are specifically involved in the clinical surveillance of the neonate with congenital malformations.

In the diagnosis communication phase, it is necessary to avoid words that can be related to the negative development of the baby and try not to give vague and approximate information. At the same time, it is not helpful to provide a long list of possible complications and comorbidities that a child could encounter over time, which only leads to parents feeling overwhelmed and powerless [15]. It is better to summarize the main features of the condition in a brief but clear way, keeping the focus on the child: every baby is unique, and it is wrong to consider him as a sum of symptoms. The discussion of the condition and the possible comorbidities should be accompanied, every time, by a description of the therapeutic possibilities that exist today and the achievable outcomes. Overall, it should be emphasized that the child will be included in follow-up programs of surveillance in a specialist center to verify the growth and identify any possible problems at an early stage to supply appropriate measures and treatments as soon as possible. In the same way, it is not necessary to give all the information at the first meeting; it is important to give more time to the couple to face problems and questions that will be debated in other subsequent meetings, where parents will be progressively informed about what they should pay attention to during the different phases of their child's life [1, 6, 7, 9].

3.8 Neonatal Care at Birth

The birth of a baby with congenital malformations is the starting point of a clinical process to reach a precise diagnosis. This leads to appropriate clinical planning and definition of prognosis and counseling to the parents. Different causal pathways may lead to a similar phenotype, and the diagnosis process may be long and difficult, requiring a follow-up survey to establish the natural history of the condition. Frequently, the evaluation process of a neonate affected by congenital malformations must proceed rapidly since decisions regarding intervention and treatment hinge on an accurate diagnosis. The diagnosis of these conditions, as said before, could be prenatally detected, but sometimes it is discovered at the moment of birth either by obstetricians on call or by the neonatologist during the first postnatal control or in connection with the resuscitation approach. All neonates have to undergo a thorough physical examination, and to reach a possible diagnosis, it is necessary to follow multiple sources of information. The methodology to approach the pathological aspects observed at birth is divided into some steps, starting from collecting as much information as possible about maternal medical history, pregnancy reproductive and delivery history, and family history, and an accurate description of the phenotype, with appropriate imaging and laboratory tests, is a relevant step too [6, 13, 25].

3.9 Maternal Medical History

Clear links exist between maternal diseases, including some specific conditions, such as myotonic dystrophy, autoimmune conditions, and diabetes mellitus type I. The incidence of major congenital anomalies among infants of diabetic mothers is four to five times higher than in the general population. It is fundamental to reach information about maternal exposure to drugs, cigarettes, alcohol, and infectious diseases. Medicament exposure during pregnancy may cause adverse pregnancy outcomes, including congenital anomalies, spontaneous abortion, fetal growth restriction, and low birth weight. It is estimated that 2–3% of birth defects are due to drug exposure during pregnancy. Ever since the thalidomide disaster occurred in the 1960s, increasing attention to medication safety in pregnancy has been paid. The proportion of pregnancies involving medication varied dramatically from 27% in the United States to 93% in countries in France. The phenomenon is more common than before because of the higher proportion of pregnancies complicated by chronic diseases and inadvertent drug use after conception. Assisted reproductive technologies (ART) are the treatment of choice for infertile couples. However these procedures are generally considered safe, children conceived by ART show a higher risk of prenatal and perinatal complications as congenital imprinting disorders like Beckwith–Wiedemann syndrome and Silver–Russel syndrome. The incidence of these syndromes in these infants is higher than general population. Human epigenome studies have generally revealed the enrichment of alteration in imprinted regions in children conceived by assisted reproductive technologies [2, 4, 11].

3.10 Pregnancy History

The pregnancy history can provide important information regarding the prenatal onset of congenital abnormalities, including information about the following

1. *Length of gestational age* (*GA*): it includes alteration in GA both before and after maturity.
2. *Fetal activity*: this includes alteration in the onset of fetal activity, which increases from

the 19th and 20th weeks of gestation and reaches a maximum between the 29th and 38th weeks and then decreases somewhat until delivery. Some structural defects are often associated with delayed onset and/or decreased intensity of fetal movement as well as the localization of fetal activity to one particular quadrant of the abdomen.

3. *Amniotic fluid (AF)*: this includes abnormalities in the amount of AF, such as oligohydramnios and polyhydramnios. During the third trimester of gestation, AF, under physiological conditions, is in a constant state of dynamic equilibrium between its production and resorption. AF is influenced by fetal urine, bronchopulmonary efflux, fetal swallowing and intramembranous and intravascular absorption. Polyhydramnios occurs if the fetus shows difficulty in swallowing AF, as in gastrointestinal or neurological abnormalities. Oligohydramnios is usually present following chronic leakage of AF or anomalies in the urinary system, as in renal agenesis, a polycystic kidney, or urethral obstruction.
4. *Ultrasound findings*: the prenatal detection of abnormalities on routine fetal ultrasound may identify abnormalities and can lead to suspect some genetic or chromosomal disorders. This detailed information regarding the pattern of events can help suspect or reach a diagnosis, also with the contribution of some prenatal genetic tests.
5. *Finding of prenatal screening*: nuchal translucency (NT) scan can detect about 80% of fetuses with trisomy 21 and other major aneuploidies, for a false positive rate of 5%. The combination of NT and maternal biochemical markers can help reach a safer diagnosis. Specifically, the dosage of maternal serum-free beta-hCG and PAPP-A improve detection to 90%. There is now evidence that the detection rate can increase to about 95%, and the false positive rate can be reduced to 3% by also examining the nasal bone, ductus venous flow, and tricuspid flow [2, 22].

3.11 Delivery History

1. *Presentation*: Breech presentation occurs in 3% of normal-term deliveries. However, it occurs much more frequently in some disorders that affect the form and/or function of the fetus. Structural anomalies such as hydrocephalus would be less compatible with vertex presentation because of the large head and joint dislocation (fetal akinesia and fetuses with multiple congenital contractures or arthrogryposis), which may reduce the ability of the fetus to modify its position. Defects of function include some conditions associated with neuromuscular disorders, such as trisomy 18, Prader–Willy syndrome, and Steinert myotonic dystrophy, among others.
2. Type of delivery: In the management of pregnancy complicated by fetal malformation, the choice of delivery method may be made on obstetrical grounds or in the belief that one method offers the fetus benefit over the other. Clear evidence of benefit from cesarean delivery is not available in the case of many malformations that are often considered for abdominal delivery. The choice must be based on the knowledge of individual malformations, fetal maturity, and presentation.
3. Growth deficiency: Growth deficit is another sign that may bring the child to the attention of the neonatologist. Small size at birth, disproportionate to gestational age, is frequently an important clue to prenatal dysmorphic processes. There is an increased incidence of malformation as the weight for gestational age decreases. In addition, there is a marked increase of disabilities in small for gestational age children who had some structural abnormalities.
4. Neonatal adaptation: The immediate postpartum period is a time of significant physiological adaptation for the baby. The neonate must adapt from being completely dependent on his mother for life-sustaining oxygen and nutrients to an independent being, a task accomplished over a period of hours to days. Successful transition from fetal to neonatal

life requires a complete interaction among the various systems: respiratory, cardiovascular, thermoregulatory, endocrinologic, and immunologic. Establishing respiration is critical to the neonate's transition as the lungs become the organs of gas exchange after separation from maternal uteroplacental circulation. Over 90% of neonates make the transition from intrauterine life to extrauterine life without difficulty, requiring little to no assistance. However, for the 10% of neonates who do require assistance, about 1% require extensive resuscitation measures to survive. Neonates with prenatal onset of structural defects frequently have problems with postnatal respiratory adaptation, which may be secondary to altered development of fetal lung or brain structure.

3.12 Family History

A careful, thorough, and fully recorded history, complete with pedigree, forms the foundation for the diagnostic process. Family history can provide a good quality of information and represent the first clue regarding the possible genetic etiology of congenital malformations. Consanguinity in the parents increases the chance of having autosomal recessive conditions as well as multifactorial disorders in their progeny.

3.13 Physical Examination

The critical aspect of a dysmorphology evaluation lies in the recognition or confirmation of major and minor structural anomalies, and therefore, a physical examination of the neonate with congenital abnormalities is the most important step. The clinical assessment of the neonate must be thorough and accurate. Some abnormalities may be quite prominent or involve large areas, while others may be rather subtle. Selected measurements of physical features are extremely useful in confirming a clinical appearance of abnormality. Standard tables and graphs by gestational age norms for many of such physical dimensions are available with the aim of providing standards, both for comparison and for improved definition of normal patterns of human development and growth at birth and late in life [26]. From the primarily qualitative description, it is necessary to pass a new step where accuracy and quantitation must be necessary. Careful documentation by measurement, in well-known conditions, will allow one to distinguish heterogeneity, learn more about natural history, and provide a basis for the future application of techniques and concepts from developmental biology and molecular genetics. The real value of a single measurement lies in a comparison with a standard, which can be either age related or familial and ethnic related.

With the parents' permission, it is useful to take photographs of the baby because photographic documentation often can be of great value and can be used to observe changes in time and to compare with other babies with a similar phenotype. A neonatologist should take care to continue to search for the less obvious anomalies even when a major malformation is present. It could be of some help to ask for advice and expertise from the geneticist with experience in the neonatal age. Peculiar phenotype change can be observed in each individual during the years from neonate to child and to adolescent to adult too. A common pitfall to avoid is the tendency to make an erroneous diagnosis of a well-known syndrome, usually not completely supported by the abnormalities observed at birth. The description of the clinical association should include, moreover, the structural defects, even neuromotor evaluation, growth development, the disorder of sexual differentiation, or pubertal development.

3.14 Surveillance After Birth

Transitional care from hospital to home represents a very critical moment. Returning home with a malformed baby can result in an emotional burden that is very challenging, not only for the parents and family but also for the family pediatrician, territorial doctors, and nursing care, who are required to acquire in a short time new knowledge and skills. Consequently, it is necessary to arrange the complexity of the care, before discharge, organizing care pathways that are in favor of the transition and integration between hospital and home. A consensus statement on birth defect surveillance (2019) proposes, among other things, "to establish a holistic, multidisciplinary and multi-sectorial approach that adequately meets the health the educational, occupational, rehabilitation and social needs of people with birth defects. Many infants with severe birth defects experience lifelong disability requiring long-term treatment or rehabilitation" (World Health Organization 2019). There are promising models for rehabilitation services for children with birth defects. These models are found in communities: hospitals, schools, other institutions, and primary health care. The more comprehensive models are in the primary care system and are centered on rehabilitation strategy. Some reports focus on the care of infants and children with birth defects and on rehabilitation programs, which are required for lifelong conditions. In many cases, appropriate education and rehabilitation for children substantially increase their ability to function independently and contribute to family and community responsibilities. The assumption is that children with disabilities have the right to live a good life. It is mandatory to offer to them and their family the clinical and the social support required their usual way of living. They should have an education like everybody else and should be able to go to school and follow a course of study, like other children. In Italy, school inclusion was regulated in 1977 (National Law n. 517, 1977), with the abolition of differential classes. Even if people learn very slowly, have problems seeing or hearing, or find it hard to move about, they still should be respected for being girls and boys. Nobody should be looked down on or treated badly because of their disability. Houses, shops, and schools should be built in such a way that everyone can easily go in and out and make use of them.

A practical example of a follow-up service to a child born with birth defects could be represented by the surveillance over time of neonates affected by trisomy 21 (T-21), well known as Down syndrome. DS is by far the most common and the best-known aneuploidy due to the nondisjunction, translocation, or mosaicism of chromosome 21. In 94–97%, the extra chromosome may be maternal or, less frequently, paternal in origin. In 3%, there is D/G translocation. Trisomy/normal (mosaicism) occurs in 1–2%. DS occurs approximately in one in every 800 live births in the Emilia-Romagna region.

Physical examination is the first step within the first hours of life, in which it is possible to feel there are enough criteria to advance the diagnosis of DS. The phenotype is characterized by several clinical features, of which the most constant and typical are neuromotor disability and craniofacial dysmorphisms, together with other variable signs and symptoms, such as cardiac malformations and growth delay. Physicians can suspect DS based on some characteristic physiognomic features of infants, and physical examination is the first essential step to reach a diagnosis Neonatologists can also use score system as Hall's ten cardinal signs or Jackson's checklist, which is a more complex scoring system, that could guide them in making diagnosis of DS. The diffusion of these scoring systems is an excellent way to bring attention to clinical and phenotypic signs of DS, contributing to a better understanding of the role of the excess chromosome 21.

When recording the history from the parents of a child with T-21, the clinician should include the following information: parental concern about hearing, vision, developmental delay, respiratory infections, and other problems. Delay in the child's cognitive abilities and motor and language development is the most frequent question from parents and the family, too, and the usual reason for their great anxiety and concern. The clinician must support the family since a diagnosis of DS is made, also if it is done during pregnancy, and has to reassure them about the great possibility for these patients to reach as well as a level of autonomy in life. To reach this result it is necessary to inform about the opportunity to assure and the necessity to implement on one hand all the best assistance for possible clinical problems in the development of the child and on the other hand to underline the strength of early surveillance of neuromotor and neuro-sensorial maturation. All this is to activate the health service of precocious sensorial and motor enabling when clinicians observe a delay or an impaired maturation. Starting from birth it is important and basic to follow the child in a longitudinal survey of all pediatric ages. Neonatologists are now referred to early intervention programs shortly after birth and inform the parents about the best way to follow and foster the growth and development of their child. The goal of intervention programs for children with Down syndrome is to maximize each child's developmental potential and improve the quality of his/her life. In the past few decades, advances in medical care have resulted in improved health and life expectancy for individuals with DS. Each clinical center involved in the clinical assistance of the child has to implement specific protocols, which are internationally defined and useful. Guidelines, produced by the American Academy of Pediatrics (AAP) and recently published (Pediatrics 2022), are a useful guide to follow and to help practitioner doctors and institutions to take care of these children starting from prenatal diagnosis, if there was, to adolescence [24]. Children with DS often have multiple health needs. It makes sense, from the family's perspective, to reduce the number of hospital visits by having multidisciplinary clinical and coordinated appointments. The Center for Rare Disease of Bologna University Hospital uses a care protocol for the survey of children with Down syndrome, which was proposed in 1984. Time after time, the survey was adopted, and the protocol used is shown in Table 3.1. During the first and subsequent visits, it is recommended to pay attention to the child's strengths and achievements, helping parents focus on the child's potential rather than weaknesses. It is also essential to keep parents in touch, if they so wish, with other families with children with DS so they can share information and experiences and expand the support network for both the family and the child.

Table 3.1 Follow-up protocol applied for Down-syndrome-specific care at the Center for Rare Disease Neonatology Dept. Bologna University Hospital

	Birth	3 m	6 m	9 m	12 m	18 m	24 m	36 m	Yearly
Anamnesis	•	•	•	•	•	•	•	•	•
Health maintening visit	•	•	•	•	•	•	•	•	•
Neurological ev.	•	•	•	•	•	•	•	•	•
Neurophiasic ev.		•			•		•	•	
Blood test + TAM	S		•		•	•	•	•	•
NBS	•								
TSH	◄		•		•		•		•
Cerebral US	•	•							
EEG + MRI (1)			•						
Abdominal US	•								
Cardiological Ex.	•				•				
Pneumological Ex (2)									•
Gastro-enter. Ex (3)					•				
ENT Ex. + BAER	S	•	•		•			•	
Ophthalmic ex.	S	•		•				•	
Dental visit			•		•		•	•	•

Cervical X-ray at 9 years (atlantoaxial stability control)
S screening, *TAM* transient abnormal myelopoiesis, *NBS* newborn screening, *TSH* thyroid stimulating hormone, *EEG* electroencephalogram, *MRI* magnetic resonance imaging, *ENT* ear nose throat, *BAER* brainstem auditory evoked response
(1) If cerebral US is pathological
(2) + Pulse-oximetric for OSAS control
(3) + Screening for celiac disease

References

1. ICBDSR, WHOICDCI. Birth defects surveillance a manual for programme managers. Geneva: World Health Organization; 2014.
2. Corsello G, Giuffrè M. Congenital malformations and syndromes: early diagnosis and prognosis. In: Neonatology. Milan: Springer; 2012. p. 31–45.
3. Cornel MC. Registration and prevention of congenital anomalies. Brussels: EUROCAT; 1993.
4. Graham JM, Sanchez-Lara PA. Smith's recognizable patterns of human deformation. Amsterdam: Elsevier Health Sciences; 2015.
5. Dyken P, Miller MD. Facial features of neurologic syndromes. St Louis: Mosby Inc.; 1980.
6. Aase JM. Dysmorphologic diagnosis for the pediatric practitioner. Pediatr Clin N Am. 1992;39(1):135–56.
7. Stevenson RE, Hall JG. Human malformations and related anomalies. Oxford: Oxford University Press; 2005.
8. Feingold M, Pashayan HM. Genetics and birth defects in clinical practice. Boston: Little Brown & Company; 1983.
9. Roberts I. Nelson's textbook of pediatrics (20th edn.), by R. Kliegman, B. Stanton, J. St. Geme, N. Schor (eds). Berlin: Springer; 2017.
10. Skotko BG, Capone GT, Kishnani PS, for the Down Syndrome Diagnosis Study Group. Postnatal diagnosis of down syndrome: synthesis of the evidence on how best to deliver the news. Pediatrics. 2009;124(4):e751–8.

11. Kalter M, Warkany J. Congenital malformation etiologic factors and their role in prevention. N Eng J Med. 1983;308(8):424–31.
12. Donnai D. Handbook of normal physical measurements. J Med Genet. 1990;27:407–8.
13. Baraitser M. Handbook of normal physical measurements-Hall, JG, Frosteriskenius, VG, Allanson, JE. Oxford: Blackwell Science Ltd; 1990.
14. Liao J, Mehta L. Molecular genetics of Noonan syndrome and RASopathies. Pediatr Endocrinol Rev. 2019;16(Suppl 2):435–46.
15. Fung A, Manlhiot C, Naik S, Rosenberg H, Smythe J, Lougheed J, et al. Impact of prenatal risk factors on congenital heart disease in the current era. J Am Heart Assoc. 2013;2(3):e000064.
16. Fuhrmann W, Vogel F. Genetic counseling. Berlin: Springer Science & Business Media; 2012.
17. Gelehrter TD, Collins FS, Ginsburg D. Principles of medical genetics. Philadelphia: Lippincott Williams & Wilkins; 1998.
18. Mastroiacovo P, Kallén K, Castilla EE. Genetic and Reproductive Epidemiology Research Society (GRANTS) Ghedini Ed. 1992.
19. Gripp KW, Slavotinek AM, Hall JG, Allanson JE. Handbook of physical measurements. Oxford: Oxford University Press; 2013.
20. Gleason CA, Juul SE. Avery's diseases of the newborn. Amsterdam: Elsevier Health Sciences; 2017.
21. Vanstone M, King C, de Vrijer B, Nisker J. Non-invasive prenatal testing: ethics and policy considerations. J Obstet Gynaecol Can. 2014;36(6):515–26.
22. Reddy UM, Filly RA, Copel JA. Prenatal imaging: ultrasonography and magnetic resonance imaging. Obstet Gynecol. 2008;112:145.
23. Ami O, Maran JC, Gabor P, Whitacre EB, Musset D, Dubray C, et al. Three-dimensional magnetic resonance imaging of fetal head molding and brain shape changes during the second stage of labor. PLoS One. 2019;14(5):e0215721.
24. Bull MJ, Trotter T, Santoro SL, Christensen C, Grout RW. Health supervision for children and adolescents with down syndrome. Pediatrics. 2022;149(5):e2022057010.
25. MacLeod PM. Implication of the child with malformations for the family and society. In: Human malformations and related anomalies. Oxford: Oxford University Press; 1993.
26. Hall J, Allanson J, Gripp K, Slavotinek A. Handbook of physical measurements. Oxford: Oxford University Press; 2006.

Part III

Frail Children

4 Frail Children with Chronic Lung Disease

Alessandro Onofri, Serena Caggiano, Claudio Cherchi, M. Beatrice Chiarini Testa, and Renato Cutrera

Abbreviations

AAD	Assisted autogenic drainage
BPD	Bronchopulmonary dysplasia
CF	Cystic fibrosis
CFTR	Cystic fibrosis transmembrane conductance regulator
chILD	Children
CPAP	Continuous positive airway pressure
CWS	Chest wall strapping
HFCWO	High-frequency chest wall oscillation
HFNC	High-flow nasal cannula
ILD	Interstitial lung disease
IPV	Intrapulmonary percussive ventilation
LTHOT	Long-term home oxygen therapy
MAC	Manually assisted cough
NIV	Non-invasive ventilation
NMDs	Neuromuscular diseases
PCF	Cough peak flow
PEP	Positive expiratory pressure

A. Onofri · S. Caggiano · C. Cherchi · M. B. C. Testa · R. Cutrera (✉)
Pediatric Pulmonology and Respiratory Intermediate Care Unit, Sleep and Long Term Ventilation Unit, Academic Department of Pediatrics (DPUO), Bambino Gesù Children's Hospital, IRCCS, Rome, Italy
e-mail: alessandro.onofri@opbg.net; serena.caggiano@opbg.net; claudio.cherchi@opbg.net; mbeatrice.chiarini@opbg.net; renato.cutrera@opbg.net

This chapter covers various aspects of chronic respiratory diseases in children, with a particular focus on the most important primitive respiratory disorders and secondary disorders with respiratory system involvement. Moreover, we analyzed the different conditions and treatments of frail children with chronic respiratory disorders.

4.1 Bronchopulmonary Dysplasia

The perinatal period, i.e., the period from birth (and especially premature birth) to the 28th day of life, is the period of greatest mortality. Preterm birth is the major determinant of neonatal mortality and morbidity. There is an increasing survival of children born at a very early gestational age with an increasing proportion of children with long-term respiratory and/or neurological impairment. The most important long-term consequence of prematurity is bronchopulmonary dysplasia (BPD). This condition is defined as oxygen dependency at 36 postmenstrual weeks. It is one of the most important complications of prematurity, with a reported incidence of 23% of infants born at 28 weeks, increasing to 73% of infants born at 23 weeks. As stated below, BPD incidence is increasing due to the increased survival of very early pre-term infants. It is characterized by prolonged respiratory support, compromised lung function and

M. Lima, M. C. Mondardini (eds.), *Frailty in Children*,
https://doi.org/10.1007/978-3-031-24307-3_4

recurrent respiratory infections during the first year of life [1]. Despite advances in early respiratory care to avoid lung injury, sometimes long-term respiratory support is needed. Prolonged care needs include tracheostomy with mechanical ventilation, high FiO_2 concentrations and multiple respiratory medications, such as intermittent corticosteroids, bronchodilators, diuretics and other drugs [2].

4.2 Interstitial Lung Diseases (ILDs)

Interstitial lung disease (ILD) in children (chILD) is a heterogeneous group of rare respiratory disorders that are mostly chronic, with complex pathogenesis characterized by an injury of the lung parenchyma with inflammation and fibrotic changes. ILDs are mostly chronic and impair the respiratory function of the lung. The heterogeneity of child conditions determines often a strong difficultly to find effective treatments. The clinical manifestations vary from asymptomatic presentation to more characteristic and severe clinical presentations with respiratory symptoms and exacerbations [3]. General measures are essential, with mainly administration of oxygen for chronic hypoxaemia and maintenance of nutrition with an adequate energy intake. Immunization with influenza vaccine on an annual basis is recommended, along with other routine immunizations against major respiratory pathogens. In addition, an aggressive treatment of intercurrent infections and a strict avoidance of tobacco smoke and other air pollutants are strongly recommended. Pharmacological therapy includes anti-inflammatory and immunosuppressive molecules. Steroids are the preferred choice, administered orally and/or intravenously [4]. New therapeutic strategies include anti-fibrotic and anti-inflammatory drugs, but lung transplantation remains the ultimate therapy for end-stage lung diseases [5].

4.3 Neuromuscular Diseases (NMDs)

Neuromuscular diseases are responsible for chronic respiratory failure and for approximately half of all long-term home ventilation in children and adolescents [56% of non-invasive ventilation (NIV) and 44% of all mechanical ventilation in children] [6].

The pathogenesis of respiratory failure consists of ventilatory insufficiency caused by weakness of the respiratory muscles, while the lungs are primarily healthy. The respiratory care of these patients must compensate for the ensuing mechanical problems of inadequate sighing, coughing, and insufficient functioning of the respiratory pump and upper airway. The patient's medical history includes a course of respiratory tract infections, symptoms of sleep-disordered breathing (snoring, observed apnoeas, abnormal sleep positions, frequent awakening in immobile patients, frequent positioning, secondary nocturnal enuresis, nycturia, night sweats, frequent nightmares, morning fatigue, morning headaches, lack of appetite, daytime fatigue, and restlessness in small children during the day), symptoms of daytime hypoventilation/hypercapnia (depressed mood, lack of drive, poor concentration, tiredness, headaches, lack of appetite, nausea, dyspnoea, tachycardia, sweating, anxiety, exhaustion), difficulty speaking (volume, shortness of breath), indications of difficulty of swallowing and aspiration, drooling, oxygen saturations in different states, changes in the patient's weight, as well as use of and problems with current treatments [7]. Children with neuromuscular diseases must undergo a complex multidisciplinary assessment. The respiratory system can be involved in different ways, depending on the time of onset, the phenotype of the disease and the comorbidities. Lung function testing (when feasible) and the assessment of sleep-disordered breathing with poly(somno)graphy and overnight carbon dioxide (CO_2) monitoring are highly recommended in these patients. Children with neuromuscular diseases resulting in symptomatic nocturnal hypoventilation or daytime hypercapnia should be provided with mechanical ventilation support [8]. Long-term ventilation is associated with an increase in survival rate. NIV is effective in correcting sleep-disordered breathing, daytime hypercapnia and the symptoms of nocturnal hypoventilation. Percentages of use for non-invasive ventilation compared to tracheostomy vary, possibly because of differences in ethical perspectives, nationality and medical staff expertise. Usually, tracheostomy is considered in cases of severe bulbar dysfunction, failure to extubate, need for long ventilatory support, NIV failure or severe mid-face hypoplasia [6, 9].

4.4 Cystic Fibrosis (CF)

Pulmonary involvement in cystic fibrosis in characterized by mucus plugging, chronic inflammation and bronchiectasis. Lung function is progressively deteriorated by airflow obstruction and parenchymal damage. The lack of a cystic fibrosis transmembrane conductance regulator (CFTR) protein causes the disease, which is multi-systemic rather than only pulmonary. As regards respiratory involvement, despite the improvement in CF care, chronic respiratory failure and end-stage lung disease develop in most of the patients [10, 11]. With the progression of pulmonary involvement and increased respiratory load, patients develop a rapid shallow breathing pattern and subsequent daytime hypercapnia. In addition, chronic alveolar hypoxia, hypercapnia, and endothelial dysfunction due to chronic inflammation may cause pulmonary hypertension. Pulmonary hypertension is inversely correlated with respiratory function and nocturnal oxygen saturation. Hypoxemia, hypercapnia and pulmonary hypertension indicate a poor prognosis and a prompt referral for lung transplantation [12, 13]. The management of the disease is multidisciplinary, and the treatment is not only symptomatic but also targeted with new effective modulator therapies [14]. Physiotherapy, mucociliary clearance therapy and antibiotics for the high prevalence of pulmonary infections are the most important intervention to avoid the deterioration of lung function. When hypercapnia takes over, non-invasive ventilation could be effective to reduce respiratory effort, improving alveolar ventilation and gas exchange [15].

4.5 Different Treatments in Children with Chronic Respiratory Disorders

4.5.1 Long-Term Oxygen Therapy

Long-term home oxygen therapy (LTHOT) has become an increasingly common practice, and many patients benefit from its use. It has several clinical and physiological benefits, as well as greater comfort for patients and significant cost reduction when compared to hospitalizations [16]. The use of LTHOT in paediatric patients has several special characteristics and important differences when compared to the use in adults. In fact, physical growth and neurological development must be considered. The evolution of some diseases that cause hypoxemia in children is generally good; many children require LTHOT only for a limited period of time [17]. BPD and CF can be mentioned to illustrate how this form of treatment is being incorporated into paediatric practice. The number of children who needs LTHOT is increasing worldwide; particularly, the great advances in neonatology have increased the survival of very premature patients who are discharged on oxygen treatment. Extremely pre-term infants with lung immaturity at higher grades, which also can develop into chronic lung disease, will be dependent on oxygen for months or years, thus making BPD the most frequent indication of LTHOT in children. The long-term prognosis of premature patients is usually good, and the time of supplemental oxygen use should be evaluated individually, ranging from a few days to months or years. Comorbidities must always be reassessed (malnutrition, heart disease, pulmonary hypertension, infection) if the oxygen requirement increases or is extended for too long [18]. In the case of CF, the evolution of treatment associated with improved nutrition has increased the survival of these patients, but some require LTHOT in the advanced stages of the disease or while waiting for a lung transplant. Episodes of hypoxia in CF patients may occur during sleep, exercise, air travel, and infectious exacerbations, and these are not limited to severe patients. Hypoxia during sleep and exercise may occur in stable patients who do not have hypoxia during the day. The deleterious effects of hypoxia in patients with CF are numerous: pulmonary hypertension, worsening of pulmonary infection and inflammation, reduced exercise capacity and muscle strength, and worsening of the quality of sleep and quality of life [19]. Bronchiolitis obliterans, usually secondary to viral infections, is a cause of severe chronic obstructive pulmonary disease in infants. It is often accompanied by hypoxemia and the need for LTHOT during varying periods. There are no established oxygen saturation levels for the start of LTHOT in these patients. The use of the same criteria applied in children with BPD (SpO_2 <93%) is suggested as it predominantly affects infants [20]. Interstitial lung diseases represent a rare and diverse group of lung diseases in children, where gas exchange is often compromised by the presence of hypoxemia. Therefore, many of these patients require LTHOT for varying periods, associated with drug therapy [21]. Pulmonary hypertension secondary to lung disease results from chronic alveolar hypoxia and considerably worsens the prognosis of the underlying disease. Chronic hypoxia leads to pulmonary vasoconstriction and endothelial dysfunction. Moreover, the pulmonary circulation is more reactive to hypoxia in children than in adults. In these cases, oxygen is the most potent pulmonary vasodilator, and LTHOT can slow down and even reverse alterations in the pulmonary vascular bed induced by hypoxia and may contribute to the improvement of survival [22]. For chronic hypoventilation, with a central or peripheral origin, the treatment of choice is NIV via a face mask or tracheostomy, but oxygen therapy can be used in milder and non-progressive cases, in cases when NIV use is impossible and in cases in which, despite NIV, patients persist with hypoxemia due to inadequate ventilation or the presence of associated lung disease. If LTHOT is used alone, CO_2 levels must be monitored [23]. It is not uncommon for children with chronic encephalopathy to develop chronic hypoxemia and a need for LTHOT. This usually stems from multiple factors: recurrent pneumonia usually related to aspiration processes secondary to gastroesophageal reflux and/or dysphagia, ineffective cough, and pulmonary restriction due to scoliosis or other chest deformities [24]. In children with terminal cancer, there are no data on the management of terminal dyspnoea, but in some cases, there may be benefits with oxygen as chronic hypoxia can cause irritability, headache and restlessness. When indicated, the use of a nasal cannula should be preferred so as not to cover the child's face with a mask. The management of these cases should be individualized, and if, together with the patient and family, symptom relief is observed, LTHOT should be used [25]. Traditional nasal cannula oxygen administration is used at low flows (0.5–6 L/min) with significant mixing from room air limiting the maximal FiO_2 delivery to 0.45. Conversely, with the use of a high-flow nasal cannula (HFNC), there is little entrapment of room air because of the high gas flow, allowing for more precise and higher FiO_2 delivery. HFNC consists of the delivery of high-flowing heated and humidified air through the nose, with FiO_2, which may be set from 21% to nearly 100%. Standard flow rates do not require humidification; HFNC requires humidification because of the drying effect of un-humidified cold oxygen on nasal secretions and the respiratory mucosa. In addition, the high gas flow flushes carbon dioxide from the upper airway, reducing the anatomical dead space and impeding expiratory flow. Thus, HFNC can create continuous positive airway pressure, although less than NIV. These factors lead to a reduction in respiratory rate, hypoxemia and the sensation of dyspnoea compared with traditional oxygen administration through a nasal cannula or face mask in patients with respiratory distress during their end-of-life period [26]. Whereas NIV can be claustrophobic and impede eating and talking, HFNC use can allow select patients to talk and eat while receiving adequate oxygenation [27]. Since its introduction as an alternative to continuous positive airway pressure (CPAP) in pre-term infants, HFNC oxygenation has been widely used for various respiratory conditions, not only as an essential intensive care device [28]. HFNC in fact is a well-tolerated treatment alternative to CPAP in infants and young children with obstructive sleep apnoea (OSA) and with poor adherence and mid-face hypoplasia risk [29]. The nasal cannula used with HFNC is less invasive and more comfortable than nasal masks or nasal prongs used for CPAP therapy and is easier to apply in the case of craniofacial malformations. HFNC may be used as a rescue therapy for children not compliant with CPAP, but an improvement in the devices currently available is also needed in order to adapt their characteristics to the needs of children with OSA [30].

4.5.2 Mechanical Ventilation

Mechanical ventilation is used in children with acute and chronic respiratory failure. We do not deal with acute respiratory failure in this chapter. As stated above, children with chronic respiratory failure and/or sleep-disordered breathing due to a broad range of diseases should require mechanical ventilatory support. The diagnosis of chronic alveolar hypoventilation rests on the identification of chronic hypercapnia. Advances in the use of long-term non-invasive ventilation (NIV) have progressively led to a reduction in the need for invasive mechanical ventilation (IMV) through tracheostomy [31–34]. We recently performed a retrospective cohort study of paediatric (within 18 years old) patients hospitalized in our paediatric tertiary center (Bambino Gesù Children's Hospital) between 1 January 2000 and 31 December 2017 using long-term NIV and intermittent mandatory ventilation (IMV). A total of 432 children were included in the study, and we found that children on ventilation suffered mainly from neuromuscular diseases or diseases of the upper airways and the central nervous system. Children invasively ventilated usually started support younger, spent more hours on ventilation and were more severely ill. Our results highlighted that along with the growing number of children on long-term ventilation, it is increasing their medical complexity and their need for high-quality health care programmes able to promote their well-being [34]. Our results are similar to those of many studies performed, especially in western and more developed and high-income countries. Logically, the percentage of use for NIV compared with IMV could vary because of differences in ethical perspectives, nationality and medical staff expertise. However, the use of long-term NIV in children is growing around the world due to improvements in technology, progressive experience by healthcare providers and increased indications in different disorders [35].

Notably, not all patients are eligible for long-term NIV. The inability to protect the lower airways, anatomic face abnormalities, severe mid-face hypoplasia, and the high need for ventilation (more than 16 h) are important contraindications of NIV. The conditions listed above may preclude the initiation of or adherence to NIV and may lead to considering alternative treatments, such as invasive ventilation via tracheostomy, in concert with the family and patient [36].

4.5.3 Tracheostomy

Over the last decade, tracheostomy has been increasingly performed in children with complex and chronic conditions for the management of upper airway obstruction, prolonged ventilation, abnormal ventilatory drive and neuromuscular conditions [37]. The range of indications for tracheostomy is reported in Table 4.1. Congenital upper airway anomalies resulting in a difficult airway that cannot be secured by other means frequently necessitate transient or permanent tracheostomy, especially in infants and young children with compromised nasal breathing. Upper airway obstruction as an indication is decreasing in frequency, and ventilator dependence is an evolving indication in developed countries. Tracheostomy can be required in neurologically compromised paediatric patients; the most common underlying neurological diagnoses

Table 4.1 Main indications for tracheostomy

Indications for tracheostomy	Examples
Upper airway obstruction	Subglottic stenosis Tracheomalacia Tracheal stenosis Craniofacial syndromes Craniofacial and laryngeal tumours Bilateral vocal cord paralysis Obstructive sleep apnoea Laryngeal trauma
Pulmonary/lung disease	Bronchopulmonary dysplasia Interstitial lung diseases
Congenital heart disease	Post-operative diaphragmatic paresis
Neurological/ neuromuscular disease	Duchenne muscular dystrophy Spinal muscle atrophy type I Congenital central hypoventilation syndrome cerebral palsy Traumatic brain and spinal injury Spina bifida
Long-term ventilation	NIV h 16–24, severe mid-face hypoplasia
Pulmonary toilet/ management of secretions	

involved are cerebral palsy [38], followed by drug-resistant epilepsy and other neurological situations characterized by ventilator dependence, inability to tolerate secretions or recurrent aspiration pneumonia, hypotonia and upper respiratory obstruction [39]. The survivability of extreme prematurity, bronchopulmonary dysplasia and other complex cardiopulmonary conditions in the neonate continues to improve. As the worldwide care for premature and medically complex newborns improves, the most common indication for paediatric tracheostomy is now the need for long-term ventilation. There are no comprehensive recommendations for an invasive versus a non-invasive mode of ventilatory support in ventilator-dependent children. Often, young age, ventilator dependency for most of the day and frequent episodes of respiratory exacerbation with a need for intubation increase the likelihood of being tracheotomized. In addition, secondary mid-face hypoplasia has emerged as a worrisome complication of long-term mask application in young children. This has a significant effect on dentition and on nasopharyngeal patency in patients susceptible to upper airway obstruction. Chronic lung disease of infancy and complex congenital heart disease are other important entities associated with the occasional need for tracheostomy in heart disease, mostly for long-term ventilation, because of ongoing cardiac failure, tracheo-bronchomalacia or post-operative diaphragmatic paresis. For many of these medically complex children, the timing of when the tracheostomy is performed and the preoperative discussion regarding ongoing care are significantly challenging [36, 40–44]. Multidisciplinary input regarding the prognosis of a tracheostomy candidate should be established with the healthcare team and family before proceeding to surgery, unless the indication for tracheostomy is urgent. The procedure is the first step in the long process of transitioning ventilatory care from the hospital to home. A well-orchestrated use of hospital services and education is necessary to facilitate this process, which places a unique burden of responsibility on patients' families. Post-operative morbidity and mortality from tracheostomy are often related to deteriorating medical comorbidities and, rarely, device-related complications [45–47]. However, there remain significant risks of improper care and monitoring of the patient with a tracheostomy, including accidental decannulation or mucus plugging of the tube. Thus, paediatric healthcare providers should familiarize themselves with routine tracheostomy care, especially in practice settings with medically complex patients. Tracheostomy care is a longitudinal investment by families, providers and institutions to prevent complications both in the hospital and at home. For example, there is no consensus regarding the frequency of tracheostomy tube changes; usually, the recommended tube change frequency is once a month or more frequently, depending on the single case; sometimes, the child presents secretions that tend to obstruct the lumen of the cannula, and in these cases, a more frequent change of the cannula is required [47]. The advantages of frequent tube changes include keeping caregivers comfortable and well practised in tube changing, the possibility of decreasing airway infection and/or airway granulomas and the possibility of reducing the incidence of tube occlusion by inspissated secretions. The disadvantages of frequent tube changes include the possible stretching of the tracheostomy stoma when cuffed. In summary, the criteria favouring tracheostomy in children are upper airway obstruction with low chances of a definitive, spontaneous resolution within a reasonable time (weeks); low probability that surgery can definitely correct the cause; high risk of critical upper airway obstruction with simple respiratory tract infections or minor bleeding (epistaxis); high risk or previous history of difficulties in airway management in the case of an emergency; and difficult-to-control gastro-oesophageal reflux. Also, other criteria included are the child requiring long-term ventilation and pulmonary toilet, having a high risk of mid-facial deformation from mask pressure, being ventilator dependent for most of the day (more than 12 h per day) or being unable to cope with a mask (full face or nasal mask); recurrent aspirations (gastro-oesophageal reflux, laryngeal incompetence) with a significant benefit from pulmonary toilet; and, finally, safety measures and local experience highly in favour of invasive ventilation. There are two fundamental criteria for decannulation in a child with a chronic tracheostomy: (1) the original need for the tracheostomy tube is no longer present, and (2) the patient is able to maintain a safe and adequate airway independent of the tracheostomy tube. The criteria for safe paediatric decannulation are graduation from the regular use of mechanical ventilation (possibly allowing for occasional backsliding during acute illness); the absence of recent known aspiration events and the completion of an endoscopic airway assessment confirming the absence of upper airway pathology, which could be masked by the tracheostomy tube (including awake flexible laryngoscopy to assess vocal fold movement); and safe daytime capping of the tracheostomy tube for several weeks. Additional optional steps may include successful weaning from supplemental oxygen, interval downsizing of the existing tracheostomy, tolerance of a Passy-Muir speaking valve, performance of a drug-induced sleep endoscopy and performance of a capped or decannulated polysomnography [42, 45].

4.6 Respiratory Physiotherapy in Children with Chronic Respiratory Disorders

Chest physiotherapy is a crucial part of the management of many respiratory diseases, in particular for children requiring mechanical ventilation and those with chronic conditions such as bronchiectasis or neuromuscular diseases. Physiotherapy often focuses on treating or alleviating generic problems that are amenable to intervention rather than being disease specific.

4.6.1 Peripheral Airway Clearance Techniques: "Sputum Mobilizing"

The term airway clearance describes the different treatment modalities performed to enhance the clearance of bronchopulmonary secretions. Peripheral airway clearance techniques aim to improve ventilation, mobilize secretions and enhance mucus transport from peripheral to central airways (12th generation of the bronchial tree and above) with higher expiratory than inspiratory airflows (called biased expiratory flow). These include *manual techniques*, *positive expiratory pressure (PEP)*, *assisted autogenic drainage (AAD)*, *high-frequency chest wall oscillation (HFCWO)*, *intrapulmonary percussive ventilation (IPV)* and *chest wall strapping (CWS)* [48].

In CF, the introduction of airway clearance techniques prior to the diagnosis of bronchiectasis is widely debated. For symptomatic patients who show evident response to treatment, a consensus is acquired; however, in the asymptomatic patient, benefits are still uncertain [49]. Routine chest physiotherapy is not needed, except for those patients with abnormal mechanisms of airway clearance. In CF, there is evidence that inflammation and infection are present early in life [48]. Airway clearance treatment options must be chosen, considering the child's age and ability to participate in the treatment. There are a wide variety of airway clearance techniques, and no single best technique has been identified [50].

4.6.2 Proximal Airway Clearance Techniques: "Cough Augmentation"

Cough is the primary defense mechanism against foreign bodies in the central airways. An effective cough is a vital mechanism to protect against respiratory tract infections, which are the main causes of hospitalization in patients affected by NMD. Progressive neuromuscular weakness can lead to the inability to take deep breaths and to cough effectively [51]. Proximal airway clearance is a technique that aims to augment the cough by assisting inspiration, expiration or both. They are often described as "cough augmentation" techniques, supporting or imitating a cough [52]. The ability to clear bronchopulmonary secretions is essential to preventing sputum retention and associated complications, including lower respiratory tract infection. Physical therapies involve measuring cough peak flow (PCF): reduced cough power is defined by values less than 270 L/min in children, and values less than 160 L/min are associated with a high risk of atelectasis and pneumonia [53]. Assisted cough techniques should be targeted to whichever component of the cough is reduced [54]. If there is only expiratory muscle weakness, then a manually assisted cough (MAC) will improve PCF by an abdominal thrust or costal lateral compression after an adequate spontaneous inspiration or maximal insufflation [55]. If there is inspiratory muscle weakness, then the inspiratory component can be supported by a maximum insufflation capacity, which is a series of deep breaths to total lung capacity (TLC) via a face mask attached to a one-way valve and Ambu bag [56]. If the cough is extremely impaired, the patient may require mechanical insufflation/exsufflation. This device enhances secretion clearance by applying positive pressure to the airway (insufflation) and then rapidly shifting to negative pressure (exsufflation). The rapid shift in pressure produces a high expiratory flow, simulating a natural cough [57].

References

1. Onland W, Offringa M, van Kaam A. Late (≥7 days) inhalation corticosteroids to reduce bronchopulmonary dysplasia in preterm infants. Cochrane Database Syst Rev. 2012;18:CD002311.
2. Thébaud B, Goss KN, Laughon M, Whitsett JA, Abman SH, Steinhorn RH, Aschner JL, Davis PG, McGrath-Morrow SA, Soll RF, Jobe AH. Bronchopulmonary dysplasia. Nat Rev Dis Primers. 2019;5(1):78.
3. Nathan N, Berdah L, Delestrain C, Sileo C, Clement A. Interstitial lung diseases in children. Presse Med. 2020;49(2):103909.
4. Clement A, de Blic J, Epaud R, Galeron L, Nathan N, Hadchouel A, Barbato A, Snijders D, Kiper N, Cunningham S, Griese M, Bush A, Schwerk N, chILD-EU collaboration. Management of children with interstitial lung diseases: the difficult issue of acute exacerbations. Eur Respir J. 2016;48(6):1559–63.
5. Richeldi L, du Bois RM, Raghu G, Azuma A, Brown KK, Costabel U, Cottin V, Flaherty KR, Hansell DM, Inoue Y, Kim DS, Kolb M, Nicholson AG, Noble PW, Selman M, Taniguchi H, Brun M, Le Maulf F, Girard M, Stowasser S, Schlenker-Herceg R, Disse B, Collard HR, INPULSIS Trial Investigators. Efficacy and safety of nintedanib in idiopathic pulmonary fibrosis [Erratum in: N Engl J Med. 2015 Aug 20;373(8):782]. N Engl J Med. 2014;370(22):2071–82. https://doi.org/10.1056/NEJMoa1402584.
6. Chatwin M, Tan HL, Bush A, Rosenthal M, Simonds AK. Long term non-invasive ventilation in children: impact on survival and transition to adult care. PLoS One. 2015;10(5):e0125839.
7. Hull J. British Thoracic Society guideline for respiratory management of children with neuromuscular weakness. Thorax. 2012;67(Suppl 1):i1–40.
8. Ward S, Chatwin M, Heather S, Simonds AK. Randomised controlled trial of non-invasive ventilation (NIV) for nocturnal hypoventilation in neuromuscular and chest wall disease patients with daytime normocapnia. Thorax. 2005;60(12):1019–24.
9. Racca F, Bonati M, Del Sorbo L, Berta G, Sequi M, Capello EC, Wolfler A, Salvo I, Bignamini E, Ottonello G, Cutrera R, Biban P, Benini F, Ranieri VM. Invasive and non-invasive long-term mechanical ventilation in Italian children. Minerva Anestesiol. 2011;77(9):892–901.
10. Proesmans M, Vermeulen F, De Boeck K. What's new in cystic fibrosis? From treating symptoms to correction of the basic defect. Eur J Pediatr. 2008;167(8):839–49.

11. Armstrong D. The use of continuous positive airway pressure or non-invasive ventilation as forms of respiratory support in children with cystic fibrosis. Paediatr Respir Rev. 2013;14:19–21.
12. Fauroux B, Hart N, Lofaso F. Non invasive mechanical ventilation in cystic fibrosis: physiological effects and monitoring. Monaldi Arch Chest Dis. 2002;57(5–6):268–72.
13. Fraser KL, Tullis DE, Sasson Z, Hyland RH, Thornley KS, Hanly PJ. Pulmonary hypertension and cardiac function in adult cystic fibrosis: role of hypoxemia. Chest. 1999;115:1321–8. https://doi.org/10.1378/chest.115.5.1321.
14. Bierlaagh MC, Muilwijk D, Beekman JM, van der Ent CK. A new era for people with cystic fibrosis. Eur J Pediatr. 2021;180(9):2731–9.
15. Atag E, Krivec U, Ersu R. Non-invasive ventilation for children with chronic lung disease. Front Pediatr. 2020;8:561639.
16. Balfour-Lynn IM, Primhak RA, Shaw BN. Home oxygen for children: who, how and when? Thorax. 2005;60:76–81.
17. Bhandari A, Panitch HB. Pulmonary outcomes in bronchopulmonary dysplasia. Semin Perinatol. 2006;30:219–26.
18. Addea FV, Alvarezb AE, Barbisanc BN, Guimarãesd BR. Recommendations for long-term home oxygen therapy in children and adolescents. J Pediatr. 2013;89(1):6–17.
19. Li YN, Liu L, Qiao HM, Cheng H, Cheng HJ. Post-infectious bronchiolitis obliterans in children: a review of 42 cases. BMC Pediatr. 2014;25(14):238.
20. Griese M. Chronic interstitial lung disease in children. Eur Respir Rev. 2018;27(147):170100.
21. Schulze-Neick I, Beghetti M. Issues related to the management and therapy of paediatric pulmonary hypertension. Eur Respir Rev. 2010;19(118):331–9.
22. Fauroux B, Khirani S, Griffon L, Teng T, Lanzeray A, Amaddeo A. Non-invasive ventilation in children with neuromuscular disease. Front Pediatr. 2020;8:482.
23. Balfour-Lynn IM, Field DJ, Gringras P, Hicks B, Jardine E, Jones RC, Magee AG, Primhak RA, Samuels MP, Shaw NJ, Stevens S, Sullivan C, Taylor JA, Wallis C, Paediatric Section of the Home Oxygen Guideline Development Group of the BTS Standards of Care Committee. BTS guidelines for home oxygen in children. Thorax. 2009;64 Suppl 2:21–6.
24. Balfour-Lynn IM. Domiciliary oxygen for children. Pediatr Clin N Am. 2009;56:275–96.
25. Ruangsomboon O, Dorongthom T, Chakorn T, Monsomboon A, Praphruetkit N, Limsuwat C, Surabenjawong U, Riyapan S, Nakornchai T, Chaisirin W. High-flow nasal cannula versus conventional oxygen therapy in relieving dyspnea in emergency palliative patients with do-not-intubate status: a randomized crossover study. Ann Emerg Med. 2020;75(5):615–26.
26. Shah N, Mehta Z, Mehta Y. High-flow nasal cannula oxygen therapy in palliative care #330. J Palliat Med. 2017;20(6):679–80.
27. Kwon JW. High-flow nasal cannula oxygen therapy in children: a clinical review. Clin Exp Pediatr. 2020;63(1):3–7.
28. Ignatiuk D, Schaer B, McGinley B. High flow nasal cannula treatment for obstructive sleep apnea in infants and young children. Pediatr Pulmonol. 2020;55(10):2791–8. https://doi.org/10.1002/ppul.25009.
29. Amaddeo A, Khirani S, Frapin A, Teng T, Griffon L, Fauroux B. High-flow nasal cannula for children not compliant with continuous positive airway pressure. Sleep Med. 2019;63:24–8.
30. Griffon L, Touil S, Frapin A, Teng T, Amaddeo A, Khirani S, Fauroux B. Home overnight gas exchange for long-term noninvasive ventilation in children. Respir Care. 2020;65(12):1815–22.
31. Amaddeo A, Fauroux B. Oxygen and carbon dioxide monitoring during sleep. Paediatr Respir Rev. 2016;20:42–4.
32. Amaddeo A, Moreau J, Frapin A, Khirani S, Felix O, Fernandez-Bolanos M, et al. Long term continuous positive airway pressure (CPAP) and noninvasive ventilation (NIV) in children: initiation criteria in real life. Pediatr Pulmonol. 2016;51:968–74.
33. Amaddeo A, Frapin A, Fauroux B. Long-term non-invasive ventilation in children. Lancet Respir Med. 2016;4(12):999–1008.
34. Pavone M, Verrillo E, Onofri A, Caggiano S, Chiarini Testa MB, Cutrera R. Characteristics and outcomes in children on long-term mechanical ventilation: the experience of a pediatric tertiary center in Rome. Ital J Pediatr. 2020;46:1–9.
35. Castro-Codesal ML, Dehaan K, Bedi PK, Bendiak GN, Schmalz L, Katz SL, MacLean JE. Longitudinal changes in clinical characteristics and outcomes for children using long-term non-invasive ventilation. PLoS One. 2018;13(1):e0192111.
36. Praud JP. Long-term non-invasive ventilation in children: current use, indications, and contraindications. Front Pediatr. 2020;8:584334.
37. Watters KF. Tracheostomy in infants and children. Respir Care. 2017;62(6):799–825.
38. Wilkinson DJ, Baikie G, Berkowitz RG, Reddihough DS. Awake upper airway obstruction in children with spastic quadriplegic cerebral palsy. J Paediatr Child Health. 2006;42(1–2):44–8.
39. Gupta A, Stokken J, Krakovitz P, Malhotra P, Anne S. Tracheostomy in neurologically compromised paediatric patients: role of starplasty. J Laryngol Otol. 2015;129(10):1009–12.
40. Friesen TL, Zamora SM, Rahmanian R, Bundogji N, Brigger MT. Predictors of pediatric tracheostomy outcomes in the United States. Otolaryngol Head Neck Surg. 2020;163:19459982091762–194599820917620.
41. Trachsel D, Hammer J. Indications for tracheostomy in children. Paediatr Respir Rev. 2006;7(3):162–8.
42. Arcand P, Granger J. Pediatric tracheostomies: changing trends. J Otolaryngol. 1988;17(2):121–4.

43. Graham RJ, Rodday AM, Parsons SK. Family-centered assessment and function for children with chronic mechanical respiratory support. J Pediatr Health Care. 2014;28(4):295–304.
44. Fuller C, Wineland AM, Richter GT. Update on pediatric tracheostomy: indications, technique, education, and decannulation. Curr Otorhinolaryngol Rep. 2021;9:188–99. https://doi.org/10.1007/s40136-021-00340-y.
45. Funamura JL, Yuen S, Kawai K, Gergin O, Adil E, Rahbar R, Watters K. Characterizing mortality in pediatric tracheostomy patients. Laryngoscope. 2017;127(7):1701–6.
46. Tsuboi N, Ide K, Nishimura N, Nakagawa S, Morimoto N. Pediatric tracheostomy: survival and long-term outcomes. Int J Pediatr Otorhinolaryngol. 2016;89:81–5.
47. Urrestarazu P, Varón J, Rodríguez A, et al. Clinical consensus statement on the care of the child with a tracheostomy. Arch Argent Pediatr. 2016;114:89–95.
48. Prasad S, Main E, Dodd M, Association of Chartered Physiotherapists. Finding consensus on the physiotherapy management of asymptomatic infants with cystic fibrosis. Pediatr Pulmonol. 2008;43:236–44.
49. Chatburn RL. High-frequency assisted airway clearance. Respir Care. 2007;52(9):1224–35.
50. Armstrong DS, Hook SM, Jamsen KM, et al. Lower airway inflammation in infants with cystic fibrosis detected by newborn screening. Pediatr Pulmonol. 2005;40:500–10.
51. Wright S, Wakeman R, Collins N, Chatwin M. 17—Physical therapies in pediatric respiratory disease, Kendig's disorders of the respiratory tract in children. 9th ed. Amsterdam: Elsevier; 2019. p. 273–288.e3.
52. Panitch HB. Respiratory implications of pediatric neuromuscular disease. Respir Care. 2017;62(6):826–48. https://doi.org/10.4187/respcare.05250.
53. Chatwin M, Toussaint M, Gonçalves MR, Sheers N, Mellies U, Gonzales-Bermejo J, Sancho J, Fauroux B, Andersen T, Hov B, Nygren-Bonnier M, Lacombe M, Pernet K, Kampelmacher M, Devaux C, Kinnett K, Sheehan D, Rao F, Villanova M, Berlowitz D, Morrow BM. Airway clearance techniques in neuromuscular disorders: a state of the art review. Respir Med. 2018;136:98–110. https://doi.org/10.1016/j.rmed.2018.01.012.
54. Cherchi C, Chiarini Testa MB, Deriu D, Schiavino A, Petreschi F, Ullmann N, Paglietti MG, Cutrera R. All you need is evidence: what we know about pneumonia in children with neuromuscular diseases. Front Pediatr. 2021;9:625751. https://doi.org/10.3389/fped.2021.625751.
55. Toussaint M, Boitano LJ, Gathot V, et al. Limits of effective cough-augmentation techniques in patients with neuromuscular disease. Respir Care. 2009;54:359–66.
56. Armstrong A. Developing a breath-stacking system to achieve lung volume recruitment. Br J Nurs. 2009;18:1166–9.
57. Hov B, Andersen T, Hovland V, Toussaint M. The clinical use of mechanical insufflation–exsufflation in children with neuromuscular disorders in Europe. Paediatr Respir Rev. 2017;17:30096–9. https://doi.org/10.1016/j.prrv.2017.08.003.

5 Frailty in Patients with Chronic Kidney Disease

Andrea Pession and Cristina Bertulli

5.1 Introduction

Chronic kidney disease (CKD) is a clinical syndrome characterized by a progressive and irreversible loss of kidney function. This condition develops into end-stage kidney disease (ESKD), the stage at which it becomes necessary to initiate renal replacement therapy (hemodialysis, peritoneal dialysis, kidney transplant) [1].

Epidemiologic data on CKD in children may be underestimated because CKD can be asymptomatic in its earlier stages, and the majority of studies only take into account patients with moderate to severe CKD. Moreover, childhood CKD registries are usually limited to small reference populations.

Kidney damage stages are the following: **Stage 1**, glomerular filtration rate (GFR) >90%; **Stage 2**, GFR 89–60%; **Stage 3**, with biochemical alterations, growth retardation, nutritional difficulties, and GFR 59–30%; **Stage 4**, with worsening of symptoms and GFR 29–15%; **Stage 5**, with end-stage kidney disease, which requires renal replacement therapy and GFR <15% or dialysis (classification of different stages of CKD according to the KDOQI guidelines [2]).

Despite these limitations, the incidence of pediatric CKD in Europe is reported to be around 11–12 per million age-related population for stages 3–5, while the prevalence is ~55–60 per million age-related population. The incidence and prevalence of CKD are greater in males than in females because the frequency of congenital abnormalities of the kidney and urinary tract (CAKUT) is higher in males.

The most frequent causes of CKD are CAKUT, steroid-resistant nephrotic syndrome (SRNS), chronic glomerulonephritis (e.g., lupus nephritis, Alport syndrome), and renal ciliopathies (e.g., autosomal dominant polycystic kidney disease), which account for approximately 50, 10, 8, and 5% of cases, respectively. These causes are significantly different from the ones responsible for CKD in adults. Structural causes (such as renal hypoplasia or posterior urethral valves) are predominant in younger patients, while the incidence of glomerulonephritis increases in those older than 12 years. Congenital malformation disorders are characterized by a slower progression to ESKD in comparison with glomerular diseases [3].

A. Pession
Paediatric Unit, IRCCS Azienda Ospedaliero-Universitaria di Bologna, Bologna, Italy

Department of Pediatrics, Sant'Orsola Hospital, IRCSS, University of Bologna, Bologna, BO, Italy
e-mail: andrea.pession@unibo.it

C. Bertulli (✉)
Paediatric Unit, IRCCS Azienda Ospedaliero-Universitaria di Bologna, Bologna, Italy

Nephrology and Pediatric Dialysis, Department of Pediatrics, Sant'Orsola Hospital, IRCSS, University of Bologna, Bologna, BO, Italy
e-mail: cristina.bertulli@aosp.bo.it

M. Lima, M. C. Mondardini (eds.), *Frailty in Children*,
https://doi.org/10.1007/978-3-031-24307-3_5

Frailty is described as a state of increased vulnerability to health problems; in the general population, it has been shown to be predictive of adverse outcomes, including hospitalization, decreased quality of life, and mortality. Frailty is common in patients with CKD and is associated with an increased risk of adverse health outcomes [4–6]. The relationship between CKD and frailty is not completely understood. Studies have shown that inflammation is associated with frailty in many chronic diseases, and this suggests a "shared pathophysiology" of frailty. Shlipak et al. demonstrated that there are raised levels of proinflammatory cytokines in CKD patients.

The causes of a chronic proinflammatory state in CKD patients are not well understood, although it is likely that they are multifactorial. The increased plasma levels of proinflammatory cytokines can be caused by both decreased renal clearance and increased cytokine production. The progressive reduction of renal function is associated with a significant increase in serum cytokine levels in CKD patients. Another important factor for the activation of the inflammatory response is the immunological effect of uremic toxins on the immune system [7].

Alterations in body composition have also emerged as another determinant of inflammation. Fat tissue is an active endocrine organ that produces several adipokines, including leptin, resistin, adiponectin, IL-6, and TNF-a. Recently, a relationship between body fat mass (particularly truncal fat mass) and inflammatory parameters in CKD patients who are starting dialysis have been established. Thus, it is likely that the fat tissue production of inflammatory markers may contribute to inflammation in CKD patients [8].

Chronic kidney disease is associated not only with the condition of chronic inflammation but also with different clinical problems, like anemia, growth retardation, malnutrition, bone mineral disease, hypertension and cardiovascular disease, reduced muscle strength, and fatigue. Patients need to attend frequent outpatient clinic visits and sometimes require long periods of hospitalization.

Anemia is a common complication in patients with CKD and is caused by decreased production of erythropoietin as well as iron dysregulation. Anemia is considered when hemoglobin falls below the age- and sex-specific fifth percentile value. The prevalence of anemia increases with advancing stages of CKD (the prevalence is 73% at stage III, 87% at stage IV, and 93% at stage V) [9, 10]. Treatment involves the administration of recombinant human erythropoietin and iron supplementation, and the treatment goal is to achieve hemoglobin levels of approximately 11 g/dL [11]. Anemia in CKD patients can cause many adverse clinical consequences, including poor quality of life, depressed neurocognitive ability, reduced exercise capacity, and the progression of cardiovascular risk factors, like left ventricular hypertrophy [12].

Growth impairment is a common complication in pediatric CKD patients. The degree of growth impairment increases as GFR declines [13]. There is an evident correlation between growth impairment and the age of CKD onset. Infants with CKD are at a higher risk of severe growth retardation, considering that one third of total growth occurs in the first 2 years of life [14]. Malnutrition, metabolic acidosis, mineral and bone disease, anemia, and fluid and electrolyte abnormalities are all factors that contribute to growth impairment [3]. After infancy and early childhood, growth failure is also due to disturbances in growth hormone metabolism. However, inadequate nutrition due to vomiting and anorexia is the most important factor causing growth retardation. Treatment with a recombinant human growth hormone is effective and does not carry the risk of major adverse events [15].

Chronic kidney disease-mineral and bone disease (CKD-MBD) is a systemic disorder of mineral and bone metabolism caused by CKD. It is defined by the presence of the following features: abnormalities in calcium, phosphorus, parathyroid hormone, or vitamin D metabolism and abnormalities in bone histology or linear growth or strength; vascular or other tissue calcification can develop if the disorder is not treated properly. The principal effect of CKD-MBD is growth retardation.

The effective treatment of CKD-MBD can reduce the development of cardiovascular disease, which can occur because of the presence of vascular calcification [16].

Supplementation with vitamin D is started in the early stages of CKD. Phosphate control is crucial and begins with dietary restriction; however, it is usually difficult for children to follow a strict diet, and phosphate binders therefore become a necessity. Compliance with phosphate binders is often poor because of their unpleasant taste and the need to take them with every meal [17].

Hypertension can be present from the earliest stages of CKD, and its prevalence increases as GFR declines [18]. Hypertension represents a potential risk factor for cardiovascular morbidity in children with CKD during adulthood. Blood pressure should be checked at every outpatient clinical visit, and an antihypertensive treatment must be started as soon as blood pressure readings are ≥90th percentile for sex and height.

Some patients with CKD have masked hypertension (normal office blood pressure but elevated ambulatory blood pressure), and for this reason, they need to undergo 24-h ambulatory blood pressure monitoring [19].

The effective control of blood pressure reduces cardiovascular morbidity and mortality and the progression of CKD. Antihypertensive therapy with renin–angiotensin–aldosterone system inhibitors is crucial, especially in proteinuric patients [20].

Children with CKD are at risk of **malnutrition and protein energy wasting** (PEW), which leads to weight loss and growth failure. In the context of CKD, the term PEW was proposed by the International Society of Renal Nutrition and Metabolism to describe a "state of decreased body stores of protein and energy fuels (body protein and fat masses)" [21]. Inadequate nutritional intake, systemic inflammation, endocrine perturbations, and abnormal neuropeptide signaling may contribute to PEW [1, 6–10]. This condition is characterized by maladaptive responses, including anorexia and increased metabolic rate, and is associated with low serum albumin and loss of body weight; muscle mass is reduced, whereas fat mass is normal or increased [22].

The pathophysiology of PEW syndrome in CKD is multifactorial, and many factors are involved, such as endocrine disorders (e.g., vitamin D deficiency), acidosis, anemia, oxidative stress, inflammatory cytokines, volume overload, anorexia, metabolic disorders, and dietary restriction.

Anorexia plays a crucial role in the development of PEW; in CKD patients, it is caused by a combination of factors, including altered taste, gastroesophageal reflux, delayed gastric emptying, and elevated levels of numerous cytokines, such as IL-1, IL-6, and TNF-α. Alterations in appetite-regulating hormones, like leptin and ghrelin, may contribute to anorexia in these patients.

Moreover, a low-protein diet is usually prescribed in the advanced stages of CKD. To obtain a reduction in protein intake, aproteic products are prescribed, but these are usually unpalatable. Compliance with these types of dietary products can be poor in children with CKD, leading to a worsening of malnutrition [23].

All these factors play a crucial role in children with CKD, who may face many issues, such as malnutrition, uremic toxins, inflammation, cachexia, and protein-energy wasting.

Muscle wasting and fatigue are caused by chronic inflammation, which is present in patients with CKD, as mentioned before. Inflammation activates the ubiquitin-proteasome system, which leads to increased muscle breakdown that is not balanced by a corresponding upregulation of anabolic pathways.

The treatment of children with CKD with a recombinant human growth hormone has been identified as an important and significant determinant of higher muscle mass relative to height [21].

5.2 Newborns and Infants with CKD

Neonatal CKD is defined as a decrease in kidney function, which manifests in the neonatal period and is lifelong. The incidence is difficult to assess because there are only a few systematic studies available in the literature.

The gender distribution (male-to-female ratio of 2.8:1) is due to the higher prevalence of obstructive uropathies (such as posterior urethral valves) in males, which are frequent causes of CKD [24]. More than 50% of infants with CKD are premature. Preterm neonates have a higher risk of CKD for several reasons. First, they are born with a smaller complement of nephrons because nephrogenesis plateaus at 36 weeks. Second, preterm neonates are frequently exposed to nephrotoxic medications and other risk factors for developing acute kidney injury [25]. Finally, CKD is more prevalent in preterm neonates because prenatal kidney disease leads to a higher risk of preterm delivery (for example, oligohydramnios).

The principal etiologies of neonatal CKD are summarized in Table 5.1 [24].

Chronic kidney disease management in newborns and infants depends on the severity of the CKD and ranges from simple long-term surveillance for mild CKD to renal replacement therapy for ESKD.

The pharmacological management of CKD centers around drugs to replace missing endogenous renal products (erythropoietin, calcitriol), drugs to mimic the homeostatic functions of the kidney (phosphorus binders, potassium binders, and bicarbonate and sodium supplementation), and the administration of vitamins/minerals which are poorly absorbed or utilized in CKD (vitamin D, iron). Other drugs are used for specific indications, such as hypertension [26].

Growth and nutrition represent the cornerstone of the management of CKD during this period of life. One of the most important reasons for paying attention to nutrition in this very young CKD population is its impact on growth. Both linear growth and neurodevelopment progress most rapidly during the first 3 years of life; therefore, inadequate nutrition during this period can cause serious growth and developmental delays that are difficult to recover later.

Table 5.1 The principal etiologies of neonatal chronic kidney disease

Etiologies of neonatal CKD	
Congenital	Acquired
Autosomal dominant polycystic kidney disease	Renal arterial thrombosis
Autosomal recessive polycystic kidney disease	
Other renal ciliopathies	
Renal dysplasia/CAKUT	Renal vein thrombosis
Posterior urethral valves	
Other forms of urinary tract obstruction	

Nutritional intake is frequently suboptimal in infants with CKD. Anorexia is the primary reason for growth failure, even in children with mild CKD. As seen before, anorexia is caused by a combination of factors, including altered taste, gastroesophageal reflux, delayed gastric emptying, and elevated levels of cytokines. Special milk formula and supplementation with maltodextrins are usually prescribed in these patients.

Gastrostomy or nasogastric feeding tubes are an essential component of the nutritional management of almost every infant on dialysis and for many with CKD [27].

In the case of ESKD, the choice of chronic renal replacement therapy usually falls on peritoneal dialysis in the neonatal population. There are some indications for hemodialysis or continuous renal replacement therapy in neonates, of which hyperammonemia is the most important.

Patients with a weight of less than 10 kg are not suitable for kidney transplantation. Considering the nutritional and growth problems seen in these infants, the target of 10 kg is not easy to reach, and patients can remain on dialysis for long periods, with consequent clinical complications due to renal replacement therapy.

Newborns and infants with CKD can require long periods of hospitalization (like in the case of congenital nephrotic syndrome), and this fact can contribute to a delay in the acquisition of neurodevelopmental skills.

Taking care of a baby with all these problems is a full-time job for the family and can become a constant burden. For this reason, families should be offered psychological support.

The most important predictor of mortality in this patient age group is the presence of nonrenal diseases, like pulmonary or cardiological complications; in fact, CKD can also be a feature of polymalformative syndromes [24].

5.3 Children and Adolescents with CKD

As mentioned before, children and adolescents with CKD are fragile subjects because of the disease itself and the complications caused by it. These patients require frequent visits to the hospital for blood exams and checkups, and this can have a negative psychological impact as they will miss school and perceive themselves as being different from their peers.

Long hospital stays can be necessary, not only in newborns but also in older patients.

Treatment compliance is another crucial aspect, especially during adolescence [28].

Patients sometimes refuse to accept the disease and decide to stop taking medications because they do not see an immediate difference in their clinical status. It is necessary to create an open and sincere line of communication between doctors and patients, especially during this crucial period.

The frequency of checkups increases during ESKD due to the fact that numerous biochemical and instrumental exams must be performed in order to schedule a living donor kidney transplant from a relative or to put the patient on the deceased donor kidney transplant waiting list. The transplant workup usually includes blood exams, virological status, echocardiography, abdominal ultrasound and Doppler, chest X-ray, ophthalmological evaluation, bone age assessment, and urological evaluations in patients with urological malformations (like vesicoureteral reflux, posterior urethral valves, neurological bladder).

5.4 Transplanted Patients

In children with ESKD, renal replacement therapy must be considered. Today, kidney transplantation is the treatment of choice and has widely substituted, when possible, both peritoneal and hemodialysis.

A recipient weight of at least 10 kg is required to minimize the risk of vascular thrombosis and to accommodate a comparatively large adult kidney [29].

It is necessary that the patient has completed the vaccination schedule for age before starting posttransplant immunosuppression therapy; this is especially so for live vaccines, which are contraindicated after transplant [30].

Recently, perioperative volume management and donor selection have significantly improved surgical outcomes; however, vascular thrombosis (3.2% of pediatric kidney transplants) remains a cause of graft loss in the pediatric population [31].

After transplantation, the patients start immunosuppressive therapy, which will be continued throughout their lives and consists of calcineurin inhibitors, antiproliferative agents, and corticosteroids. These therapies expose the patients to opportunistic infections.

Another problem for transplanted patients is posttransplant lymphoproliferative disease (PTLD): the most frequent types of cancers are skin cancers, particularly squamous cell carcinoma and melanoma; anogenital/gynecologic cancers; Kaposi's sarcoma; sarcoma; thyroid tumors; hepatobiliary tumors; leukemia; and brain tumors. The recommended strategies for the prevention and monitoring of secondary malignancies are virological monitoring, vaccination, education, and routine cancer surveillance. A higher incidence is seen in Epstein-Barr virus (EBV)-negative recipients at 5 years posttransplant, compared with EBV-positive recipients [32].

Persistent posttransplant hypertension is a common complication and a risk factor for adverse cardiovascular outcomes. Left ventricular hypertrophy serves as an intermediate endpoint for cardiovascular disease risk stratification. The aggressive treatment of high blood pressure is crucial for reducing cardiovascular disease. The treatment goal is to obtain a blood pressure around the 50th percentile for sex and height [33, 34].

Age at transplantation (prepuberal or puberal), allograft function, and corticosteroid therapy are the main factors that influence growth after kidney transplant. After transplant, growth velocity can improve if attention is paid to conservative measures, particularly in younger children, such as adequate nutritional intake, correction of metabolic acidosis, prevention of renal osteodystrophy, and steroid reduction or avoidance.

Graft survival has progressively improved over the last two decades, thanks to increased awareness regarding donor source and recipient age. Data collected from 2006 to 2010 showed that living donor graft survival of pediatric patients at 1 and 5 years was 96.5% and 86.1%, respectively, while deceased donor recipients have lower graft survival rates of 96.3% and 77.5%, respectively [35]. Adolescents have the poorest 5-year results of any age group, including adults; this can be explained by the reduced compliance to therapy seen in this age group, which can lead to graft loss in some cases. During adolescence, patients tend to compare themselves to their peers, and even the presence of abdominal scars or other feeding or dialysis devices placed within the body can represent a problem and a limitation for the socialization of the patient.

Another crucial point that can influence graft survival is the transition into adult care. Early preparation of the family, with the patient; the use of checklists to document maturing transition skills, and a gradual transition instead of an abrupt transfer are necessary. It is crucial to create a multidisciplinary team, which includes a pediatric nephrologist, an adult nephrologist, and pediatric and adult psychologists, who work together with the family and the patients and participate in clinical outpatient visits during the months before the transition [36].

Even considering the improvements in pediatric kidney transplant over the last few years, we must bear in mind that transplantation is not a curative treatment, and subsequently, the ongoing chronic illness persists in terms of daily immunosuppressive treatment and its potentially unpleasant side effects, the fear of organ dysfunction, and the need for continuous medical supervision.

5.5 Health-Related Quality of Life and Psychological Aspects

Medical and surgical advances have changed the physical outcomes and survival rates of children with CKD drastically.

However, a chronic disease like CKD remains demanding, time-consuming, and invasive, placing high demands on children and their families; these patients deal with a life of limitations, and their quality of life is significantly impaired. Chronic kidney disease affects many aspects of the life of these children: they are subjected to daily dietary and fluid restrictions, difficult and invasive treatments with complex drug regimens, and even hospitalization; they can have devices in their bodies for feeding or dialyzing. All these aspects influence their physical, emotional, and sexual growth. Data in the literature have shown that these emotional alterations in patients with CKD and their caregivers can also persist into adulthood [37].

Chronic kidney disease also places particular demands on a child's social life. Children need to be with their peers in and out of school, playing sports and participating in other activities with classmates and friends. Medical appointments, dialysis sessions, and home medication therapies significantly reduce social time. These children may become more and more isolated, making peer acceptance a bigger issue. Data from the literature have demonstrated that children undergoing dialysis have worse emotional performance in comparison to those undergoing conservative treatment and transplanted patients. Data on school performance have shown that children with CKD are at risk of impairment [38].

The management of these patients represents a challenge for the healthcare team and for the patients and their caregivers.

References

1. Levey AS, Eckardt K-U, Tsukamoto Y, Levin A, Coresh J, Rossert J, Zeeuw DDE, Hostetter TH, Lameire N, Eknoyan G. Definition and classification of chronic kidney disease: a position statement from Kidney Disease: Improving Global Outcomes (KDIGO). Kidney Int. 2005;67(6):2089–100.
2. K/DOQI Clinical Practice Guidelines. K/DOQI clinical practice guidelines for chronic kidney disease: evaluation, classification, and stratification. Am J Kidney Dis. 2002;39:S1–S266.
3. Becherucci F, Roperto RM, Materassi M, Romagnani P. Chronic kidney disease in children. Clin Kidney J. 2016;9(4):583–91.
4. Nixon AC, Bampouras TM, Pendleton N, Mitra S, Dhaygude AP. Diagnostic accuracy of frailty screening methods in advanced chronic kidney disease. Nephron. 2019;141:147–55.

5. Nixon AC, Bampouras TM, Pendleton N, Woywodt A, Mitra S, Dhaygude A. Frailty and chronic kidney disease: current evidence and continuing uncertainties. Clin Kidney J. 2018;11:236–45.
6. Sgambat K, Matheson MB, Hooper SR, Warady B, Furth S, Moudgil A. Prevalence and outcomes of fragility: a frailty-inflammation phenotype in children with chronic kidney disease. Pediatr Nephrol. 2019;34(12):2563–9.
7. Shlipak MG, Fried LF, Crump C, Bleyer AJ, Manolio TA, Tracy RP, Furberg CD, Psaty BM. Elevations of inflammatory and procoagulant biomarkers in elderly persons with renal insufficiency. Circulation. 2003;107(1):87–92.
8. Pecoits-Filho R, Sylvestre LC, Stenvinkel P. Chronic kidney disease and inflammation in pediatric patients: from bench to playground. Pediatr Nephrol. 2005;20(6):714–20.
9. KDOQI; National Kidney Foundation. KDOQI clinical practice guidelines and clinical practice recommendations for anemia in chronic kidney disease. Am J Kidney Dis. 2006;47(5 Suppl 3):S11–145.
10. Atkinson MA, Warady BA. Anemia in chronic kidney disease. Pediatr Nephrol. 2018;33(2):227–38.
11. Port RE, Mehls O. Erythropoietin dosing in children with chronic kidney disease: based on body size or on hemoglobin deficit? Pediatr Nephrol. 2009;24:435–7.
12. Mitsnefes MM, Kimball TR, Kartal J, Witt SA, Glascock BJ, Khoury PR, Daniels SR. Progression of left ventricular hypertrophy in children with early chronic kidney disease: 2-year follow-up study. J Pediatr. 2006;149(5):671–5.
13. Rodig NM, McDermott KC, Schneider MF, Hotchkiss HM, Yadin O, Seikaly MG, Furth SL, Warady BA. Growth in children with chronic kidney disease: a report from the chronic kidney disease in children study. Pediatr Nephrol. 2014;29(10):1987–95.
14. André JL, Bourquard R, Guillemin F, Krier MJ, Briançon S. Final height in children with chronic renal failure who have not received growth hormone. Pediatr Nephrol. 2003;18(7):685–91.
15. Rees L. Growth hormone therapy in children with CKD after more than two decades of practice. Pediatr Nephrol. 2016;31(9):1421–35.
16. Wesseling-Perry K. Bone disease in pediatric chronic kidney disease. Pediatr Nephrol. 2013;28(4):569–76. https://doi.org/10.1007/s00467-012-2324-4.
17. Kidney Disease: Improving Global Outcomes (KDIGO) CKD-MBD Work Group. KDIGO clinical practice guideline for the diagnosis, evaluation, prevention, and treatment of chronic kidney disease-mineral and bone disorder (CKD-MBD) (including 2017 update). Kidney Int Suppl. 2009;113:S1–130.
18. Barletta GM, Pierce C, Mitsnefes M, Samuels J, Warady BA, Furth S, Flynn J. Is blood pressure improving in children with chronic kidney disease? A period analysis. Hypertension. 2018;71(3):444–50.
19. Mitsnefes M, Flynn J, Cohn S, Samuels J, Blydt-Hansen T, Saland J, Kimball T, Furth S, Warady B, CKiD Study Group. Masked hypertension associates with left ventricular hypertrophy in children with CKD. J Am Soc Nephrol. 2010;21(1):137–44.
20. Hsu TW, Liu JS, Hung SC, Kuo KL, Chang YK, Chen YC, Hsu CC, Tarng DC. Renoprotective effect of renin–angiotensin–aldosterone system blockade in patients with predialysis advanced chronic kidney disease, hypertension, and anemia. JAMA Intern Med. 2014;174(3):347–54.
21. Mak RH, Cheung WW, Zhan JY, Shen Q, Foster BJ. Cachexia and protein-energy wasting in children with chronic kidney disease. Pediatr Nephrol. 2012;27(2):173–81.
22. Mak RH, Cheung W, Cone RD, Marks DL. Mechanisms of disease: cytokine and adipokine signaling in uremic cachexia. Nat Clin Pract Nephrol. 2006;2:527–34.
23. Mak RH, Cheung W, Cone RD, Marks DL. Leptin and inflammation-associated cachexia in chronic kidney disease. Kidney Int. 2006;69:794–7.
24. Misurac J. Chronic kidney disease in the neonate: etiologies, management, and outcomes. Semin Fetal Neonatal Med. 2017;22(2):98–103.
25. Sutherland MR, Gubhaju L, Moore L, Kent AL, Dahlstrom JE, Horne RS, Hoy WE, Bertram JF, Black MJ. Accelerated maturation and abnormal morphology in the preterm neonatal kidney. J Am Soc Nephrol. 2011;22(7):1365–74.
26. Zaritsky JJ, Warady BA. Chronic kidney disease in the neonate. Clin Perinatol. 2014;41:503–15.
27. KDOQI Work Group. KDOQI clinical practice guideline for nutrition in children with CKD: 2008 update. Executive summary. Am J Kidney Dis. 2009;53:S11–104.
28. Warady BA, Chadha V. Chronic kidney disease in children: the global perspective. Pediatr Nephrol. 2007;22:1999–2009.
29. Jalanko H, Mattila I, Holmberg C. Renal transplantation in infants. Pediatr Nephrol. 2016;31(5):725–35.
30. Kroger AT, Duchin J, Vázquez M. General best practice guidelines for immunization: best practices guidance of the Advisory Committee on Immunization Practices (ACIP). Washington, DC: Centers for Disease Control and Prevention; 2017.
31. Irtan S, Maisin A, Baudouin V, et al. Renal transplantation in children: critical analysis of age related surgical complications. Pediatr Transplant. 2010;14(4):512–9.
32. Hebert SA, Swinford RD, Hall DR, Au JK, Bynon JS. Special considerations in pediatric kidney transplantation. Adv Chronic Kidney Dis. 2017;24(6):398–404.
33. Hamdani G, Nehus EJ, Hanevold CD, Sebestyen Van Sickle J, Woroniecki R, Wenderfer SE, Hooper DK, Blowey D, Wilson A, Warady BA, Mitsnefes MM. Ambulatory blood pressure, left ventricular hypertrophy, and allograft function in children and young adults after kidney transplantation. Transplantation. 2017;101(1):150–6.
34. Flynn JT, Kaelber DC, Baker-Smith CM, Blowey D, Carroll AE, Daniels SR, de Ferranti SD, Dionne

JM, Falkner B, Flinn SK, Gidding SS, Goodwin C, Leu MG, Powers ME, Rea C, Samuels J, Simasek M, Thaker VV, Urbina EM, Subcommittee on Screening and Management of High Blood Pressure in Children. Clinical practice guideline for screening and management of high blood pressure in children and adolescents. Pediatrics. 2017;140(3):e20171904.

35. Organ Procurement and Transplantation Network (OPTN) and Scientific Registry of Transplant Recipients (SRTR). OPTN/SRTR 2015 Annual Data Report. 2016.
36. Scarponi D, Cammaroto V, Pasini A, La Scola C, Mencarelli F, Bertulli C, Busutti M, La Manna G, Pession A. Multidisciplinarity in transition pathways for patients with kidney disease: the current state of play. Front Pediatr. 2021;20(9):689758.
37. Heath J, Mackinlay D, Watson AR, Hames A, Wirz L, Scott S, Klewchuk E, Milford D, McHugh K. Self-reported quality of life in children and young people with chronic kidney disease. Pediatr Nephrol. 2011;26(5):767–73.
38. Duvant P, Fillat M, Garaix F, Roquelaure B, Ovaert C, Fouilloux V, Tsimaratos M, Auquier P, Fabre A, Baumstarck K. Quality of life of transplanted children and their parents: a cross-sectional study. Orphanet J Rare Dis. 2021;16(1):364.

Children with Chronic Liver Disease

6

Giuseppe Maggiore, Claudia Della Corte, Daniela Liccardo, Antonella Mosca, and Andrea Pietrobattista

A child with a chronic liver disease (CLD) is a frail child, exposed to the several consequences of chronic liver damage, such as malnutrition, sarcopenia, fat-soluble vitamin deficiency, gastrointestinal bleeding related to portal hypertension, and reduced synthesis of clotting factors, also due to vitamin K deficiency, ascites, and severe pruritus disturbing the night sleep (Fig. 6.1). These conditions make the quality of life of these children very poor. Moreover, chronic and active liver damage progressively lead to cirrhosis and end-stage liver disease (ESLD).

In the recent years, for the majority of these frail children with CLD, liver transplantation (LT) has become a powerful therapeutic option with a high rate of success and with a dramatic improvement of their quality of life [1].

The principal causes of frailty in children due to chronic liver diseases are: (1) cholestatic liver disorders, (2) inflammatory liver diseases, (3) metabolic liver disorders (MLD), and nutritional metabolic liver damage.

G. Maggiore (✉) · C. D. Corte · D. Liccardo · A. Mosca · A. Pietrobattista
Hepatogastroenterology, Nutrition, Digestive Endoscopy and Liver Transplant Unit, IRCCS Ospedale Pediatrico Bambino Gesù, Rome, Italy
e-mail: giuseppe.maggiore@opbg.net; claudia.dellacorte@opbg.net; daniela.liccardo@opbg.net; antonella.mosca@opbg.net; andrea.pietrobattista@opbg.net

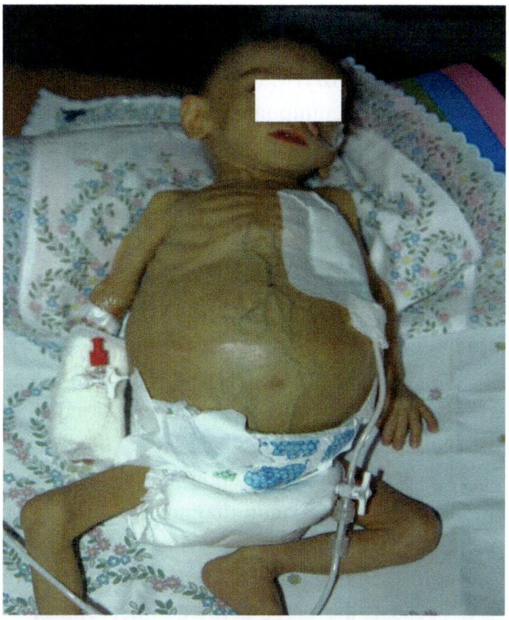

Fig. 6.1 The frail infant with biliary cirrhosis and end-stage liver disease

6.1 The Frail Infant/Child with a Cholestatic Liver Disease

Neonatal jaundice is a common and benign condition. However, a minority of infants (1:2500) can present, within the first 3 months of life, with prolonged jaundice caused by a reduction of bile flow with accumulation in the liver and

M. Lima, M. C. Mondardini (eds.), *Frailty in Children*,
https://doi.org/10.1007/978-3-031-24307-3_6

in extrahepatic tissues of substances normally excreted in the bile, such as bilirubin, cholesterol, and bile acids. This condition is defined as neonatal cholestasis (NC). NC is characterized by a conjugated hyperbilirubinemia (direct bilirubin levels >1.0 mg/dL or >17 mmol/L for total serum bilirubin of up to 5 mg/dL and a direct bilirubin fraction of more than 20% of the total bilirubin for values greater than 5 mg/dL). NC may be the presenting sign of severe hepatobiliary or metabolic diseases causing end-stage liver disease (ESLD) and death [2]. Cholestasis refers to a defect in intrahepatic production or the transmembrane transport of bile components or a mechanical obstruction causing abnormal bile flow. The most common causes of NC are biliary atresia (BA) (25–40%) and an array of individually uncommon monogenetic disorders (25%). Other causes of cholestasis are related to preterm birth (10%), infectious diseases (1–9%), biliary sludge (2%), and, finally, idiopathic cases (13–30%) [2]. Often, the etiology is unknown; however, recently, the rate of patients designated as having "idiopathic neonatal hepatitis" continues to decline with advancements in the discovery of new etiologies, mostly with the increasing use of available next-generation DNA sequencing (NGS) technologies. Once NC is diagnosed, an extensive systematic approach is crucial to promptly achieve a rapid diagnosis so a specific and often life-saving therapy can be started.

Rapid diagnosis is essential, particularly for BA, because the early surgical intervention of hepatoportoenterostomy (Kasai procedure) before 2 months of age correlates with better long-term outcomes with a native liver. Unfortunately, the diagnosis of BA is often delayed, and for this reason, the value of direct bilirubin should be systematically determined in any infant presenting with prolonged jaundice lasting longer than 14 days of age for term and 21 days for preterm infants with or without depigmented stool [3]. Overall, the NC diagnostic approach is challenging since the differential diagnosis is broad. The number of unique disorders presenting with cholestasis in the first months may be greater than at any other time in life and includes a wide range of causes. The mandatory diagnostic workup should include extensive biochemical, radiological, and clinical investigations. In 2017, the North American and the European Society for Pediatric Gastroenterology, Hepatology and Nutrition published a common guideline for the evaluation of cholestatic infants, where, however, it is clearly stated that these guidelines are intended to be flexible and tailored to the individual patient and local practice and are not meant to determine standards of care for all infants [4]. All infants with NC will benefit from both early nutritional interventions with medium-chain triglyceride (MCT)-containing formula and fat-soluble vitamin supplementation to enhance growth and prevent intestinal malabsorption, which can result in malnutrition and frailty [5]. Infantile cholestatic disorders might be progressive, and thus medical management should include the treatment of possible complications, such as pruritus, portal hypertension, and bacterial cholangitis, which can further concur to the concept of frailty.

6.1.1 Principal Causes of Neonatal Cholestasis

6.1.1.1 Biliary Atresia

Biliary atresia is a rare obliterative cholangiopathy of unknown origin involving intra- and extrahepatic biliary structures. Its prevalence in Europe and the USA varies from 1:5000 to 1:20,000 live-born. BA spontaneously progresses to cirrhosis and ESLF in the first years of life. Its treatment is principally surgical and is based on two sequential procedures: the Kasai portoenterostomy (KP), corresponding to a bilio-digestive anastomosis between the *porta hepatis* and an intestinal Roux loop, and, in the case of failure of this procedure, LT [6]. BA is the main indication of the need for pediatric liver transplants worldwide [7]. BA presents, most commonly, with cholestasis between 2 and 5 weeks of life; the etiology is unknown, and theories on his pathogenesis include genetic contributions to bile duct dysmorphogenesis, viral infection, toxins, or chronic inflammatory or immune-mediated bile duct injury [8]. BA does not seem to be a single entity but appears to be a pathological phenotype caused by different etiologies, including a perinatal insult that triggers an immune-mediated obliteration of the extrahepatic bile duct lumen or an embryonic or fetal defect in the normal morphogenesis of the biliary tree [9]. Two clinical phenotypes of BA exist: "classical," which is not associated with extrahepatic congenital anomalies, and "BA associated with splenic malformation," which includes other congenital anomalies, such as, most frequently, *situs inversus*, asplenia, polysplenia, preduodenal portal veins, cardiac malformations, and intestinal malrotation [10]. The success of hepatoportoenterostomy depends on the precocity of the diagnosis and surgery [11]. Unfortunately, in the early phase of the disease, a newborn with BA appears healthy, meconium is rarely discolored, stools are only moderately discolored, and jaundice is mild. In regions with a high prevalence of BA, such as Taiwan (1:2700), a strategy based on universal screening using a stool color card has been successfully developed [12]. Abdominal Doppler ultrasound is noninvasive and is early recommended during NC diagnostic workup. It can detect abnormalities in the liver and gallbladder suggesting BA. Infants with BA often suffer from the absence of the gallbladder or from a small contracted gallbladder; however, a normal gallbladder does not rule out BA. The presence of a triangular or tubular echogenic cord of fibrous tissue at the *porta hepatis* representing the biliary remnant, described as the "triangular cord sign," has a diagnostic sensitivity for BA of 70% [2]. A definitive diagnosis of BA relies on liver biopsy and intraoperative cholangiography. The classic histologic findings are enlarged portal tracks with fibrosis, bile plugs, and bile duct proliferation, while intraoperative cholangiography documents the lack of a patent extrahepatic bile duct.

The current standard treatment for BA is based on KP, which aims to obtain successful bile drainage and the clearance of jaundice. If KP is performed within the first 60 days of life, 70% of patients will establish bile flow, while after 90 days of life, less than 20% of patients will have bile flow. Management of patients with a late diagnosis (>90 days) of BA is still controversial about indication to perform KP or directely shift to liver transplantation. The overall outcome of KP is related to the clearance of bilirubin, and avoidance of ascending cholangitis, which are both supposed to improve survival with native liver and delay of LT. KP is a palliative surgery and resolves cholestasis in about half of patients; however, in 70% of patients, hepatic fibrosis will progress to cirrhosis (Fig. 6.2), and these patients will require LT. Exactly for this purpose and despite some differences among various centers, post-KP standard protocol treatment has been always based on long-term prophylactic antibiotics and adjuvant steroid therapy [13]. Cholangitis is a common complication of KP, with an incidence variable between 40 and 93% [14]. In most case series, more than half of patients have their first episode of cholangitis within the first 6 months, and several postoperative antibiotic prophylaxes have been used to reduce this complication. Adjuvant steroids have been used empirically for many years after KP to reduce the risk of fibrosis, treating inflammation at the porta hepatis. However, both treatments reached just controversial results in the literature [15, 16].

The outcome of KP depends on early surgery performed before the age of 6 weeks and on the caseload of the center performing the primary surgery. Long-term results of KP show a survival rate with the native liver at 10 years in about 30% of patients and at 20 years of about 25%. At present, sequential treatment for biliary atresia results in long-term survival, with a good quality of life, in more than 90% of treated patients.

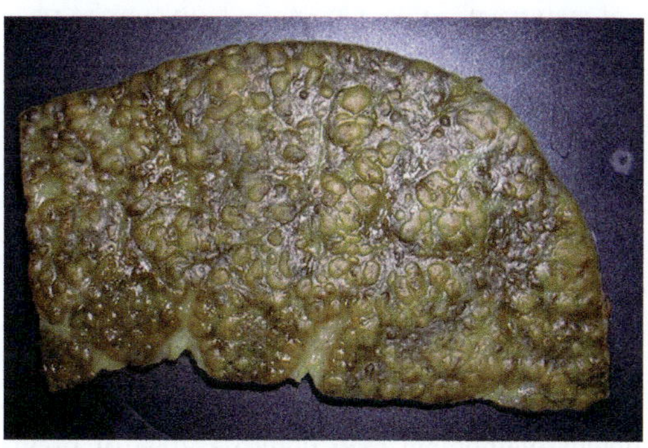

Fig. 6.2 Macroscopic features of biliary cirrhosis in biliary atresia

6.1.1.2 Genetic Cholestasis

Progressive Familial Intrahepatic Cholestasis (PFIC)

PFIC is a heterogeneous group of rare autosomal recessive liver disorders of childhood characterized by mutations in genes encoding proteins involved in the hepatocellular transport system and bile formation (Table 6.1). The exact prevalence remains unknown, but the estimated incidence varies between 1:50,000 and 1:100,000 births. The pathogenesis of cholestasis in PFIC includes defects in canalicular transport, tight junction integrity, nuclear signaling, vesicular trafficking, and membrane maintenance, which cause the loss of bile acids and lipid homeostasis [17]. Historically PFIC1, PFIC2, and PFIC3 are the principal subtypes of PFIC, but with the use of NGS, other inherited cholestatic liver diseases have been detected. Both PFIC1 and PFIC2 are caused by impaired bile salt secretion due to defects in ATP8B1 encoding the FIC1 protein and in ABCB11 encoding the bile salt export pump (BSEP) protein, respectively [18]. Patients with PFIC1 present recurrent episodes of jaundice within the first few months of life and develop short stature, deafness, pancreatitis, and persistent diarrhea later. In PFIC2, the disruption of BSEP results in the accumulation of bile acids within the hepatocytes, causing severe cholestasis, potentially progressive to ESLD within the first few years of life. Children with PFIC2 also have an increased risk of developing hepatocellular carcinoma. Defects in ABCB4, encoding the multidrug resistance 3 protein (MDR3), impair biliary phospholipid secretion, resulting in PFIC3. The bile of infants with PFIC3 has insufficient phospholipid concentration, making the micelles unstable and toxic to bile ducts, which ultimately produce intra and lobular cholangiopathy [19]. Over the past years, the PFIC group is expanding with new subtypes. Tight junction protein 2 (TJP2) deficiency has been identified and included [19]. MYO5B deficiency, which impairs the targeting of BSEP to the canalicular membrane, may underlie 20% of previously undiagnosed low gamma-glutamyl transferase (GGT) cholestasis without intestinal involvement [20]. More recently, the homozygous loss of the farnesoid X receptor (FXR) function due to NR1H4 mutations has been described as a new low GGT form of severe PFIC [21]. FXR plays an important role in bile acid homeostasis and is involved in the regulation of other known cholestasis genes. Early-onset vitamin-K-independent coagulopathy and markedly elevated AFP levels may help distinguish FXR deficiency from other forms of PFIC.

The main clinical features of PFIC include cholestasis, jaundice, and pruritus, which can evolve into ESLD and death or to rescuing LT from infancy to adulthood. Diagnosis is made by a genetic test, together with a detailed history, physical examination, laboratory tests (mainly serum bile acids that are high), imaging, or histological evaluations if needed, as well as specific tests to exclude other causes of childhood cholestasis. The medical management of PFIC initially is based on nutritional support to optimize the absorption of fat and fat-soluble vitamins and achieve weight gain in the presence of intestinal malabsorption due to profound cholestasis. Pruritus often requires aggressive treatment with multiple therapies, including ursodeoxycholic acid (UDCA), cholestyramine, rifampin, and opioid antagonists. In medically refractory cases or in the presence of advanced liver disease, treatment may include surgical biliary diversions and LT. A new medical approach, includes the use of inhibitors of the ileal apical sodium-dependent bile acid transporter (ASBTi), which block BA enterohepatic recirculation (IBATi) [4]. Noteworthy, the prognosis and outcome after LT may vary depending on the PFIC subtype. In the scope of cholestasis with normal GGT, the differential diagnosis should always include a high suspicion of PFIC.

6.1.1.3 Alagille Syndrome (ALGS)

ALGS is a multisystem disease that includes chronic cholestasis due to the progressive paucity of interlobular bile ducts. ALGS is an autosomal dominant disease, with gene mutations within the Notch signaling pathway; JAGGED1 (JAG1) accounts for 95% of cases and NOTCH2 for 2–3%. JAG1 is expressed early in the development

Table 6.1 Summary of the typical clinical features and specific gene target of progressive familial intrahepatic cholestasis

Type	Phenotype (cholestasis in all)	GGT	Surgical options	Post-LT	Gene	Protein function
PFIC1	– Diarrhea – Hearing loss – Pancreatitis – BRIC1	Low/normal	– Biliary diversion – LT	– Diarrhea – Metabolic acidosis – Steatosis	ATP8B1	Phosphatidylserine translocates phospholipids across the canalicular membrane
PFIC2	– Early cirrhosis – HCC risk – BRIC2	Low/normal	– Biliary diversion – LT	– Risk of alloimmune BSEP dysfunction	ABCB11	ATP-dependent canalicular BA export pump
PFIC3	– Cholelithiasis – Potential ESLD – Risk of HCC and CCA	High	– LT		ABCB4	Transport of phosphatidylcholine into canaliculi
PFIC4	– Rapid progression – HCC risk – Neurological and respiratory symptoms	Low/high	– LT		TJP2	Regulates passage of molecules between hepatocytes and prevents BA reflux
PFIC5	– Fast evolution to ESLD – Deep coagulopathy – High AFP	Low/normal	– LT	– Possible steatosis	NR1H4 (FXR)	Nuclear BA receptor and the control of BA homeostasis
PFIC6	– Episodic cholestasis – Intestinal involvement in some cases	Low/normal	– LT	– Possible steatosis	MYO5B	Cell polarization and trafficking of BSEP

AFP alpha-fetoprotein, *BA* bile acids, *BSEP* bile salt export pump, *ESLD* end-stage liver disease, *GGT* gamma-glutamyl transferase, *LT* liver transplantation, *PFIC* progressive familial intrahepatic cholestasis of the cardiopulmonary system, biliary system, kidney, and brain [22]. There is great variability in the penetrance of disease even in the same family. Due to the variable clinical presentation of ALGS, it is difficult to know the exact incidence and prevalence. It is estimated that the prevalence of ALGS varies from 1:30,000 to 1:100,000 [2]. Extrahepatic manifestations include vascular, facial, ocular, cardiac, vertebral, and renal anomalies; therefore, a multidisciplinary approach is mandatory for its medical management. ALGS is diagnosed when an individual has three out of seven major clinical features (Table 6.2). Bile duct paucity on liver histology is no longer considered mandatory for the diagnosis; the presence of chronic cholestasis with a genetic test can be used instead. Liver function tests usually show elevated direct bilirubin, serum aminotransferases, GGT, serum bile acids, and cholesterol levels [23]. Severe hypercholesterolemia can lead to the development of xanthomas. Growth failure, delayed puberty, and malnutrition are common in children with ALGS. Children with ALGS, probably because of their genetic defects, have poorer growth than children with other types of CLD. The treatment of liver involvement in ALGS is mainly supportive, trying to ameliorate severe pruritus and xanthomas with agents that reduce cholestasis (UDCA, naltrexone, rifampin, and cholestyramine). Surgical biliary diversion techniques have been used for this purpose, without changing overall disease progression. LT for end-stage liver disease has an 80% 5-year survival rate, improving liver function and catch-up growth [24]. One of the life-threatening complications of ALGS is related to cerebral vascular anomalies, which can lead to strokes, and intracranial or internal carotid artery aneurysms, which can result in catastrophic bleeding [2]. The potential for vascular anomalies is particularly concerning in the setting of LT, and it is recommended that children with ALGS who are being evaluated for transplantation have magnetic resonance imaging with angiogram to screen for intracranial and intra-abdominal vascular anomalies. As for the PFIC group, also in ALGS, new therapies that target the enterohepatic circulation of bile acids have been proposed, targeting the symptom of pruritus [4]. A recent placebo-controlled trial of an IBATi for pruritus in ALGS revealed decreases in caregiver and clinician "itch scores" and serum bile acid concentration in the IBATi group [25].

Table 6.2 Clinical characteristics and diagnostic criteria for ALGS

Organ/system	Presentation
Liver/cholestasis	Neonatal onset of conjugated hyperbilirubinemia, elevated total serum bile acids with or without pale stools
Dysmorphic facies	Broad forehead, deep-set eyes, prominent ears, straight nose with a bulbous tip, and pointed chin (triangular face appearance)
Congenital heart disease	Most frequently peripheral pulmonary artery stenosis but also pulmonary atresia, atrial septal defect, ventricular septal defect, and tetralogy of Fallot
Vertebral anomalies	"Butterfly" vertebrae
Eye	Posterior embryotoxon
Renal	Heterogenic group of renal abnormalities (renal cyst, dysplasia, uteropelvic junction obstruction)
Vascular	Abdominal and cerebral vascular anomalies (Moyamoya syndrome)

6.2 The Frail Child with an Inflammatory Chronic Liver Disease

Chronic inflammatory liver diseases in children, because of the widespread vaccination against the hepatitis B virus and the low rate and recent efficacious treatment of hepatitis C virus (HCV) infection, are mostly represented by autoimmune liver diseases (AILD). AILD belong to a wide spectrum of inflammatory hepatic disorders of unknown etiology, in which liver damage is likely to arise from an autoimmune attack that, if untreated, can evolve into irreversible derangement of the liver architecture and the loss of function.

In pediatric patients, three main types of autoimmune disorders are described based on the main target of inflammatory damage

- Autoimmune hepatitis (AIH), in which hepatocytes represent the principal target involved in liver damage
- Autoimmune sclerosing cholangitis (ASC), in which cholangiocytes and biliary structures are mainly affected
- "AIH/ASC overlap syndromes," in which hepatocytes and cholangiocytes are equally and simultaneously damaged

6.2.1 Autoimmune Hepatitis

AIH is characterized by high serum activity of transaminases, elevated immunoglobulin G levels, and the presence of specific autoantibodies. Depending on the autoantibody pattern, two types of AIH are defined in children: AIH type 1, with seropositivity for smooth muscle antibodies (SMA) and/or antinuclear antibodies (ANA), and AIH type 2, with positivity for anti-liver kidney microsome type 1 antibody (anti-LKM1) and/or anti-liver cytosol type 1 antibody (anti-LC1) [26]. These two types of AIH differ in age at onset, the type of presentation, and the response to treatment withdrawal, as reported in Table 6.3. Moreover, in 10–15% of cases, no antibodies are detected in the blood; even the histological features and response to therapy are identical to those in the classic forms of AIH; these forms are called "seronegative autoimmune hepatitis" [27].

Table 6.3 Clinical characteristics of autoimmune hepatitis

	AIH type I (ANA/ASMA +)	AIH type II (LKM +)
Age of onset	Children to adulthood with two reported peaks, at 10–20 years and 45–65 years	Children, median age 10 years
Gender (F, M)	4:1	9:1
Clinical presentation	Variable	Generally severe
Response to treatment	Generally good	Generally good but high risck of fulminant hepatic failure at onset
Risk of recurrence after treatment withdrawal	High	High
Prognosis	Good	Good

The prevalence of AIH is unknown and probably underestimated. It varies between different geographical areas, but generally, it is about two to three cases per 100,000 pediatric patients, with a higher prevalence in girls. Recent data showed an increase in the prevalence of this disease from 3 to 12% in the last decade in the pediatric population attending a tertiary center.

The etiology of AIH is unknown, even if both genetic and environmental factors are involved in its pathogenesis. In fact, in genetically predisposed individuals, environmental factors, not yet identified, trigger an inappropriate response to certain antigens causing hepatic damage. Susceptibility to AIH is linked to genes in the human leukocyte antigens that are involved in antigen presentation to CD4 T cells [28].

The clinical spectrum of AIH is particularly variable, and sometimes it can be completely asymptomatic, and the diagnosis is made following an incidental finding of raised hepatic aminotransferases and/or the finding of hepato- and/or splenomegaly on routine evaluation (20% of cases). The most frequent possible clinical presentations are the following:

- Acute hepatitis (the most frequent, 70% of cases), characterized by nonspecific symptoms (fatigue, malaise, nausea/vomiting, abdominal pain), followed by more specific signs, such as jaundice, pale stools, and dark urine; in some cases, an evolution to fulminant hepatic failure is reported.
- Insidious onset (10% of cases), with fatigue, weight loss, and relapsing jaundice, lasting several months before diagnosis.
- Complications of undiagnosed cirrhosis with portal hypertension (<1% of cases), such as ascites or gastrointestinal bleeding.

As described in the case of other autoimmune disorders, also AIH, in association with other extrahepatic autoimmune diseases, can occur in nearly 20% of cases.

Table 6.4 Diagnostic criteria for AIH in children

Laboratory findings	Hypertransaminasemia +/− hyper GGT +/− hyper-IgG
Autoantibodies	ANA/ASMA/LKM/LC-1 >1:20
Liver biopsy	Interface hepatitis and other histological features associated with AILD (lymphoplasmacytic infiltrate, rosette formation, etc.)
Exclusion of other chronic liver disorders	Wilson disease, viral hepatitis, metabolic diseases, alpha1-antitrypsin deficiency

Because of the absence of a unique diagnostic biomarker and various clinical and laboratory presentations, the diagnosis of AIH can be insidious. The diagnosis is based on a combination of clinical, laboratory, histological, and imaging findings when other chronic liver diseases are ruled out by appropriate tests (Table 6.4). To support clinicians in the diagnostic workup, the International Autoimmune Hepatitis Group (IAIHG) has proposed a scoring system, which includes the activity of transaminases, IgG levels, liver-specific autoantibodies, other autoimmune disorders, and characteristic histological features, giving a final value indicative of probable or definite AIH. Liver biopsy is useful in the diagnostic workup of AIH, and it should be done if clotting tests are normal. The typical histological finding is *interface hepatitis*, characterized by a dense mononuclear and plasma cell infiltration of the portal area, damaging the limiting plate. Hepatic regeneration with *rosette* formation may also be present [29, 30].

The cornerstone of AIH treatment is immunosuppression, which is effective in approximately 90% of cases. The "conventional" schedule of treatment consists of prednisone at the dose of 1–2 mg/kg/die (maximum 60 mg/die), which is progressively reduced on the basis of biochemical response to the lowest dose compatible with biochemical remission, associated with azathioprine as a steroid-sparring agent. Azathioprine may be used at diagnosis or added after a few weeks at a starting dose of 0.5–1 mg/kg/die and is increased up to 2.0–2.5 mg/kg/day [31].

Usually, in the first 6 months of treatment, 75–90% of patients normalize their liver function tests, inducing a phase of remission of liver disease. Unfortunately, in a subgroup of patients (about 10%), standard immunosuppression is unable to induce and maintain stable remission or is not well tolerated long term because of its side effects. In these patients, other immunosuppressive agents are needed, aiming to prevent progression to ESLD.

The most frequent side effects of steroid therapy are represented by cushingoid features, with weight gain, *facies lunaris*, dorsal hump, cutaneous *striae*, acne, and hirsutism, which often lead to poor compliance, particularly in adolescent girls. Severe but less frequent adverse effects are osteopenia with the risk of vertebral collapse, diabetes, cataracts, and hypertension, which usually occur after prolonged therapy at a high dosage. The main alternative treatments are based on the use of cyclosporine (Cys A) and mycophenolate mofetil (MMF) [32]. Several studies reported the efficacy and safety of Cys A as a first-line option to induce remission in selected subsets of patients in which side effects due to conventional schedule are to be avoided or in patients with frequent relapses during standard therapy. MFM is another second-line option for AIH patients who are nonresponders or intolerant to conventional treatment with azathioprine. In difficult-to-treat patients, who are resistant or intolerant to conventional treatments, the use of the most powerful calcineurin inhibitors, such as tacrolimus, should be considered. LT may become necessary in 5–10% of patients with AILD, or in case severe acute onset forms unresponsive to rescue therapies or in cases with poor control evolving to cirrhosis and end-stage liver disease. AIH recurs frequently after LT in approximately 20–40% of cases.

6.2.2 Autoimmune Sclerosing Cholangitis (ASC)

ASC is characterized by a chronic inflammatory liver damage involving intra and extrahepatic bile ducts associated with autoimmune features. The diagnosis is based on biliary imaging demonstrating typical large and medium size bile ducts alteration such as stricture, dilatation, and irregularity of bile duct profile and by liver biopsy revealing pathognomonic features of inflammatory cholangiopathy, as fibrous obliterative cholangitis of small bile ducts. As previously stated, ASC may demonstrate features akin to AIH, with the simultaneous autoimmune aggression of hepatocytes and cholangiocytes. This condition, called "overlap syndrome," is today referred to as ASC. Moreover, a possible evolution from AIH to ASC in the same patient exists, confirming that these entities are part of the same pathogenetic process [32].

ASC frequently occurs in association with other immune-mediated disorders and, in particular, with chronic inflammatory bowel diseases. In fact, several studies have demonstrated that the progression of biliary disease may be linked to persistent inflammatory bowel damage. Children with ASC are treated with the same schedule used in AIH patients, to which is added UDCA at the dose of 15–20 mg/kg/die. The prognosis of ASC is worse than AIH because disease progression to irreversible liver damage requiring LT is described in 50% of cases despite adequate treatment. ASC also may recur in liver grafts.

6.2.3 Giant Cell Hepatitis Associated with Autoimmune Hemolytic Anemia (GCH-AHA)

GCH-AHA is a rare form of AILD typical of infancy, characterized by a severe course and poor response to conventional immunosuppressive therapies. GCH-AHA presents generally in the first year of life, with autoimmune hemolytic anemia associated with acute liver injury histologically defined by widespread giant cell transformation. This liver disease has a less favorable response to immunosuppressive treatment compared to classical AILDs and shows high mortality despite and recurrence after liver transplant [33].

6.3 The Frail Infant/Child with a Metabolic Liver Disease (MLD)

Inborn metabolic disorders comprise a wide group of diseases caused by enzyme defects affecting amino acids, carbohydrates, metal and lipid metabolism, as well as mitochondrial defects [34, 35]. The newborn screening allows identifying a wide number of these inherited metabolic disorders, and it is a useful tool to reduce morbidity and mortality rates.

MLD represents about 10–15% of acute liver failure in infants and children and approximately 10% of pediatric liver transplants. In some centers, MLD is the second most common indication of pediatric LT after BA [36]. This percentage increases from 30 to 50% for children under the age of 3 years. The precocity of the diagnosis influences the prognosis of these children as it allows the timely undertaking of specific therapies aimed to avoid irreversible damage in treatable diseases. For these reasons, the diagnostic approach to children with MLD requires an accurate clinical and anamnestic evaluation as well as specific biochemical investigations (Table 6.5).

Table 6.5 First- and second-line investigations in evaluating a patient with a liver disease

First-line investigations
Alanine and aspartate aminotransferases (transaminases)
Alkaline phosphatase, lactate dehydrogenase, cholinesterase
Gamma-glutamyl transpeptidase, bilirubin, conjugated and unconjugated
Serum bile acids, alfa-fetoprotein
Coagulation studies: PT, PTT, factors V, VII, and XI
Glycemia, albumin, prealbumin
Urea, creatinine, uric acid, CK
Ammonia
Hepatitis A, B, C; cytomegalovirus; EBV; herpes simplex; toxoplasmosis; HIV
Bacterial cultures of blood and urine
Second-line investigations in suspected metabolic liver disease
Plasma/serum
Copper, ceruloplasmin
Serum iron and ferritin, transferrin, and transferrin saturation
Galactose-1-phosphate uridyltransferase (galactosemia)
Lactate, pyruvate, 3-hydroxybutyrate, acetoacetate
Free fatty acids, very-long-chain fatty acids (peroxisomal disorders)
Amino acids, transferrin isoelectric focusing (CDG syndromes)
Free and total carnitine, acylcarnitine profile
A1-antitrypsin activity and PI phenotyping

(continued)

Table 6.5 (continued)

Second-line investigations in suspected metabolic liver disease
Lysosomal enzymes
Urine
Amino acids, ketones
Reducing substances/sugars (galactosemia, fructose intolerance)
Individual bile acids (bile acid synthesis defects)
Organic acids (incl. specific assays for orotic acid and succinylacetone)
Copper in 24 h urine

PT prothrombin time, *PTT* partial thromboplastin time, *EBV* Epstein-Barr virus, *HIV* human immunodeficiency virus

6.3.1 Inborn Errors in Protein Metabolism

6.3.1.1 Urea Cycle Defects (UCDs)

UCDs are rare inherited defects in the urea cycle enzymes, leading to a reduced ability to convert ammonia to urea in the liver [37]. They are caused by a deficiency of one of the six enzymes of the urea cycle: three mitochondria—*N*-acetyl glutamate synthase, carbamoyl phosphate synthase 1, and ornithine transcarbamylase (OTC)—and three cytoplasmic—arginine succinate synthase, arginine succinate lyase, and arginase 1. These metabolic pathways are located mainly or exclusively in the liver. All these deficiencies are inherited in an autosomal recessive (AR) manner, except for OTC deficiency, which is inherited in an X-linked recessive way.

The excess in circulating ammonia leads to central nervous system toxicity and irreversible neurologic damage. Clinical findings depend on the deficient enzyme and the gene mutation leading to its inactivation, but, anyway, all these defects may lead to death in the first years of life if not promptly recognized. Medical management is complex, and it includes ammonia scavengers, such as sodium phenylbutyrate, and a diet restrictive of protein combined with essential amino acid supplementation. However, these patients remain at risk for metabolic decompensation. Severe hyperammonemia may require dialysis to reduce ammonia levels. Because of the poor outcome of these inherited urea cycle enzymes defects, LT is indicated in patients with a recurrent or poorly controlled disease to avoid long-term exposure to high ammonia levels and the development of disabilities. LT provides a replacement for the deficient enzyme, and plasma ammonia levels normalize within 24 h from transplantation [38]. For the best neurological outcomes, early diagnosis and aggressive management are essential.

6.3.1.2 Hereditary Tyrosinemia Type 1 (HT-1)

HT-1 is a rare AR disorder with an incidence of 1:100,000–1:120,000 and is characterized by deficient activity of fumaryl acetoacetate hydrolase, the last enzyme in the tyrosine catabolic pathway, which results in the accumulation of toxic metabolites, such as fumaryl acetoacetate and maleylacetoacetate, which are alkylating agents that cause damage to the deoxyribonucleic acid (DNA), resulting in a predisposition to hepatocellular carcinoma (HCC) [39]. One of these metabolites is succinyl acetone, which serves as the diagnostic marker for HT-1. The clinical spectrum of the disease is wide: the acute form is characterized by an early and severe acute liver failure, while the chronic form appears later with growth failure, neurologic crisis, renal tubular acidosis, cirrhosis, and HCC. Until 1992, the only treatment for this disease was LT; since then, NTBC/nitisinone (2-(2-nitro-4-trifluoromethylbenzol)-1,3-cyclohexendiome) has been successfully used in combination with diets low in phenylalanine and tyrosine, but patients remain at risk of developing HCC. LT is indicated in case of HCC, decompensated cirrhosis or patients without compliance to medical therapy and acute liver failure (ALF). The long-term outcome of these patients is excellent (85–100%), but there is a minimal risk of recurrence of HCC in the transplanted liver so that strict surveillance is required [40].

6.3.1.3 Maple Syrup Urine Disease (MSUD)

MSUD is an AR disorder of branched-chain amino acids (BCAA) due to the impaired activity of the branched-chain acid dehydrogenase complex (BCKD). If left untreated, MSUD can result in mental illness and even death. The clinical phenotype is dependent on the degree of residual enzyme activity.

Classical MSUD, seen in infants with less than 2% of BCKD activity, causes an increase in BCAA from birth. By age 2 days, if untreated, infants develop irritability, lethargy, and dystonia. Of note is the absence of significant hyperammonemia. Infants may develop lethargy, apnea crisis, seizures, and cerebral edema. Emergency treatment includes the removal of neurotoxins through dialysis. The initiation of treatment before 72 h of age greatly reduces morbidity and mortality. Long-term management includes the aggressive management of episodic metabolic decompensation and dietary restriction in BCAA.

Long-term dietary management can be difficult and does not prevent metabolic decompensation in the case of intercurrent illness. Although BCKD is expressed in many tissues, LT prevents metabolic decompensation and allows for dietary freedom [41]. Because BCKD is also expressed in other tissues, the liver removed from patients with MSUD, in the case of LT, may be considered for use as domino grafts [42]. Following LT, the level of toxic amino acids normalizes and remains stable during intercurrent illnesses. In addition, the complications of MSUD, including cognitive, behavioral, and motor impairments, slowly improve.

6.3.1.4 Methylmalonic and Propionic Acidemias

Methylmalonic acidemia (MMA) and propionic acidemia (PA) are the two commonest organic acidemias, rare disorders of BCAA metabolism [43]. PA is caused by a deficiency in propionyl-CoA carboxylase, a downstream enzyme in the catabolism of isoleucine, valine, methionine, threonine, and odd-chain fatty acids, which converts propionyl CoA in methylmalonyl CoA. MMA is caused by a defect in methylmalonyl CoA mutase or its coenzyme adenosylcobalamin, both resulting in the defective conversion of methyl malonyl CoA in succinyl CoA. Metabolic control is difficult, and many patients develop multiple decompensations, progressive neurological deterioration, and cardiac and renal complications. Acute management is aimed to remove toxic intermediates from the body, through a combination of dialysis and medical therapy based on supplementation with L-carnitine and vitamin B12. The aim of nutritional support is to reduce kidney, heart, and brain damage and to achieve a normal developmental status. More recently, LT has become a possible alternative therapy to conventional dietary management for MMA and PA patients. LT improve overall survival of patients who benefit of an improved quality of life because of unrestricted diet and drastic decrease hospitalization time recovering from decompensation [44]. Normal growth and acceptable psychomotor and neurological development may be achieved by LT.

6.3.2 Inborn Errors in Carbohydrate Metabolism

6.3.2.1 Hereditary Fructose Intolerance (HFI)

HFI is an AR disorder caused by aldolase B deficiency, which blocks the metabolism of fructose-1-phosphate into di-hydroxy acetone phosphate and D-glyceraldehyde [45]. The accumulation of fructose-1-phosphate can cause hypoglycemia due to the inhibition of glycogen phosphorylase and the inability to condense glyceraldehyde-3-phosphate and di-hydroxy acetone phosphate. In addition, amounts in excess of fructose-1-phosphate lead to adenosine triphosphate (ATP) depletion, which is thought to lead to impaired protein synthesis and, ultimately, liver and renal dysfunction.

Patients with HFI are asymptomatic until fructose, sucrose, or sorbitol is introduced into the diet in the form of fruits or vegetables. Presentation can include hypoglycemia with lactic acidosis and ketosis, nausea, vomiting, abdominal pain, and lethargy. HFI is one of the causes of infantile ALF, but it can also lead to cirrhosis in early childhood. Patients who remain undiagnosed may experience failure to thrive, chronic liver damage, and renal tubular dysfunction [46]. Generally, these patients develop aversion to sweet food and instinctively self-impose a fructose-free diet.

6.3.2.2 Galactosemia

Classical galactosemia is caused by a deficiency in the galactose-1-phosphate uridylyltransferase (GALT) gene. The most common mutation is Q188R, which occurs in 70% of patients [47]. The incidence is 1 in 45,000 live births. GALT-1 blocks the metabolism of galactose-1-phosphate to uridine diphosphate (UDP) galactose. The buildup of galactose-1-phosphate further disrupts glucose metabolism and leads to lethargy, hypotonia, vomiting, and diarrhea within hours of milk ingestion. Continued galactose ingestion leads to severe liver damage with jaundice, hemolysis, lactic acidosis, and renal tubular acidosis. Failure to thrive, hepatomegaly, splenomegaly, cirrhosis, and cataracts characterize the more chronic course. Despite aggressive management, long-term complications occur frequently and can include mental retardation and ovarian dysfunction in females. LT is rarely indicated and is performed only in progressive liver dysfunction despite a galactose-free diet.

6.3.3 Inborn Errors of Lipid Metabolism

6.3.3.1 Familial Hypercholesterolemia (FH)

FH is an autosomal dominant inherited disorder characterized by markedly elevated plasma concentration of low-density lipoprotein (LDL) cholesterol and tendon and skin xanthomas associated with a high risk of cardiovascular complications [48]. Life-long treatment includes dietary fat restriction, statins, and recurrent apheresis to reduce plasma LDL cholesterol. Currently, the only effective treatment for this disease is LT, which alone or in association with medications normalizes the plasma cholesterol level [49].

6.3.3.2 Lysosomal Acid Lipase (LAL)

LAL deficiency, previously referred to as cholesteryl ester storage disorder, is a lysosomal storage disorder characterized by the accumulation of cholesteryl esters [50]. It has a heterogeneous clinical phenotype, and end-stage liver disease may occur. LT may be necessary for LAL-D-associated liver failure but is not sufficient to prevent disease progression or liver disease recurrence. Enzyme replacement therapy addresses systemic disease and potentially improves LT outcomes.

6.3.4 Inborn Errors in Metals Metabolism

6.3.4.1 Wilson Disease (WD)

WD is an AR disorder causing ALF, acute-on-chronic liver failure, or cirrhosis in children, with an average prevalence of 1 in 30,000 individuals worldwide [51]. A genetic defect in ATP7B leads to defective excretion of copper from the liver, leading to its toxic accumulation in liver and various extrahepatic tissues, such as brain, kidney, and joint. Wilson's disease may present symptomatically at any age, although the majority presents between ages 5 and 35. Clinical presentation can vary widely; therefore, diagnosis is not always straightforward. The key features of Wilson disease are liver disease and cirrhosis, neuropsychiatric disturbances, Kayser–Fleischer ring, and acute episodes of hemolysis, often in association with ALF.

WD is one of the few metabolic liver disorders where a definitive medical therapy in the form of chelation can be offered. Medical therapy with *d*-penicillamine or trientine is effective for most patients, and patients with even advanced liver disease due to WD can reverse hepatic fibrosis with medical treatment. LT can rescue those with ALF or those with advanced liver disease who fail to respond to or discontinue medical therapy [52]. Treatment monitoring must be done at regular intervals and includes clinical evaluation, liver tests and blood counts, and copper metabolic parameters.

6.4 The Frail Children with Fatty Liver Disease

Nonalcoholic fatty liver disease (NAFLD) is the most common cause of chronic liver disease in children and adolescents. The exact prevalence of pediatric NAFLD is unknown, but available data describe a prevalence ranging from 3 to 12% in the general pediatric population, with a peak of 70% in obese children. In Western countries, the prevalence of NAFLD in children is estimated to be around 20–46%, while in Asian children, the prevalence is lower (5–18%) [53]. These ethnic differences may be related to genetic, environmental, or sociocultural factors as well as differences in body composition, insulin sensitivity, and the adipocytokine profile.

NAFLD is characterized by the accumulation of fat in the hepatocytes (at least 5%) in the absence of other causes of liver steatosis, such as Wilson's disease, deficiency in alfa-1-antitrypsin, celiac disease, HCV infection, metabolic disorders, and alcohol or drug consumption. Simple hepatic steatosis is usually a benign condition, but in some cases, it progresses to more advanced forms of liver injury, characterized by the presence of inflammation [nonalcoholic steatohepatitis (NASH)] and various degrees of fibrosis up to cirrhosis, predisposing to liver failure and/or hepatocellular carcinoma (HCC) [54]. Several studies identified insulin resistance, with or without obesity, as the underlying mechanism associated with NAFLD and identified NAFLD as the hepatic expression of a metabolic syndrome. In fact, a proposal has been recently made to change the term NAFLD to MAFLD (metabolic-associated fatty liver disease), assigning the disease a name linked to its pathogenesis. However, the new nomenclature, especially in the pediatric field, is not yet accepted by scientific societies [55].

6.4.1 Pathophysiology

In the last two decades, several advances have been made in the knowledge of the pathogenesis of NAFLD. The "two-hit" hypothesis has been exceeded by the "multi-hit" theory, in which several factors have been identified as contemporary actors in the onset and progression of liver injury. In this theory, the starting point is represented by hepatic steatosis, which can be the result of several possible factors, such as dietary habits, environmental and genetic factors, insulin resistance, obesity with adipocyte proliferation, and changes in the composition of intestinal microbiota. Adipose tissue is a metabolically active endocrine organ that causes the release of proinflammatory cytokines, such as TNF-α and IL-6, whereas beneficial adipokines are suppressed. This situation leads to the development of peripheral insulin resistance and hyperinsulinemia and increased fatty acid delivery to the hepatocyte. The disruption of normal insulin signaling in the hepatocyte and an increased abundance of fatty acids lead to disordered lipid metabolism, characterized by the overactivation of de novo lipogenesis (DNL) transcriptional factors, causing more fatty acid and glucose products to be shunted into these lipogenic pathways [56]. The role of intestinal microbiota has been recently considered within this metabolic dysregulation. An "obesogenic" diet (rich in fats and lipids) increases intestinal bacteria products (i.e., endotoxins, proteins, metabolites, lipopolysaccharides (LPS) with the subsequent activation of the Toll-like receptor (TLR) pathway, acting as a promoter of inflammation and the progression of hepatic steatosis to NASH and fibrosis. Moreover, in other pediatric studies, it was shown that intestinal bacterial permeability is modulated by the intestinal farnesoid X receptor (FXR), which regulates the transcription of genes involved in the synthesis and transport of bile acids, lipogenesis, and glucose homeostasis, directly or indirectly, through the release of fibroblast growth factor-19 (FGF19) [57]. Another role of single nucleotide polymorphisms (SNPs) in genes involved in lipid metabolism [lipin 1 (LPIN1), patatin-like phospholipase domain-containing 3 (PNPLA3)], oxidative stress [superoxide dismutase 2 (SOD2)], insulin signaling [insulin receptor substrate-1 (IRS-1)], and fibrogenesis [Kruppel-like factor 6 (KLF6)] has been associated with the severity of liver damage in NAFLD patients. Moreover, a very interesting interaction has recently been reported between genetic risk factors (PNPLA3 I148M) and the severity of steatosis and fibrosis [58]. PNPLA3, also known as adiponutrin, is a member of the patatin-like phospholipase family. The rs738409 C>G single-nucleotide polymorphism (SNP), encoding the Ile 148Met variant protein of PNPLA3, is described as a genetic determinant of hepatic steatosis. Several studies have established a strong link between PNPLA3 and the development of NAFLD. NASH was more frequently observed in GG than in CC homozygous; the rs738409-GG genotype, versus the CC genotype, was associated with a 3.24-fold greater risk of higher necroinflammatory scores and a 3.2-fold greater risk of developing fibrosis [59].

6.4.1.1 Diagnosis

Since NAFLD is the most common cause of chronic liver damage in children, it is essential to identify it as soon as possible in order to intervene promptly, changing the natural evolution of the disease and preventing complications. The main problem in the diagnostic approach to NAFLD is represented by the poverty of suggestive clinical signs. In fact, the diagnosis of NAFLD is often made following an occasional finding of the elevation of liver enzymes, in particular aminotransferases. In the literature, there is a lack of consensus as to what screening tool is more effective for identifying the pathology in subjects at risk. The European Society of Pediatric Gastroenterology Hepatology and Nutrition (ESPGHAN) suggests both measuring the serum ALT concentration and using liver ultrasound (US) as screening methods; the North American Society of Pediatric Gastroenterology Hepatology and Nutrition (NASPGHAN) recommends using ALT and not US, while the National Institute for Health Care (NICE) suggests using US and not ALT. Screening should be initiated between 9 and 11 years of age in obese or overweight children with a cardio-metabolic risk factor and repeated every 2–3 years if the risk factors remain unchanged [54]. The differential diagnosis of these conditions must consider the patient's anamnestic and clinical characteristics, as well as the outcome of laboratory tests, imaging studies, and liver biopsy.

6.4.1.2 Ultrasonography (US)

Because of its availability, security, and relatively low cost, US is the most common imaging technique used to diagnose NAFLD. Hepatic steatosis is characterized by an imaging of liver echotexture more reflective (hyperechoic) when compared to that of the right kidney (bright liver), moreover the liver may appear increased in size. However, US may be unreliable in evaluating severely obese patients or when liver fatty liver infiltration is <30% [60].

6.4.1.3 Elastography

The term elastography refers to a series of imaging techniques that allow the estimation of liver tissue rigidity by measuring the propagation of specific elastic waves (shear waves, S-waves) emitted by the probe. Elastography imaging can be US based (e.g., Fibroscan®) or magnetic resonance based [e.g., magnetic resonance elastography (MRE)]. These methods have proven effective in distinguishing NAFLD from NASH and in highlighting the presence and severity of fibrotic infiltration in the liver, especially in studies conducted in the adult population. The absence of certain cutoff values and the relatively poor diffusion of the equipment currently limit their use [61].

6.4.1.4 Magnetic Resonance (MRI)

Magnetic resonance imaging (MRI) is considered the most accurate imaging technique to assess liver fat storage in NAFLD patients because it can differentiate tissues containing only water from those containing both fat and water. MR spectroscopy (MRS) is a novel variant of the classical MRI, which quantifies triglyceride accumulation within hepatocytes through the measurement of acyl groups within the selected liver region of interest. MRS can discriminate healthy patients from those with NAFLD with a sensitivity of 92.6% and a specificity of 95.7%. In younger children, the correct execution of MR requires the sedation of the patient. This element, associated with a relatively high cost and the need for specific expertise for MRS, limits the application of MRI in everyday clinical practice.

6.4.1.5 Liver Biopsy

Liver biopsy (LB) is considered the gold standard for NAFLD diagnosis and the only method that

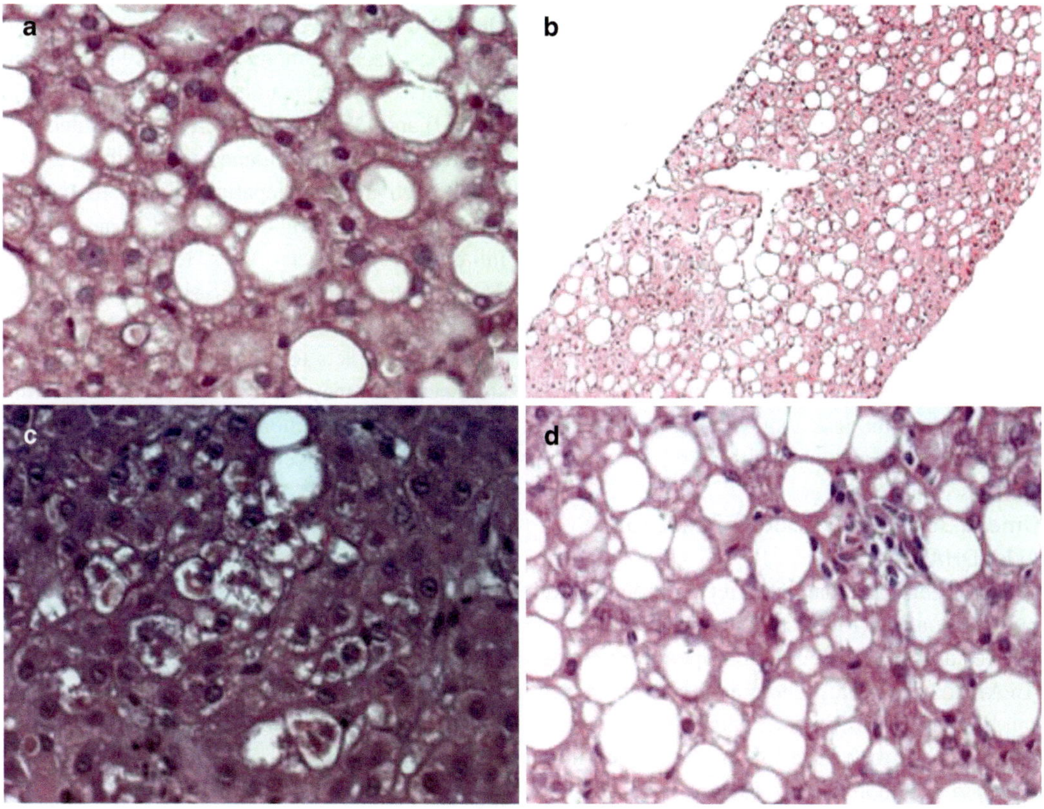

Fig. 6.3 Histological features of pediatric NAFLD/NASH. Steatosis is evident in (**a**) [40 × magnification, EE (eosin hematoxylin)] and (**b**) (10 × EE); ballooning and lipogranulomas are present in (**c**) and (**d**), respectively, (40 × EE)

can distinguish NAFLD from NASH and provide a reliable scoring system designed to estimate the severity of the disease (Fig. 6.3). Also, it may help in the differential diagnosis workup and in detecting coexisting liver diseases. In 2015, ESPGHAN defined indications for LB in NAFLD pediatric patients: it is important to highlight that LB should not be considered a screening method [62]. LB is burdened with some limitations: it is an invasive technique with minor and major complication risks. Pain and bleeding are the most common complications (84% and 2.8%, respectively). Other reported complications are infections, visceral perforation, arteriovenous fistula, pneumothorax, hemothorax, and death (0.6%). Due to such limitations and the invasiveness of LB, in recent years, new research strands have been developed to identify safe and equally effective methods for diagnosing and staging NAFLD, but to date, biopsy remains the "imperfect reference standard." In recent years, three principal scoring systems have been used in clinical and research activities: the Brunt system, the Pediatric NAFLD Histological Score (PNHS), and the NASH Clinical Research Network (CRN) system, which is validated as a histological score. The NAFLD Activity Score (NAS) is based on the evaluation of three parameters, each of which is assigned a score: steatosis, 0–3; lobular inflammation, 0–3; and ballooning, 0–2; NAS results from the unweighted sum of these parameters, for a total score ranging from 0 to 8. A NAS $\geq$5 is suggestive of NASH, while a NAS $\leq$3 excludes NASH [63].

6.4.1.6 Therapy

Diet and Physical Activity

Dietary improvements and increasing physical activity, which are intended as lifestyle modifications, are currently the primary treatment for pediatric NAFLD due to its strong association with overweight and obesity [64]. The NASPGHAN recommendations indicate that a healthier diet with avoidance of sugar-sweetened beverages, an increase from moderate- to high-intensity physical activity, and limiting screen activities to <2 h per day are the main cornerstone for both preventing and treating pediatric NAFLD. More deeply, the authors specify that small weight reduction (3–5% weight loss) can reduce hepatic steatosis, but a greater degree of weight loss (not less than 7%) is required to improve hepatic steatohepatitis.

Omega-3 Fatty Acids-Docosahexaenoic Acid (DHA)

Omega-3 fatty acids are a variety of polyunsaturated fatty acids (PUFAs). The most studied ω-3 fatty acids in humans are eicosapentaenoic acid (EPA) and docosahexaenoic acid (DHA), which can be found in fish, algae, and fish oil. Ω-3 are modulators of the transcription of genes regulating lipid metabolism and they provide an anti-inflammatory and insulin-sensitizing systemic activity. DHA shows anti-inflammatory effects being activated through GPR120 (G-protein-coupled receptor) and PPAR-γ. Both these receptors control inflammatory signaling. The activation of DHA has many effects: (1) it inhibits macrophage and lymphocyte T proliferation (decreasing the production of IL-2); (2) it reduces NFκB activation in response to endotoxins probably acting on MyD88; and (3) via PPAR-γ (together with the inactivation of NFκB), it reduces the production of inflammatory cytokines TNF, IL-6, and IL-1β. In a randomized controlled trial (RCT) by Nobili et al. NAFLD children on an 18-month regimen of daily DHA had histologically proven improvement in hepatic steatosis, ballooning, inflammation, NAS (NAFLD Activity Score), and PNHS (Pediatric NAFLD Histological Score) and showed a reduction in ductular reaction and hepatic stem/progenitor cells (HSCs) as well as the amelioration of laboratory biomarkers such as transaminase, insulin, and HOMA-IR. However, no effect on fibrosis was noted [65].

DHA and Vitamin D

In the past decades, many studies have pointed out the utility of a therapeutic approach with vitamin D (VD) and DHA. It has been demonstrated that VD receptor (VDR) ligands inhibit the TGFβ1/SMAD activation of hepatic stellate cells (HSCs) and that DHA binding to the GPR120 has an anti-inflammatory effect. After the activation of TGFβ1, the translocation of SMAD in the nucleus activates HSCs in response to a hepatic injury. This pathway acts to regulate hepatic fibrogenesis. There are many pieces of evidence suggesting that VD has a beneficial effect on fibrogenesis, improving fibrosis score, especially in children, even though it does not affect the lipid profile, insulin resistance markers, and inflammation. A recent RCT tested the combination of DHA/VD in improving the whole spectrum of NAFLD, showing that the association of DHA/VD caused an improvement in insulin resistance, the reduction of serum triglyceride concentration, and a reduction in ALT serum activity. Amelioration of the fibrosis score and reduction of the activation of hepatic stellate cells were also noted [66].

Probiotics

The role of intestinal microbiota in the pathogenesis of NAFLD has been widely discussed. Various are the mechanisms explaining the interaction between microbiota and NAFLD:

- Increased extraction of energy from the diet due to the ability of the microbiota to digest complex polysaccharides, resulting in the formation of short-chain fatty acids (SCFA)
- Intestinal epithelial damage due to the bacterial production of hepatotoxic products
- Translocation of bacterial endotoxins into the portal circulation, and the consequent hepatic damage through signaling and the activation of TLR
- Altered metabolism of choline with a consequent decrease of the liver exports of very-low-density lipoprotein (VLDL) and altered modulation of bile acid synthesis

It was recently shown that in obese children with NAFLD, bifidobacteria have a protective role against the development of NAFLD. In fact, *Bifidobacterium* spp. was prevalent in the control group, while *Lactobacillus* spp. was increased in NAFLD, NASH, and obese children. To date, two RCTs were conducted in children: one to evaluate the influence of a single strain (*Lactobacillus rhamnosus* GG) and another to evaluate the mixture of eight probiotics (VSL#3) on hepatic biomarkers. The *Lactobacillus rhamnosus* GG study did not report any effect on liver echogenicity, but it achieved a significant decrease in ALT in treated children compared to placebo. In contrast, the second RCT found that VSL#3 supplementation reduced, on ultrasound evaluation, the severity of steatosis [67].

6.4.1.7 Novel Treatments

The increase in the prevalence of NAFLD, associated with the absence of effective pharmacological treatments, has led to the study of new molecules to counteract NAFLD.

The farnesoid X receptor (FXR) is a nuclear receptor, expressed primarily in the liver and intestine, which binds to bile acids. When activated, FXR migrates into the cell nucleus and modulates the transcription of specific genes involved in the regulation of inflammation and glucose and lipid metabolism. Numerous studies, mostly based on animal models, have shown that the use of FXR agonists (e.g., obeticholic acid) could improve hepatic steatosis and steatohepatitis.

Liraglutide is an analog of glucagon-like peptide 1 (GLP-1), a gut-derived incretin hormone that induces weight loss and insulin sensitivity. In 2016, the Lifestyle, Exercise and Nutrition (LEAN) Study, conducted on 52 adult patients with NASH, showed that liraglutide led to a histological resolution of steatohepatitis.

In conclusion, the actual ideal pharmacological approach for NAFLD treatment is represented by a "combination therapy," by a mix of available agents (antioxidants, probiotics, anti-inflammatory molecules), aiming to block and revert liver damage in the treated patients. The ideal treatment should be given in a patient-tailored manner based on the evaluation of each patient and taking into account the different histological features of NAFLD (ballooning, steatosis, inflammation, fibrosis) and the main metabolic alterations in order to combine different therapeutic effects for the achievement of the best result.

References

1. Grimaldi C, Spada M, Maggiore G. Liver transplantation in children: an overview on organ allocation and surgical management. Curr Pediatr Rev. 2021;17(4):245–52. https://doi.org/10.2174/1573396317666210604111538.
2. Lane E, Murray KF. Neonatal cholestasis. Pediatr Clin N Am. 2017;64:621–39.
3. Fawaz R, Baumann U, Ekong U, et al. Guideline for the evaluation of cholestatic jaundice in infants: joint recommendations of the North American Society for Pediatric Gastroenterology, Hepatology, and Nutrition and the European Society for Pediatric Gastroenterology, Hepatology, and Nutrition. J Pediatr Gastroenterol Nutr. 2017;64:154–68.
4. Ranucci G, Della Corte C, Alberti D, et al. Diagnostic approach to neonatal and infantile cholestasis: a position paper by the SIGENP liver disease working group. Dig Liv Dis. 2021;54(1):40–53.
5. Feldman AG, Sokol RJ. Recent developments in diagnostics and treatment of neonatal cholestasis. Semin Pediatr Surg. 2020;29:150945.
6. Chardot C. Biliary atresia. Orphanet J Rare Dis. 2006;26:1–28.
7. Shneider BL, Brown MB, Haber B, Biliary Atresia Research Consortium, et al. A multicenter study of the outcome of biliary atresia in the United States 1997 to 2000. J Pediatr. 2006;148:467–74.
8. Hartley JL, Davenport M, Kelly DA. Biliary atresia. Lancet. 2009;374:1704–13.
9. Petersen C, Davenport M. Aetiology of biliary atresia what is actually known? Orphanet J Rare Dis. 2013;8:128.
10. Asai A, Miethke A, Bezerra JA. Pathogenesis of biliary atresia: defining biology to understand clinical phenotypes. Nat Rev Gastroenterol Hepatol. 2015;12:342–52.
11. Serinet MO, Wildhaber BE, Broué P, et al. Impact of age at Kasai operation on its results in late childhood and adolescence: a rational basis for biliary atresia screening. Pediatrics. 2009;123:1280–6.
12. Hsiao CH, Chang MH, Chen HL, et al. Universal screening for biliary atresia using an infant stool color card in Taiwan. Hepatology. 2008;47:1233–40.
13. Meyers R, Book LS, O'Gorman MA, et al. High-dose steroids, ursodeoxycholic acid, and chronic intravenous antibiotics improve bile flow after Kasai procedure in infants with biliary atresia. J Pediatr Surg. 2003;38:406–11.
14. Decharun K, Leys CM, West KW, et al. Prophylactic antibiotics for prevention of cholangitis in patients

with biliary atresia status post-Kasai portoenterostomy: a systematic review. Clin Pediatr (Phila). 2016;55:66–72.
15. Davenport M, Stringer MD, Tizzard SA, et al. Randomized, double-blind, placebo-controlled trial of corticosteroids after Kasai portoenterostomy for biliary atresia. Hepatology. 2007;46:1821–7.
16. Bezerra JA, Spino C, Magee JC, Childhood Liver Disease Research and Education Network (ChiLDREN), et al. Use of corticosteroids after hepatoportoenterostomy for bile drainage in infants with biliary atresia: the START randomized clinical trial. JAMA. 2014;311:1750–9.
17. Bull LN, Thompson RJ. Progressive familial intrahepatic cholestasis. Clin Liver Dis. 2018;22:657–69.
18. Jacquemin E. Progressive familial intrahepatic cholestasis. Clin Res Hepatol Gastroenterol. 2012;36(Suppl 1):S26–35.
19. Vitale G, Gitto S, Raimondi F, Mattiaccio A, et al. Cryptogenic cholestasis in young and adults: ATP8B1, ABCB11, ABCB4, and TJP2 gene variants analysis by high-throughput sequencing. J Gastroenterol. 2018;53:945–58.
20. Gonzales E, Taylor SA, Davit-Spraul A, et al. MYO5B mutations cause cholestasis with normal serum gamma-glutamyl transferase activity in children without microvillous inclusion disease. Hepatology. 2017;65:164–73.
21. Gomez-Ospina N, Potter CJ, Xiao R, et al. Mutations in the nuclear bile acid receptor FXR cause progressive familial intrahepatic cholestasis. Nat Commun. 2016;7:10713.
22. Warthen DM, Moore ED, Kamath BM, et al. Jagged1 (JAG1) mutations in Alagille syndrome: increasing the mutation detection rate. Hum Mutat. 2006;27:436–43.
23. Kamath BM, Baker A, Houwen R, et al. Systematic review: the epidemiology, natural history, and burden of Alagille syndrome. J Pediatr Gastroenterol Nutr. 2018;67:148–56.
24. Fujishiro J, Suzuki K, Watanabe M, et al. Outcomes of Alagille syndrome following the Kasai operation: a systematic review and meta-analysis. Pediatr Surg Int. 2018;34:1073–7.
25. Shneider BL, et al. Placebo-controlled randomized trial of an intestinal bile salt transport inhibitor for pruritus in Alagille syndrome. Hepatol Commun. 2018;2:1184–98.
26. Liberal R, Vergani D, Mieli-Vergani D. Pediatric autoimmune liver disease. Dig Dis. 2015;33S2:36–46.
27. Maggiore G, Socie G, Sciveres M, et al. Seronegative autoimmune hepatitis in children: spectrum of disorders. Dig Liver Dis. 2016;48:785–91.
28. Longhi MS, Ma Y, Mieli-Vergani G, Vergani D. Aetiopathogenesis of autoimmune hepatitis. J Autoimmun. 2010;34:7–14.
29. Mieli-Vergani G, Vergani D, Baumann U, et al. Diagnosis and management of pediatric autoimmune liver disease: ESPGHAN hepatology committee position statement. J Pediatr Gastroenterol Nutr. 2018;66:345–60.
30. Mileti E, Rosenthal P, Peters MG. Validation and modification of simplified diagnostic criteria for autoimmune hepatitis in children. Clin Gastroenterol Hepatol. 2012;10:417–421.e1.
31. Sciveres M, Nastasio S, Maggiore G. Novel diagnostic and therapeutic strategies in juvenile autoimmune hepatitis. Front Pediatr. 2019;7:382.
32. Di Giorgio A, Vergani D, Mieli-Vergani G. Cutting edge issues in juvenile sclerosing cholangitis. Dig Liver Dis. 2021;54:417–27. https://doi.org/10.1016/j.dld.2021.06.028.
33. Nastasio S, Matarazzo L, Sciveres M, Maggiore G. Giant cell hepatitis associated with autoimmune hemolytic anemia: an update. Transl Gastroenterol Hepatol. 2021;6:25.
34. Darwish AA, McKiernan P, et al. Paediatric liver transplantation for metabolic disorder. Part 1: liver-based metabolic disorders without liver lesions. Clin Res Hepatol Gastroenterol. 2011;35:194–203.
35. Darwish AA, McKiernan P, et al. Paediatric liver transplantation for metabolic disorder. Part 2: metabolic disorders with liver lesions. Clin Res Hepatol Gastroenterol. 2011;35:271–80.
36. Sze YK, Dhawan A, Taylor RM, Bansal S, Mieli-Vergani G, Rela M, Heaton N. Pediatric liver transplantation for metabolic liver disease: experience at King's College Hospital. Transplantation. 2009;15(87):87–93.
37. Häberle J, Boddaert N, Burlina A, et al. Suggested guidelines for the diagnosis and management of urea cycle disorders. Orphanet J Rare Dis. 2012;29:7–32.
38. Yu L, Rayhill SC, Hsu EK, Landis CS. Liver transplantation for urea cycle disorders: analysis of the united network for organ sharing database. Transplant Proc. 2015;47:2413–8.
39. Morrow G, Tanguay RM. Biochemical and clinical aspects of hereditary tyrosinemia type 1. Adv Exp Med Biol. 2017;959:9–21.
40. McKiernan P. Liver transplantation for hereditary tyrosinemia type 1 in the United Kingdom. Adv Exp Med Biol. 2017;959:85–91.
41. Mazariegos GV, Morton DH, Sindhi R, et al. Liver transplantation for classical maple syrup urine disease: long-term follow-up in 37 patients and comparative united network for organ sharing experience. J Pediatr. 2012;160:116–21.
42. Badell IR, Hanish SI, Hughes CB, Hewitt WR, Chung RT, Spivey JR, Knechtle SJ. Domino liver transplantation in maple syrup urine disease: a case report and review of the literature. Transplant Proc. 2013;45:806–9.
43. Fraser JL, Venditti CP. Methylmalonic and propionic acidemias: clinical management update. Curr Opin Pediatr. 2016;28:682–93.
44. Barshes NR, Vanatta JM, Patel AJ, et al. Evaluation and management of patients with propionic acidemia undergoing liver transplantation: a comprehensive review. Pediatr Transplant. 2006;10:773–81.
45. Bouteldja N, Timson DJ. The biochemical basis of hereditary fructose intolerance. J Inherit Metab Dis. 2010;33:105–12.

46. Wong D. Hereditary fructose intolerance. Mol Genet Metab. 2005;85:165–7.
47. Elsas LJ, Langley S, Steele E, et al. Galactosemia: a strategy to identify new biochemical phenotypes and molecular genotypes. Am J Hum Genet. 1995;56:630–9.
48. Tada H, Takamura M, Kawashiri MA. Familial hypercholesterolemia: a narrative review on diagnosis and management strategies for children and adolescents. Vasc Health Risk Manag. 2021;17:59–67.
49. Ishigaki Y, Kawagishi N, Hasegawa Y, et al. Liver transplantation for homozygous familial hypercholesterolemia. J Atheroscler Thromb. 2019;26:121–7.
50. Pastores GM, Hughes DA. Lysosomal acid lipase deficiency: therapeutic options. Drug Des Dev Ther. 2020;14:591–601.
51. Socha P, Janczyk W, Dhawan A, et al. Wilson's disease in children: a position paper by the Hepatology Committee of the European Society for Paediatric Gastroenterology, Hepatology and Nutrition. J Pediatr Gastroenterol Nutr. 2018;66:334–44.
52. Dhawan A, Taylor RM, Cheeseman P, De Silva P, Katsiyiannakis L, Mieli-Vergani G. Wilson's disease in children: 37-year experience and revised King's score for liver transplantation. Liver Transpl. 2005;11:441–8.
53. Hadžić N, Baumann U, McKiernan P, McLin V, Nobili V. Long-term challenges and perspectives of pre-adolescent liver disease. Lancet Gastroenterol Hepatol. 2017;2:435–45.
54. Vajro P, Lenta S, Socha P, et al. Diagnosis of nonalcoholic fatty liver disease in children and adolescents: position paper of the ESPGHAN Hepatology Committee. J Pediatr Gastroenterol Nutr. 2012;54:700–13.
55. Furthner D, Weghuber D, Dalus C, Lukas A, Stundner-Ladenhauf HN, Mangge H, Pixner T. Nonalcoholic fatty liver disease (NAFLD) in children with obesity: narrative review and research gaps. Horm Res Paediatr. 2021;95:167–76. https://doi.org/10.1159/000518595.
56. Mann JP, Raponi M, Nobili V. Clinical implications of understanding the association between oxidative stress and pediatric NAFLD. Expert Rev Gastroenterol Hepatol. 2017;11:371–82.
57. Nobili V, Alisi A, Mosca A, et al. Hepatic farnesoid X receptor protein level and circulating fibroblast growth factor 19 concentration in children with NAFLD. Liver Int. 2018;38:342–9.
58. Carpino G, Pastori D, Baratta F, et al. PNPLA3 variant and portal/periportal histological pattern in patients with biopsy-proven non-alcoholic fatty liver disease: a possible role for oxidative stress. Sci Rep. 2017;7:15756.
59. Mangge H, Baumgartner BG, Zelzer S, et al. Patatin-like phospholipase 3 (rs738409) gene polymorphism is associated with increased liver enzymes in obese adolescents and metabolic syndrome in all ages. Aliment Pharmacol Ther. 2015;42:99–105.
60. Di Martino M, Koryukova K, Bezzi M. Imaging features of non-alcoholic fatty liver disease in children and adolescents. Children (Basel). 2017;4:73.
61. Garcovich M, Veraldi S, Di Stasio E, et al. Liver stiffness in pediatric patients with fatty liver disease: diagnostic accuracy and reproducibility of shear-wave elastography. Radiology. 2017;283:820–7.
62. Dezsőfi A, Baumann U, Dhawan A, et al. Liver biopsy in children: position paper of the ESPGHAN Hepatology Committee. J Pediatr Gastroenterol Nutr. 2015;60:408–20.
63. Alkhouri N, De Vito R, Alisi A, et al. Development and validation of a new histological score for pediatric non-alcoholic fatty liver disease. J Hepatol. 2012;57:1312–8.
64. Vos MB, Abrams SH, Barlow SE, et al. NASPGHAN clinical practice guideline for the diagnosis and treatment of nonalcoholic fatty liver disease in children: recommendations from the Expert Committee on NAFLD (ECON) and the North American Society of Pediatric Gastroenterology, Hepatology and Nutrition (NASPGHAN). J Pediatr Gastroenterol Nutr. 2017;64:319–34.
65. Nobili V, Bedogni G, Alisi A, Pietrobattista A, Risé P, Galli C, Agostoni C. Docosahexaenoic acid supplementation decreases liver fat content in children with non-alcoholic fatty liver disease: double-blind randomised controlled clinical trial. Arch Dis Child. 2011;96:350–3.
66. Della Corte C, Carpino G, De Vito R, et al. Docosahexanoic acid plus vitamin D treatment improves features of NAFLD in children with serum vitamin D deficiency: results from a single centre trial. PLoS One. 2016;11:e0168216.
67. Alisi A, Bedogni G, Baviera G, et al. Randomised clinical trial: the beneficial effects of VSL#3 in obese children with non-alcoholic steatohepatitis. Aliment Pharmacol Ther. 2014;39:1276–85.

7 The Surgical Management of Children with Intestinal Failure

Adrian Bianchi

Foreword A multidisciplinary specialist approach and appropriate parenteral and enteral nutrition have increased survival with a better-quality life for children with intestinal failure. Such skilled care is difficult and expensive, placing a major emotional and financial burden on the family, the local carers, and national health services. Some governments will not support expensive parenteral nutrition, and others will offer only a one-off intestinal transplant, forcing families into the permanent torment of having *allowed a precious child to die because of their inability to provide appropriate care!* It is a heavy consideration for professionals when advising complex forms of management that may not be practical or affordable. It is therefore imperative to support clinical and research programmes for the prevention of intestinal failure and to maximize the vast potential of autologous bowel, with the backdrop of transplantation although still at considerable risk and expense.

In presenting controversial concepts and experiences, this chapter seeks to stimulate discussion and therapeutic change for a 'better deal' for children and families confronted with the short bowel state (SBS) and intestinal failure (IF).

A. Bianchi (✉)
The Royal Manchester Children's Hospital, Manchester, UK

The Neonatal Surgical Unit, St Mary's Hospital, Manchester, UK

7.1 Aetiology

IF has been defined as 'the reduction of gut function below the minimum necessary for the absorption of macronutrients and/or water and electrolytes, such that IV supplementation is required to maintain health and/or growth' [1]. The causes of intestinal failure in children vary from an inability to absorb because of an intrinsic mucosal problem, such as chronic villous atrophy, allergies, chronic diarrhoea, and enzyme deficiencies, as in cystic fibrosis, to those relating to impaired intestinal neuromuscular function, such as aganglionosis (Hirschsprung's disease), and chronic idiopathic intestinal pseudo-obstruction. Others are due to insufficient tissue for absorption, as in short bowel; to altered bowel anatomy as for strictures and massive bowel dilatation; or to damaged mucosa following ischaemic injury from recurrent volvulus in malrotation and gastroschisis. Despite considerable adaptation, it remains relevant to keep in mind the irreplaceable functions specific to different parts of the gastrointestinal tract and to limit surgical resections to absolute necessity. These aetiologies can be regarded as 'medical', when there is no surgical solution, and 'surgical' (the subject of this chapter), when the solution may lie wholly or partly within surgical reconstruction. The

M. Lima, M. C. Mondardini (eds.), *Frailty in Children*,
https://doi.org/10.1007/978-3-031-24307-3_7

management of IF in children commences with 'prevention and preservation', for which an understanding of the conditions leading to IF and SBS is essential.

7.2 Surgical Necrotizing Enterocolitis (S-NEC)

Premature babies, especially those below 1 kg, are vulnerable to S-NEC. This surgical condition, of yet uncertain aetiology, develops within the first days after birth and is associated with early enteral feeding and bowel distension. The previously active and stable child becomes quiet and generally unwell with apnoeic events, vomiting, acidosis, and electrolyte disturbance. Abdominal examination elicits generalized tenderness and increasing bowel distension (Fig. 7.1) with eventual diaphragmatic splinting requiring ventilatory support.

Perforation releases gas, infected necrotic material, and undigested milk curds into the peritoneal space, with sepsis that demands supportive therapy with antibiotics, fluids, blood and platelet transfusions, and inotropes. The surgeon is often first called to a severely ill child in an unstable general condition with advanced intra-abdominal sepsis and who is classed as 'unable to be moved', thereby forcing desperate surgery in unsatisfactory conditions on the neonatal unit! At laparotomy there is generalized tense small bowel distension with long segments of dubious viability also involving the colon, as well as necrosis, particularly on the antimesenteric aspect of the loops (Fig. 7.2).

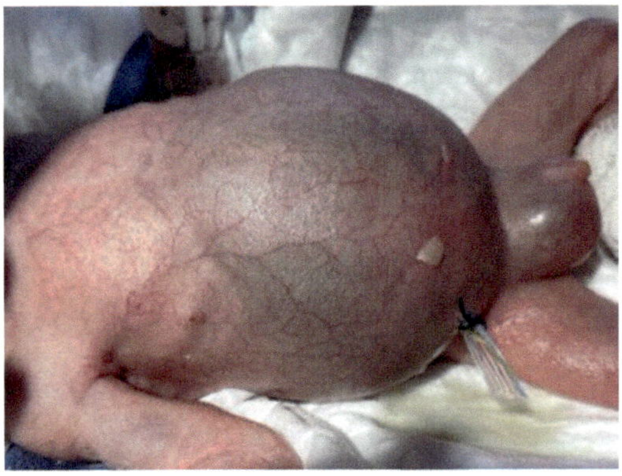

Fig. 7.1 S-NEC with abdominal distension and perforation

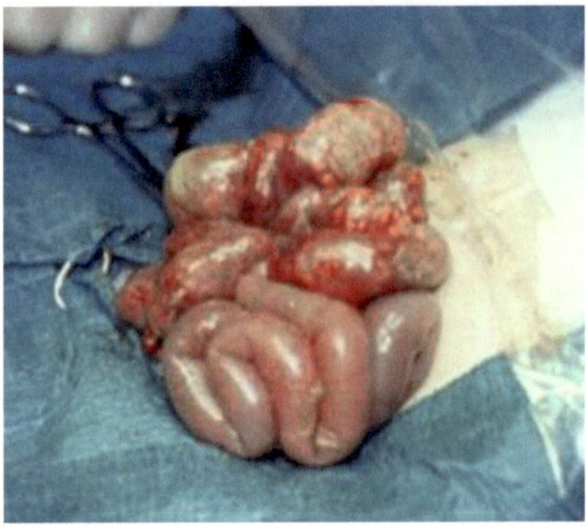

Fig. 7.2 Pre-perforation S-NEC bowel with mucosal necrosis

'Re-look' surgery for the assessment of areas of dubious viability, and further extensive gut resections are undertaken to salvage the child's life. Survivors often suffer from significant complications of prematurity, and from sepsis-induced low blood pressure and coagulopathy that cause cerebral ischaemia and haemorrhage. All S-NEC patients require a long-term central venous catheter and total parenteral nutrition with their own potential hazards, while the gastrointestinal tract attempts recovery. Additional surgery is necessary to resect strictures (Fig. 7.3) and for bowel continuity following temporary stomas.

Many suffer intestinal failure from extensive bowel loss and/or impaired absorption from ischaemic mucosal injury. S-NEC is a *potentially avoidable condition* carrying 30–50% mortality and major morbidity that figures significantly in the aetiology of SBS and IF, for which a better approach is long overdue.

The Challenges S-NEC presents the obstetrician and the multidisciplinary neonatal team (MDNT) of neonatologist, neonatal surgeon, and neonatal anaesthetist with the challenge *of managing pregnancy to eliminate premature birth.* Until such time, babies will continue to deliver prematurely with an immature bowel and immune system.

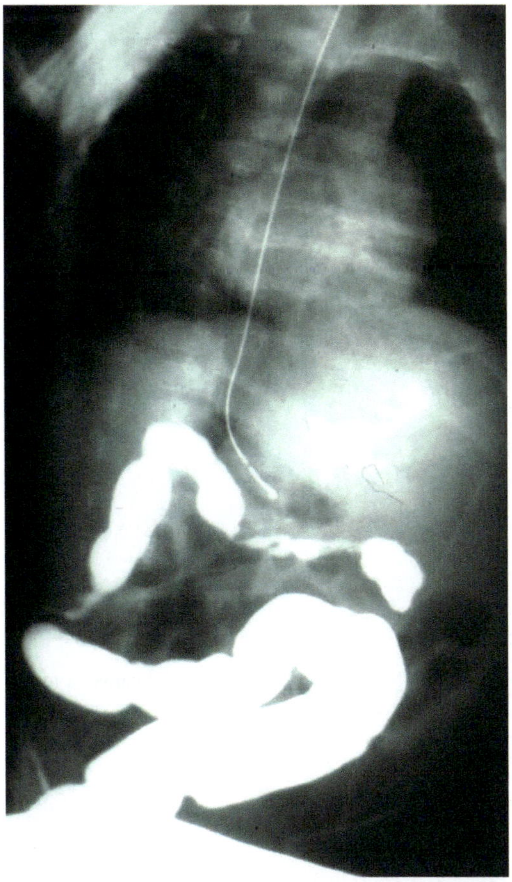

Fig. 7.3 Post S-NEC strictures

Currently a suspicion of S-NEC initiates resuscitative and supportive medical management with a 'watch-and-wait' policy based on Bell staging [2], in the hope of avoiding surgery for the premature child until there are definite signs of bowel injury, peritonitis, or perforation. Such delay invariably ends with extensive surgery for a septic, acidotic, hypotensive child with coagulopathy and a depressed immune response, showing the Y-sign of absent antimesenteric bowel perfusion on Doppler ultrasound scan [3]. The premature baby comes to surgery far too late during S-NEC, and radically different management is necessary.

Physiologically Immunity During the first 3–5 days after birth, the baby's immune system is challenged by ingested bacteria, largely acquired from the mother, which are essential for the stimulation of the gut-related immune cells on the mucosal villi, and by physiological bacteraemia, which activates systemic immunity. During this period of absent/reduced immunity, the mother produces colostrum that contains a high concentration of protective immunoglobulins (IgA, IgM, IgG). By the third to 15th day, the child's gut-related and systemic immune systems are activated and protective, and the mother's milk alters towards nutrition as well as immune protection.

Physiology-Based Management The resuscitative and early management of the premature 'at risk' child should seek to avoid predisposing factors for S-NEC and take cognition of normal physiology:

(a) **Bowel distension**: resuscitation and ventilation should avoid gaseous bowel distension, which raises intraluminal tension and reduces bowel wall circulation.
(b) **Colostrum and curd-free fresh-milk whey**: undigestible milk curds lead to lower ileal obstruction, and fermentation gases raise intraluminal pressure, causing ischaemic necrosis and perforation primarily at the antimesenteric aspect of the loop. For the first days after birth, the 'at risk' child should be enterally fed only with FRESH, preferably maternal, immune-protective colostrum. Subsequent enteral feeding continues with *immune-protective FRESH-milk whey*, obtained by treating FRESH expressed breast milk with chymotrypsin to coagulate and filter out undigestible milk curds.
(c) **The microbiome**: it is relevant to encourage the rapid development of a normal microbiome containing essential 'helpful gut flora' usually acquired from maternal contact at vaginal delivery and subsequently at the breast. Thus, following sterile caesarean section and/or isolation in an incubator, it is logical to actively inoculate the child's skin, pharynx, and gut with maternal bacteria. Particular care should be taken with antibiotics that eliminate essential 'helpful' organisms and favour potential antibiotic-resistant pathogens.

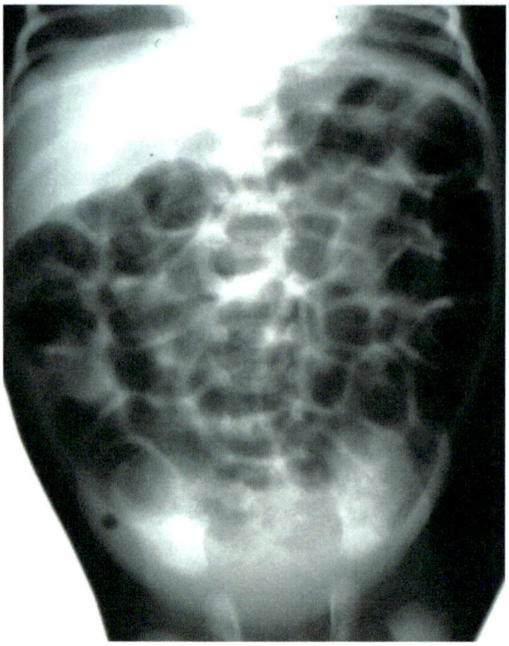

Fig. 7.4 Early S-NEC with increasing bowel distension

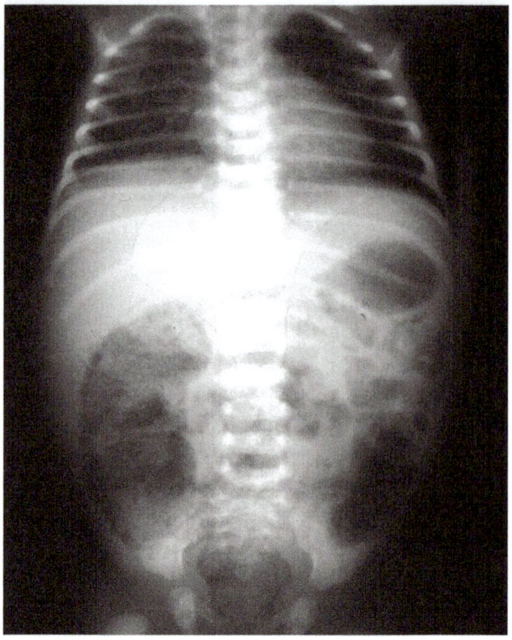

Fig. 7.5 S-NEC with intramural gas indicative of mucosal ulceration and necrosis

(d) **Early surgery**: the MDNT must be constantly alert to early alterations in the child's general condition, to abdominal tenderness and bowel distension (Fig. 7.4), and to the Doppler US ring sign of hyperaemia in oedematous inflamed bowel [3].

It is inadvisable to await definitive but late evidence of 'gut injury', such as static bowel loops, intramural gas on X-ray (Fig. 7.5), and rectal bleeding.

The critical time for bowel salvage occurs during early S-NEC when clinical, radiological, and ultrasonological features are not marked [3] but when *the bowel is still viable and when the child is in good condition* with a stable circulation, a reactive bone marrow, and an activating immune system. Through an ileal enterotomy, ALL distended bowel is collapsed to allow the return of circulation (Fig. 7.6) and washed out with a warm soap-air-isotonic saline solution (1.36% dialysis solution with 4 mmol/L potassium).

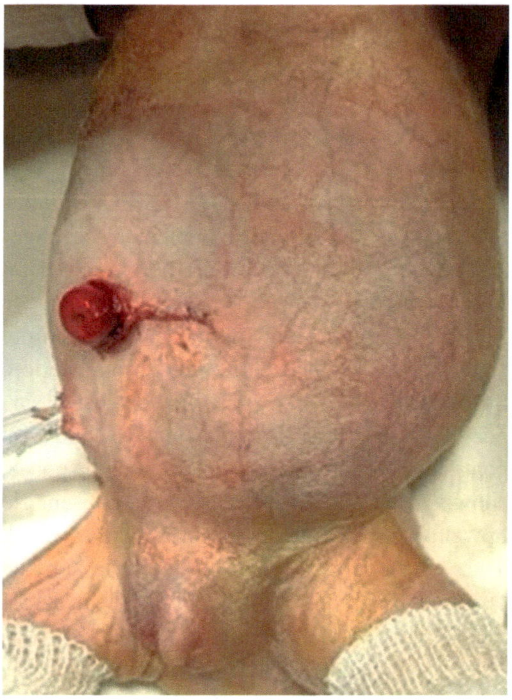

Fig. 7.6 A well child with viable bowel after early surgery

The placement of a stoma is optional, but ample abdominal drainage is relevant. With modern neonatal anaesthesia and surgery, children DO NOT DIE from an early operation, and desperate surgery on an 'unstable child' implies missed safer opportunities. Well-judged EARLY surgery increases child survival with sufficient functional bowel for a good-quality life.

7.3 Gastroschisis

Gastroschisis is likely the result of gene interaction with environmental factors, which leads to a failure of intra-abdominal midgut migration and fixation during the first 8 weeks of pregnancy. The condition affects younger mothers from less affluent backgrounds and is associated with an otherwise normal smaller baby at 34–36 weeks gestation. The bowel that lies outside the abdomen is supplied through a narrow-based superior mesenteric pedicle that passes through a 2–4 cm diameter umbilical port that is expanded to the right of a splayed umbilical cord at its left rim (Fig. 7.7). A narrow diameter umbilical port may seem to strangle a precarious midgut mesenteric pedicle.

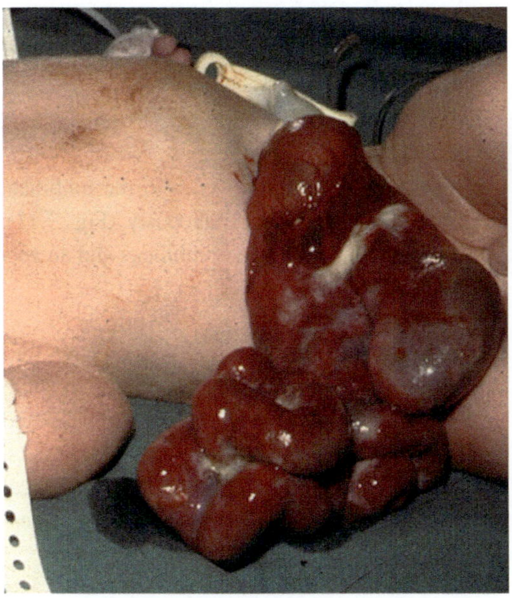

Fig. 7.7 Baby with gastroschisis and 'peel' covered bowel

The liver and spleen are always at their normal intra-abdominal location, and no other organs are extruded except for the body of the stomach, a testicle or fallopian tube, and the dome of the bladder. There is no membrane or sac, and the extruded bowel is freely bathed with liquor, becoming coated with a fibrinous 'peel' (Fig. 7.7) during the last weeks of the pregnancy. Within the thickened mass, the bowel commonly retains its structure and function. Once the 'peel' spontaneously resolves normal enteral nutrition can be expected. There is no loss of abdominal wall tissue, but the lack of bowel within the abdomen leads to a reduced intra-abdominal domain that is too small to accommodate the extruded midgut without some tension.

Antenatally, the heavy midgut on its narrow pedicle is constantly at risk from volvulus with resorption of dead bowel and closure of the umbilical port. At laparotomy, the midgut supplied by the superior mesenteric pedicle is absent, and there is only a high jejunal atresia with some 20–40 cm of dilated jejunum, and transverse and left colon (Fig. 7.8).

Recurrent episodes of volvulus may cause repetitive ischaemic injury with loss of absorptive function in the surviving bowel.

Gastroschisis can be diagnosed by antenatal ultrasound scan during early pregnancy, such that there is an opportunity for antenatal counselling, and the possibility for antenatal intervention to

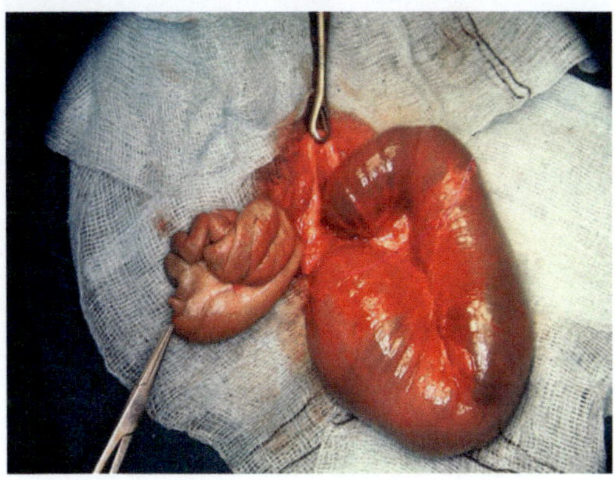

Fig. 7.8 Antenatal midgut volvulus. Resorbing bowel and jejunal atresia

prevent volvulus. Since midgut volvulus and 'peel' tend to occur later in pregnancy, premature delivery has been proposed from around the 30th week to allow easier intra-abdominal placement of more pliable bowel. However, this must be weighed against the risks of prematurity (immature lungs, cerebral bleeding, ophthalmic issues) and possible S-NEC. Presently, most gastroschisis pregnancies come to spontaneous or induced labour closer to the 36th week. There is no risk to the extruded bowel from vaginal delivery, and there is no need for a caesarean section. At birth, the child, usually in good condition and not requiring intubation or ventilation, should be nursed well over on his right side, with the unkinked mesentery and bowel flowing into a plastic bag to avoid drying and to reduce heat loss (Fig. 7.9).

A wide-bore nasogastric tube (8–10 F) on frequent suction is relevant to prevent vomiting and aspiration as well as gaseous bowel distension. Intravenous fluids are those appropriate for daily requirements and to replace stomach aspirates and serous exudates from extruded bowel. Excess fluids and colloids cause unwanted systemic and bowel oedema. Antibiotics are not relevant and favour resistant pathogens. The baby should be allowed to rest, and painless reduction of the bowel that is insensitive to handling is undertaken electively within the first 24 h, in the incubator (Fig. 7.10) and without anaesthesia or sedation [4].

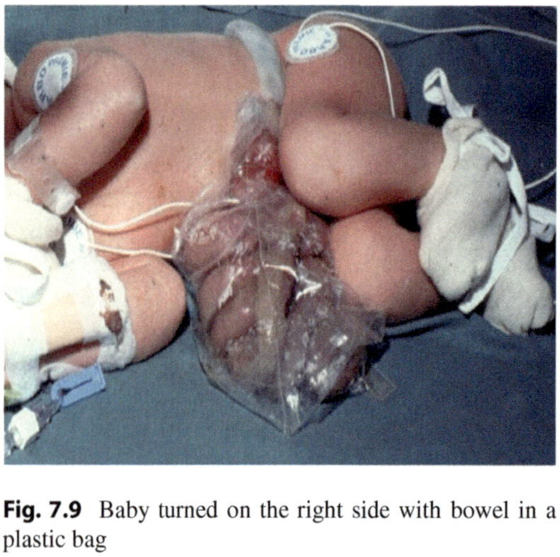

Fig. 7.9 Baby turned on the right side with bowel in a plastic bag

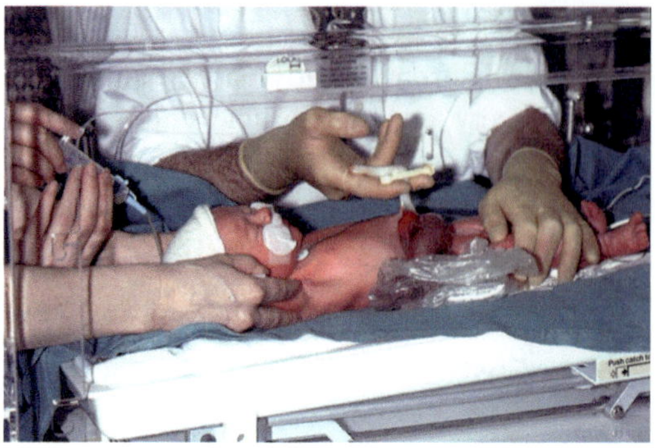

Fig. 7.10 Bowel replacement without anaesthesia or sedation

The reactions of the fully awake baby are essential to guide the surgeon through a steady reduction over 30–45 min. The baby is placed supine, and with the abdomen stabilized by upward cord traction, the bowel loops are passed into the abdominal space, loop by loop alternately to right and left, always avoiding torsion on the mesentery. The midgut should be returned to an unrotated position, with the small bowel passing to the right side and the caecum coming to overlie the stomach in the left hypochondrium. Excess intra-abdominal tension leads to diaphragmatic splinting and respiratory concerns, impacts significantly on the bowel blood supply, causes inferior vena cava compression, and interferes with renal function [5], such that it is better to accept an initial partial reduction and later completion once the abdominal domain and returned bowel have become more compliant. The umbilical port is covered over with the umbilical cord and left to close spontaneously (Fig. 7.11), leading to a centrally placed umbilicus and an aesthetic scarless abdomen.

Bowel Reduction by Gravity When excess tension is unavoidable, the bowel is placed in a silo or bag that is hung vertically above the baby and is allowed to enter the abdomen by gravity over a period of hours or days (Fig. 7.12). The umbilical port is allowed to close spontaneously or is aesthetically sutured.

Reduction Under Anaesthesia Bowel reduction under anaesthesia with a fully relaxed baby

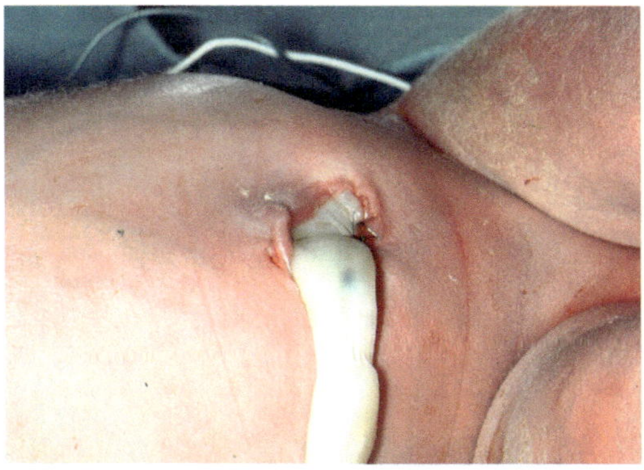

Fig. 7.11 Gastroschisis port closed with the umbilical cord

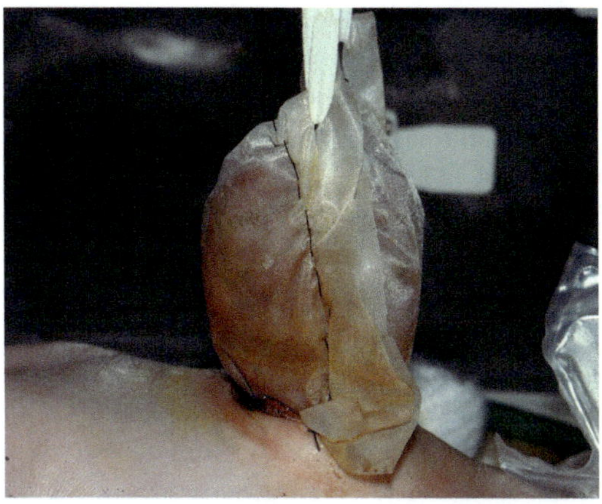

Fig. 7.12 Suspended silo and gravity reduction

requires particular attention to avoid excessive intra-abdominal tension. It is better to place a silo for slow 'gravity' reduction rather than to risk compromise of bowel blood supply, diaphragmatic splinting with difficult ventilation, and/or inferior vena cava compression and renal impairment.

Gastroschisis features strongly in the aetiology of IF because of midgut loss from antenatal volvulus and absorptive dysfunction from repetitive ischaemic injury, as well as tragically from avoidable bowel necrosis following ill-judged tense midgut reduction. Presently, antenatal intervention to prevent volvulus remains theoretical; however, postnatal bowel loss lies within the surgeon's expertise!

7.4 Non-fixation and Malrotation

Failure of intra-abdominal migration, rotation, and fixation of the bowel during the first 8 weeks of pregnancy lead to a narrow-based superior mesenteric pedicle. Undetected malrotation with midgut non-fixation is a life-threatening 'ticking time bomb' awaiting volvulus. In the absence of volvulus, the child is entirely normal at birth, and there are no pointers to the non-rotated state.

Plain abdominal X-ray (Fig. 7.13) and upper gastrointestinal contrast studies show an S-shaped duodenum with the small bowel passing to the right side and a high caecum just below the liver or towards the left hypochondrium.

Copious clean bilious vomiting in a previously well patient of any age, with a flat non-tender abdomen and a featureless abdominal X-ray (Fig. 7.14a), is pathognomonic and of the utmost surgical emergency (Fig. 7.14b). Rectal bleeding is an ominous sign that is indicative of bowel congestion and compromised circulation. At laparotomy, the volvulus is derotated, usually in an anticlockwise direction; the mesentery splayed widely open and 'roughened'; and the

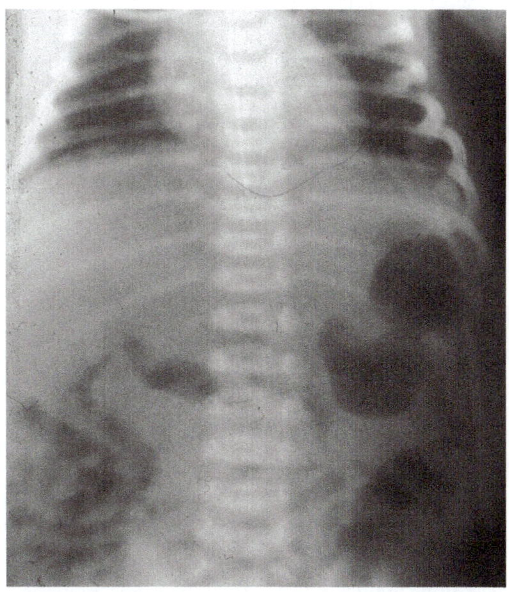

Fig. 7.13 Plain X-ray showing a non-rotated midgut

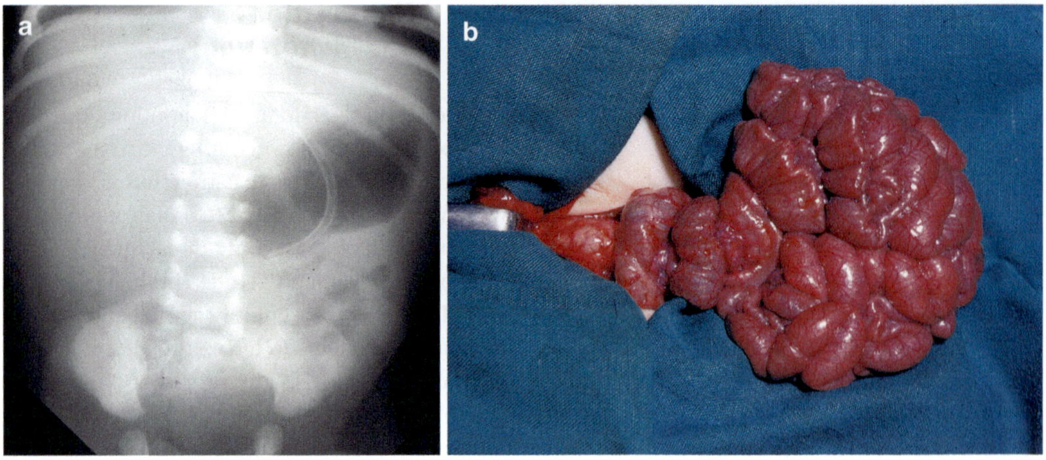

Fig. 7.14 (**a**, **b**) Featureless abdominal X-ray indicative of midgut volvulus

bowel replaced in the non-rotated position with the small bowel towards the right side and the caecum, with the appendix devascularized and inverted or removed, coming to lie high in the left hypochondrium. A laparoscopic approach must ensure a 'roughening' of the mesentery to stimulate fixative adhesions and to prevent recurrent volvulus. The patient must be made fully aware of the post-operative configuration of the bowel and of the absence of the appendix.

In A child having had an in utero volvulus with total loss of the midgut will present as a normal child with a high jejunal atresia, short bowel, and IF.

7.5 Meconium Ileus—Cystic Fibrosis

Cystic fibrosis is due to a specific autosomal recessive genetic mutation, largely affecting the Caucasian population. Delta F508, the commonest of the 1500 know mutations, configures for an abnormal cystic fibrosis transmembrane conductance regulator (CFTR), which is a channel-shaped protein that controls the passage of chloride ions and water across the cell membrane. Alterations in the CFTR lead to a viscid and salty mucus and secretions, which mainly affect the lungs, pancreas, liver, and male reproductive organs. The thick salty mucus (mucoviscidosis) predisposes to repeated bronchial infections with eventual antibiotic-resistant bacteria and progressive lung damage with respiratory failure. Thick pancreatic secretions fail to pass into the bowel, impairing normal digestion, growth, and general health. Thick biliary secretions cause stasis within the intrahepatic bile ducts and liver failure. Recurrent pancreatic damage may lead to type-1 diabetes.

Autosomal recessive transmission carries a 1:4 chance for subsequent pregnancies so that early amniocentesis and foetal gene sequencing offer the option of termination. There is presently no cure for cystic fibrosis, and life expectancy remains limited to the 30 s. Cystic fibrosis should be considered in any child with recurrent chest infections and growth failure. The child's sweat tastes markedly salty, and faeces may be particularly smelly, fatty, and tenacious. Diagnosis can be confirmed by excessive salt on a sweat test and by genetic sequencing for the abnormal mutation. Medical management with intensive chest physiotherapy and antibiotics attempts to clear tenacious mucus and limit bronchial infection. Research is directed at drugs that restructure the mutant CFTR towards normal for less viscid secretions. Nutritional and growth failure are addressed with pancreatic enzymes that are necessary throughout life, with dietary supplements and relevant vitamins, such as vit B_{12}, following the loss of ileum, and insulin management for type 1 diabetes. Future hope lies in gene replacement therapy.

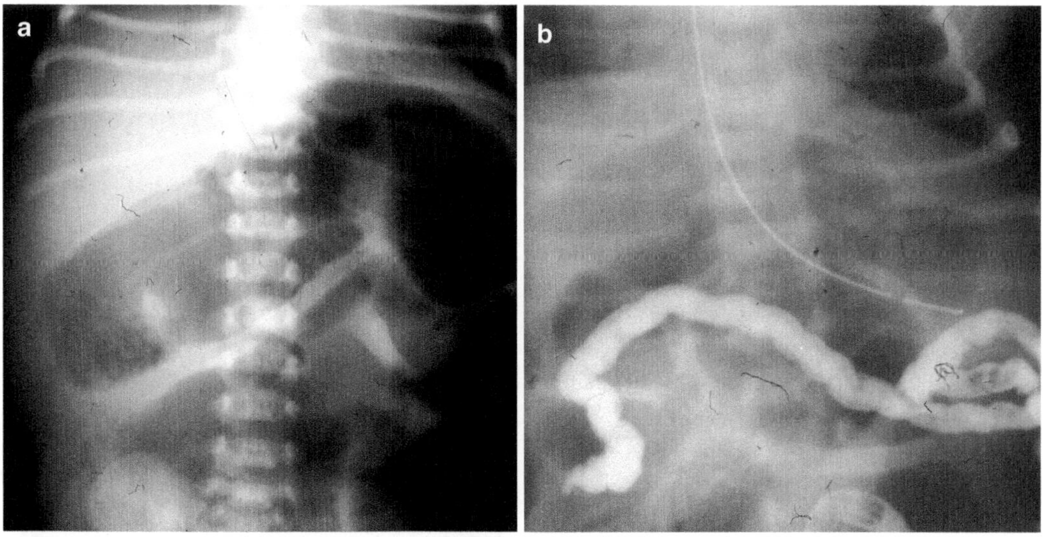

Fig. 7.15 (**a**) Neuhauser's sign. (**b**) Micro-colon with pellets

Cystic fibrosis can be detected antenatally because of large loops of meconium-filled bowel on ultrasound scan. The child is born with a non-tender distended abdomen containing palpable meconium-filled indentable loops that present a ground-glass appearance on X-ray, known as Neuhauser's sign (Fig. 7.15a), and eventually mid-to-distal small bowel obstruction.

A dilute gastrografin contrast enema reveals a micro-colon filled with tenacious 'pellets' (Fig. 7.15b). Repeated retrograde gastrografin washouts often fail to reach and clear the tenacious obstructive meconium in the dilated ileum.

Antenatal volvulus of the heavy meconium-filled loops and resorption of the dead bowel present as small bowel atresia. The autolyzing mass may form a large intra-abdominal pseudocyst with surrounding calcification (Fig. 7.16).

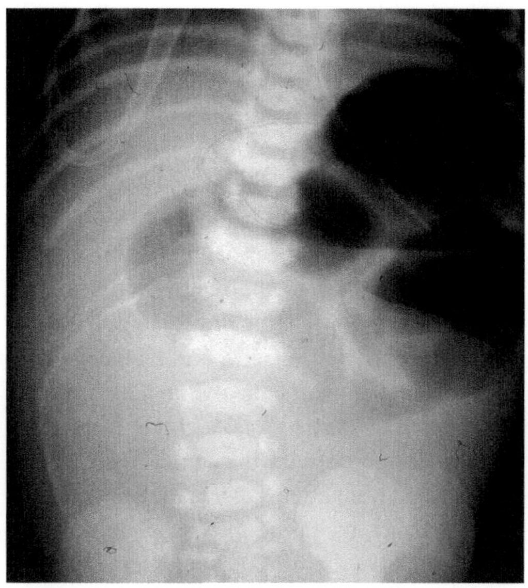

Fig. 7.16 Pseudocyst with surrounding calcification

Laparotomy is required for the clearance of the pseudocyst, the resection of all large thick-walled meconium-obstructed ileal loops, and size-matched end-to-end ileo-ileal anastomosis. The micro distal ileum, ileocaecal (IC) valve, and micro-colon should be retained and cleaned out by a gentle massage with soap and air mixture, and a record kept of the residual small bowel length measured along the antimesenteric border. Post-operative bowel patency may be delayed; however, a proximal defunctioning protective ileostomy or a Bishop-Koop stoma is not necessary and necessitates additional surgery for closure. There is commonly sufficient normally functional and adaptive small bowel to avoid SBS or IF so that long-term parenteral nutrition is not required. Intestinal failure in cystic fibrosis relates to thick pancreatic secretions that are unable to reach the bowel as well as to progressive pancreatic destruction. Surgery and nutritional management with pancreatic enzymes, dietary additives and vitamins, and insulin address the gastrointestinal issues.

The life-limiting factor for patients with cystic fibrosis is the progressive loss of lung function from mucoviscidosis and infection, and eventual respiratory failure, which requires lung transplantation. Bowel or pancreatic transplantation is not a common consideration, but liver transplantation may be relevant in the event of liver failure. To this end, careful gastroenterological management is pertinent to maintain excellent general health.

7.6 Aganglionosis—Hirschsprung's Disease

Hirschsprung's disease (HD) or aganglionosis is a complex genetic condition causing a failure of proximal-to-distal migration of ganglion cells from the neural crest to Auerbach's and Meissner's plexi, such that aganglionic bowel is aperistaltic and non-absorptive. There is a 4:1 preponderance for males, other family members may be affected, and there is a 10–15% link to other genetic conditions, such as Down's and Wardenberg's syndromes. Around 70% of aganglionosis is limited to the rectosigmoid region, but longer colonic lengths or all the colon (total colonic aganglionosis) may be involved. Long-segment aganglionosis involving long tracts of small bowel presents a short bowel state when ganglia are limited to the most proximal jejunum. The extreme form affects the whole of the gastrointestinal tract, including the oesophagus, and is only manageable by life-long parenteral nutrition or total gastrointestinal transplantation.

Hirschsprung's disease should be suspected because of developing abdominal distension and a failure to pass meconium within the first 48 h *after birth*. Rectosigmoid aganglionosis responds to internal sphincter digital dilatation with the explosive passage of faeces and flatus. Presentation may be acute and life-threatening from enterocolitis (Fig. 7.17) and septicaemia.

Less acute forms can present at a later age because of failure to thrive and with chronic con-

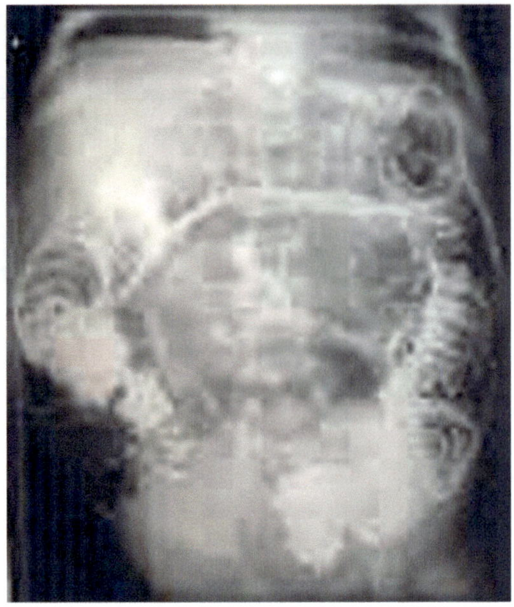

Fig. 7.17 Hirschsprung's related enterocolitis

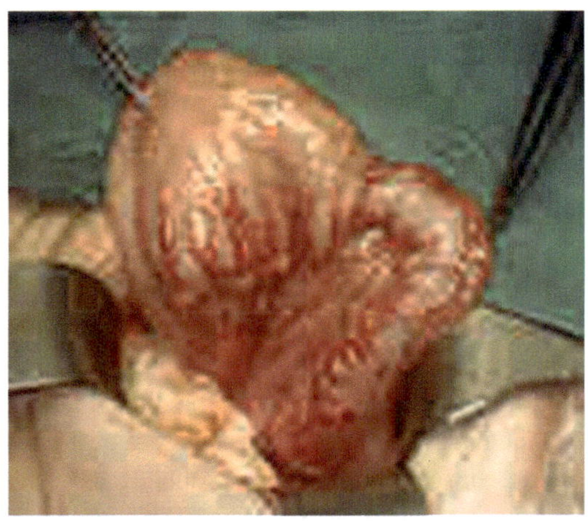

Fig. 7.18 Cone-shaped transition zone in Hirschsprung's disease

stipation. Non-peristaltic aganglionic bowel causes obstruction at the cone-shaped 'Transition Zone' (Fig. 7.18) between the ganglionic dilated proximal bowel and the collapsed distal aganglionic bowel.

Definitive diagnosis is made on a histopathological examination of mucosal and submucosal suction rectal biopsy by an absence of nerve ganglia, a proliferation of nerve fibres in Auerbach's and Meissner's plexi, and raised acetylcholinesterase levels on histochemistry. Identification of the transition zone is essential to reconstruction and requires serial bowel wall biopsies, progressing proximally to normal consistency bowel containing normal ganglia and nerve trunks. Such staging biopsies can be undertaken by an experienced pathologist at a frozen section study during a one-stage definitive surgical procedure or may be the initial 'mapping' phase of a two-stage surgical approach.

Non-surgical management of HD attempts to establish regular bowel evacuation until the planned surgical reconstruction. Failure to establish a successful evacuation pattern, a two-stage surgical approach, and enterocolitis are frequently managed with temporary colostomy in biopsy-confirmed ganglionic peristaltic bowel proximal to the transition zone. Definitive surgical reconstruction involves the resection of all the aganglionic segments and the 'pull-through' of normal diameter ganglionic peristaltic bowel to the anus. Experienced neonatal surgical units offer a one-stage definitive 'pull-through' with serial frozen section control and without colostomy during the first admission within days of birth. The Swenson (author's preference), Soave, or Duhamel pull-through procedures can be undertaken at open laparotomy, laparoscopically, or entirely transanally without an abdominal phase. The devascularized aganglionic segment is intussuscepted through the anus and resected externally, with a wide oblique colo-anal anastomosis of histologically verified ganglionic bowel returned through the anus. Continence outcomes are good, with only an occasional child continuing to have problems with constipation or poor anal control. Down's syndrome children may experience a delay in establishing full continence, but otherwise, there is no difference in outcome.

Total colonic aganglionosis requires the resection of all the colon. An ileoanal anastomosis often leads to urgency and major soiling, and an ileal J-pouch requires major attention to complete emptying to avoid enterocolitis and is more suited to the mature patient. It is better, during childhood, to accept a terminal ileostomy that is 'controllable with a stoma bag' and that allows relatively normal activities.

Long-segment aganglionosis extending high into the small bowel presents a state of intestinal failure and short bowel. A high jejunostomy has large stoma losses, and management involves complex fluid and electrolyte replacement. A controllable tube-jejunostomy (discussed later) is preferable. Survival and growth require long-term parenteral nutrition to supplement enteral intake. Autologous gastrointestinal reconstruction of the residual ganglionic bowel offers a reduction in parenteral nutrition dependence and a better-quality life. Intestinal transplantation is increasingly an option.

7.7 Ischaemic Injury, Surgical Resection, and Diversion

Ischaemic injury from vascular emboli, accidental or child-abuse-related non-accidental abdominal trauma, abdominal seatbelt compression, and knife or gunshot wounds may cause midgut loss from obstruction or disruption of the superior mesenteric pedicle or extensive bowel loss from tearing of mesenteric vessels. Extensive ill-judged resection may lead to unnecessary bowel loss during elective surgical procedures and, particularly, during emergency surgery when post-operative quality of life may take second place to immediate survival. It is imperative that surgeons appreciate the diverse functions and the consequences of the loss of the different parts of the gastrointestinal tract and develop a culture of preservation, limiting resection and diversion to absolute necessity. Digestion and absorption commence at the stomach and duodenum, with the intermix of ingested food, saliva, acid, bile, and pancreatic enzymes. The jejunum contributes considerable volumes of fluid (6–10 L) and electrolytes and is responsible for the absorption of major nutrient components (carbohydrates, proteins). It possesses marked adaptive capabilities and is particularly responsive to glucagon-like peptide 2 (GLP-2), which is produced at the caecum and right colon. The ileum has specific binding sites for the absorption of vit B_{12}, for bile salts that are relevant to fat absorption, oxalate binding, and bile salt recycling. Its adaptive capabilities are far greater than those of the jejunum, and it can increase absorption by over 500 times to compensate for small bowel loss. The distal ileum contributes a YY factor, which reduces motility and, with the ileocaecal valve, aids in slowing transit and increasing contact time for absorption. The caecum and ascending colon are the sources of GLP-2, which is the most powerful known stimulant for mucosal adaptation, and the distal colon resorbs fluid and electrolytes, thereby greatly reducing losses and leading to formed faeces that are stored in the colorectum until regular evacuation. The loss or diversion of any part of the gastrointestinal tract can have significant consequences on metabolism, fluid and electrolyte balance, and the quality and volume of the faeces.

7.8 The Short Bowel State and Intestinal Failure

IF may be temporary or long-term, and complete or partial, depending on the underlying cause and the type, length, anatomy, and absorptive capability of the residual bowel. Thus, after antenatal segmental or midgut volvulus, the residual bowel is usually peristaltic, absorptive, and adaptive but will require remodelling of the dilated proximal segment to avoid stasis with bacterial overgrowth and sepsis and for effective propulsion. The impact of ischaemia in association with gastroschisis and S-NEC may lead to severe bowel loss and/or damaged non-absorptive mucosa. It cannot be overstressed that all potentially viable and functional bowels should be preserved, limiting resection and avoiding diversion. Even multiple short segments (2–5 cm) of the neonatal small bowel, when linked together, can lead to a prognosis-altering length. After each operative procedure, the patient should be given an accurate record of the nature and length of the residual bowel, which are relevant to autologous bowel reconstruction.

The Specialist Multidisciplinary Team, Social Services, and Respite Key to the management of the short bowel state is the multidisciplinary team (MDT) of medical and surgical clinicians, psychologists, nurses, and support staff within the specialist hospital, whose role commences with stable venous access and the stabilization of the child on parenteral nutrition, and who instruct the parents for early transfer to home care assisted by the community nursing team. The long-term 'Comprehensive Health Care Package' must attend to the child's physical and mental health and must also encompass the psychological concerns (fears, worries, stress), practical issues (baby supplies, food, clothing), and financial needs of all the family members, who must significantly alter their lives, their jobs, and their aspirations. Financial support must cater for home alterations, travel for hospital visits, admissions for central venous catheter care and reconstructive bowel surgery, and for sibling support and respite care for the family as a unit. The mother, commonly the main carer, often suffers feelings of 'guilt' and diminished self-respect, and the impact on her personal life, her relationships, and her career outside the home, which are essential to her well-being and to the family finances, must be addressed to avoid resentment towards the affected child and family breakdown.

The Intestinal Failure Hub-and-Spoke Model The multidisciplinary services in a dedicated specialist centre are often far from the child's home. Management that addresses the child's mental and psychological development is best delivered by early transfer to the home, with the child able to attend school and peer-related activities. The 'hub-and-spoke model' provides for home care, supported by local services and guided by the specialist IF unit and its outreach IF team.

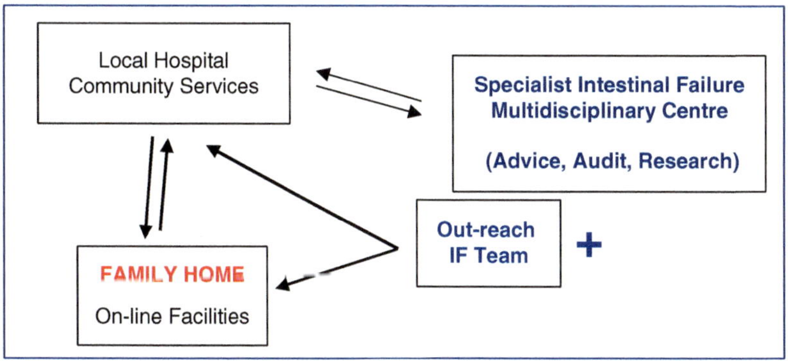

The Hub-and-Spoke Model

The specialist centre sets up and monitors the care plan and undertakes investigations, central venous catheter and autologous bowel surgery, transplantation, audit, and research. The local hospital and community health services, supported by the outreach IF team, are responsible for daily care. Online computer facilities help the family to keep abreast of IF developments and to interact with their careers and other IF families.

7.9 Medical Management

Parenteral Nutrition The central venous catheter and parenteral nutrition are the patient's lifeline until the residual bowel has adapted to sustain life and growth. A significant loss of stable venous access from sepsis or catheter breakage or blockage is an indication for bowel transplantation. Regular modifications to parenteral nutrition are specific to each patient and vary with enteral losses and bowel adaptation. Parenteral nutrition should be delivered over the night hours to allow for a rest period and for normal daytime activities. The intricacies of parenteral nutrition and intravenous access are available in the literature and will not be discussed. However, deserving of special mention is the severe hepatotoxicity induced by plant phytosterols in soya-based lipid emulsions that cause rapid liver failure, particularly in the neonate and young baby. Fat emulsions should contain no more than 1–1.5 g/kg/day of soya-based lipids. SMOF, a mixture of lipids from soya, medium-chain triglycerides, olive oil, and fish oil, is less hepatotoxic and is the presently recommended intravenous lipid emulsion. Increasing mucosal adaptation and enteral absorption allow a reduction in parenteral nutrition, which reduces liver injury and improves quality of life.

Oral and Enteral Feeding The best long-term solution for intestinal failure is *enteral nutrition by autologous bowel.* Oral enteral feeding is also particularly relevant to physiological neonatal brain learning for food experience to avoid later food aversion and phobia. Mucosal adaptation depends on regular contact with enteral fluids that contain bile, salivary and pancreatic enzymes, and food, which should be normal, varied, and taken intermittently at mealtimes with the rest of the family. Rapid transit and limited mucosal contact from short bowel limit absorption so that enteral medications such as antibiotics, loperamide, and clonidine require an increased dosage. Similarly, more concentrated solids and food thickeners are beneficial from an early stage; however, liquids should be given intermittently in small volumes and limited to the daily fluid requirements to avoid a washout effect. Constant nasogastric or gastrostomy drip-feeding should be avoided since it bypasses brain learning and does not allow 'rest periods' for the adapting bowel. It is important to reconstruct dilated bowel to avoid stasis and mucosal inflammation with bacterial translocation and sepsis. Until bowel continuity is established, enteric fluids collected from the proximal bowel should be infused into the disconnected distal bowel during the night-time hours to avoid disuse atrophy and enhance enteral absorption, at a rate and volume that allows normal stools and avoids a washout effect.

7.9.1 Autologous Gastrointestinal Reconstruction (AGIR)

Bowel length virtually doubles during the third trimester of pregnancy [6]. Thus, even short lengths of neonatal bowel (2–5 cm segments) represent a significant absorptive potential. Bowel growth is marked during the early years and continues until adulthood. Adaptation is lifelong, although finite and determined by the type of mucosa. The normal 3.5 kg neonate averages a small bowel of 1.5–2 cm diameter and a length of around 350 cm measured along the antimesenteric border from the ligament of Treitz to the ileocaecal valve, with a complete colon. After bowel loss or resection a residual jejuno-ileal length of 60–100 cm of propulsive diameter with an intact ileocaecal valve and all the colon, can be expected to adapt sufficiently and without significant long-term nutritional deficits. The loss of the ileum, IC valve, and ascending colon will require a greater length of small bowel, emphasizing the importance of preserving the IC valve and GLP-2-producing ascending colon.

Bowel Preservation At presentation and after each operative intervention, *it is essential*, for reconstruction and audit, to record and photograph or video the type, length as measured along the antimesenteric border, and diameter of all residual bowel. The massive proximal loop dilatation associated with small bowel atresia leads to a mismatched dysfunctional 'big-to-small' anastomosis with failure of propulsion, stasis, and bacterial translocation despite active peristalsis. It is necessary to resect back and/or tailor the dilated bowel along the antimesenteric border towards a better-matched (<3:1) end-to-end anastomosis. When even this extent of small bowel loss is inadvisable, *no resection or tailoring should be undertaken. ALL bowels should be preserved for reconstruction and the child referred to the specialist IF centre.*

Tube-Stomata for Enhanced Absorption and Bowel Expansion A high small bowel abdominal wall stoma causes uncontrollable enteral losses, painful skin excoriation, and difficulty with stoma bag adhesion. At first surgery, it is better to construct a *controllable tube-jejunostomy* (Fig. 7.19) with a large Foley or Malecot catheter (18–24 F), which is brought through the abdominal wall and held within the dilated proximal loop with a double purse-string suture that is drawn up against the peritoneum.

A similar separate smaller tube-ostomy is placed in the distal bowel (ileum or colon) for the infusion of the proximal bowel effluent to develop the defunctioned distal bowel until bowel continuity. Once the tube-stomata are established, daytime oral feeding with the family and night-time distal bowel infusions commence.

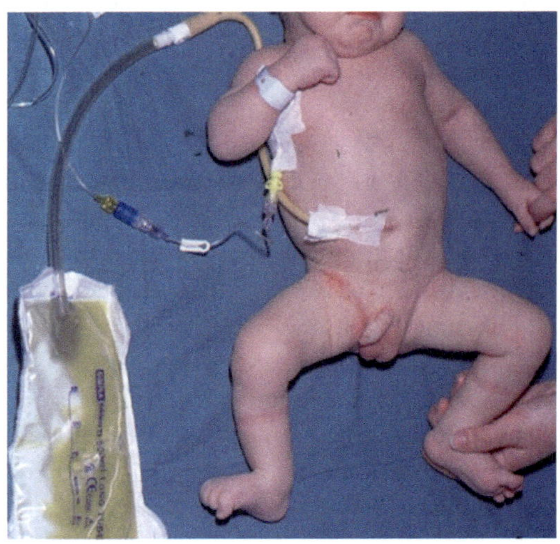

Fig. 7.19 Controllable tube-jejunostomy

Bowel Expansion Over some 6–12 months, the tube-jejunostomy is occluded intermittently and for lengthening periods to reduce losses and prolong nutrient-to-mucosa contact for enhanced absorption and adaptation. Peristalsis against occlusion forces bowel elongation and dilatation, creating additional tissue for reconstruction (Fig. 7.20).

Initial proximal tube occlusions for 5 min periods are progressively increased to tolerance (30–180 min) and alternate with similar periods of drainage to avoid stasis and bacterial overgrowth. Vomiting and discomfort from loop contractions against the occluded tube subside within a short time. The effectiveness and progress of the bowel expansion process is assessed by the child's weight gain from increasing absorption and by loop dilatation and elongation (Fig. 7.20). It is relevant to avoid excessive weight gain!, by reducing parenteral nutrition. This onerous but effective management continues for several months and until the proximal bowel dilates and elongates sufficiently for 'bowel remodelling and lengthening'.

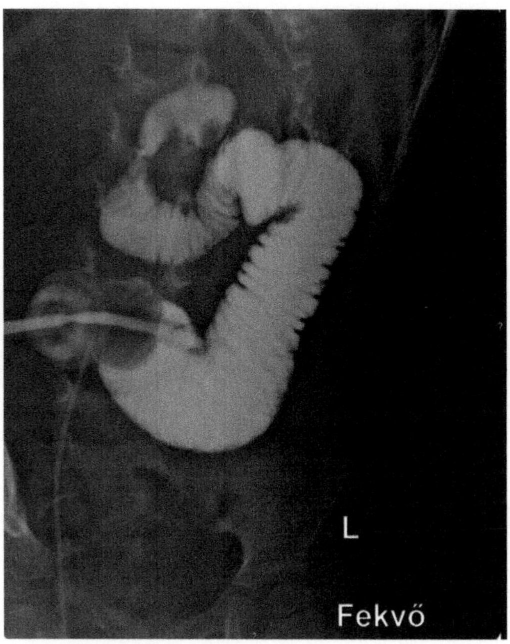

Fig. 7.20 Bowel expansion by occlusion of tube-jejunostomy

7.10 Autologous Bowel Lengthening Procedures

Longitudinal Intestinal Lengthening and Tailoring (LILT) The first bowel lengthening procedure was reported by Bianchi [7] in 1980 and first applied clinically with positive results in 1981 by Boeckman and Traylor [8]. The dilated loop is divided longitudinally, passing between the mesenteric vessels, and the two vascularized hemi-loops of half diameter (Fig. 7.21a) are anastomosed isoperistaltically in an S-shaped or spiral fashion and to the distal bowel for complete bowel continuity.

Bipolar cut-coagulation diathermy with needlepoint forceps virtually eliminates blood loss (Fig. 7.21b), and manual suturing (author's preference) ensures accurate hemi-loop construction and anastomoses. LILT retains relatively normal intestinal muscle configuration, with effective peristalsis and forward propulsion, with a return of bowel function within 3–7 days. The reduced loop diameter avoids stasis and promotes a healthy adapting mucosa with increasing absorption over a longer length. Post-operative complications such as bowel necrosis, suture line dehiscence and leakage, fistula, and stenosis have been minimal and a consequence of faulty surgical techniques.

Serial Transverse Enteroplasty (STEP) Published in 2003 by Kim et al. [9], STEP uses a mechanical stapler, passed transversely between consecutive sets of mesenteric vessels and alternating serially along the mesenteric and antimesenteric aspects, to reduce loop diameter and increase bowel length (Fig. 7.22). Particular attention is necessary to avoid leakage at the tips of the staple lines.

The disruption to the intestinal muscle anatomy is marked and could potentially reduce effective peristalsis. In most instances, healing is uneventful, and patients have progressed to full enteral autonomy and weaned from parenteral feeding. Redilatation after LILT or STEP can be

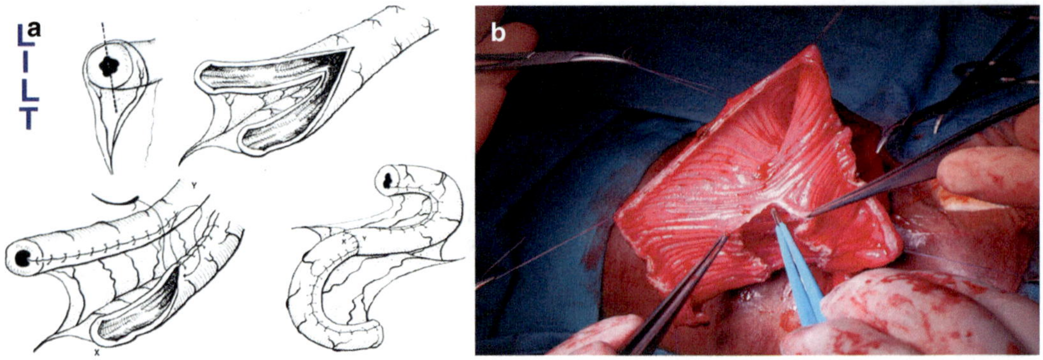

Fig. 7.21 (a) LILT (author's property). (b) Cutting bipolar diathermy

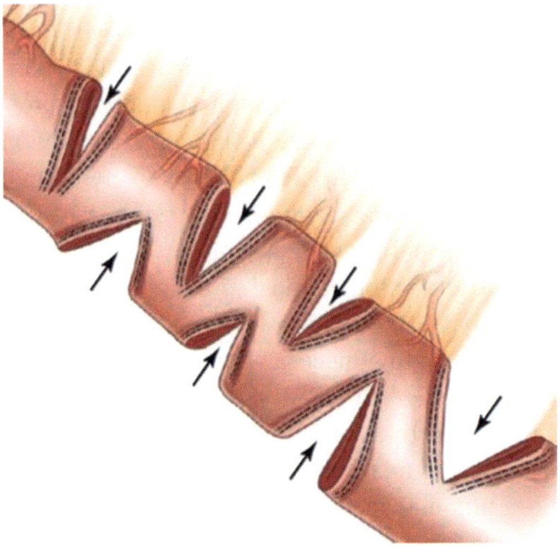

Fig. 7.22 (Author's property): Serial transverse enteroplasty (STEP)

managed by a 'second STEP' [10]. However, further significant disruption to the intestinal muscle may cause incoordinate or ineffective peristalsis.

Spiral Intestinal Lengthening and Tailoring (SILT) In 2013, Cserni et al. [11] proposed SILT to retain a more normal intestinal anatomy and avoid dissection within the mesentery. SILT cuts the dilated bowel spirally along its circumference, passing between the mesenteric vessels (Fig. 7.23). Bipolar cut-coagulation diathermy with needlepoint forceps ensures a clean bloodless cut. Longitudinal distraction and manual suture achieve a 60% isoperistaltic elongation and a significant reduction in loop diameter.

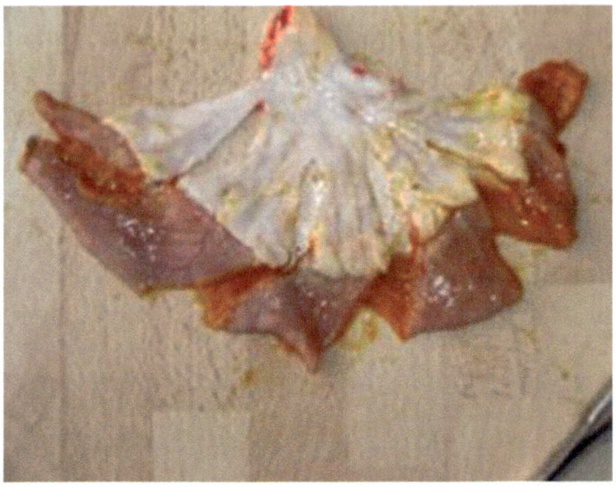

Fig. 7.23 Spiral enteroplasty—SILT

SILT respects intestinal muscle configuration and is well tolerated. It is particularly useful instead of LILT or STEP when bowel dilatation is not sufficient or can be combined with LILT or STEP during the same bowel reconstructive procedure.

Small Bowel Reversed Anteperistaltic Segments A single small bowel reversed(antiperistaltic) segment can slow transit and increase mucosal contact time and absorption while still avoiding bacterial overgrowth [12, 13]. The length of a reversed segment varies with the child's age and the nature of the residual bowel. Around 10–15 cm is a suitable length for a single reversed segment that is placed towards the distal end of the small bowel (Fig. 7.24).

Multiple judiciously spaced segments can further enhance absorption. Reversed segments can

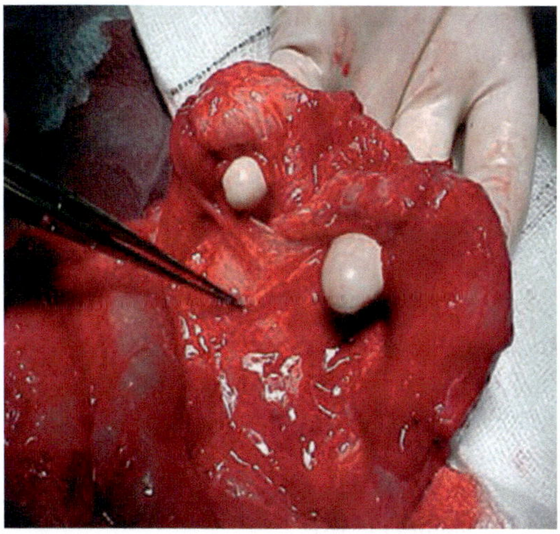

Fig. 7.24 12 cm small bowel reversed segment

be used alone or combined with lengthening procedures but are more often considered for persisting dependence on parenteral nutrition following reconstruction.

Long-Term Outcome from Bowel Reconstruction Extensive experience [14, 15] since 1981 confirms that bowel tailoring and lengthening procedures preserve all viable bowels, eliminate propulsive dysfunction and stasis, and promote effective isoperistalsis and a clean adaptive absorptive mucosa, such that many patients will dispense with parenteral nutrition and convert to full enteral nutrition within 3–12 months. The critical length of the dilated segment that can be expected to lead to enteral autonomy after lengthening is around 25–30 cm with at least half the colon. Shorter lengths also benefit from greater enteral absorption and a reduction in parenteral support and an improved quality of life. Some patients will achieve nutrient independence but continue to require fluid and electrolyte supplements. The longer-term outcome depends on the nature, adaptive potential, and specific functions of the residual bowel. An absence of ileum inevitably requires lifelong vit B_{12} supplements, and the lack of ileal-bile-salt-binding sites necessitates an oxalate reduced/free diet to limit the absorption and urinary excretion of unbound oxalates and the formation of urinary calculi. The ongoing attention of a specialist gastroenterologist is relevant throughout life to ensure normal growth and avoid nutritional deficiencies.

7.11 Pharmacological Management

(a) **Oral rehydration solution (ORS)**: rapid transit time with marked fluid and electrolyte losses causes dehydration and electrolyte imbalance, driving the kidneys towards fluid and electrolyte conservation. ORS provides additional fluid and a higher concentration of electrolytes to enhance hydration and renal function.
(b) **Opioids and cholestyramine**: loperamide and codeine slow propulsion, and cholestyramine, by binding diarrhoea-inducing bile salts, help towards increasing nutrient contact time and absorption. Higher oral doses are necessary to compensate for rapid transit through shorter bowel.
(c) **Clonidine**, given orally or by skin patch, can markedly improve absorption, significantly reduce losses, and favour enteral autonomy. A higher oral dose is necessary to compensate for rapid transit, and although both oral and patch doses are minimal, it is best to titrate the clonidine dose against any potential effect on blood pressure.
(d) **Glucagon-like peptide 2**: GLP-2, produced by the caecum and ascending colon, is a powerful mucosal stimulant that leads to an increased villus length with a greater number of cells per villus. Despite reduced single-cell absorption, the overall effect of the greater number of cells per villus is a major increase in nutrient absorption. Although GLP-2 analogues are highly effective during administration, the impact on the mucosa and on absorption is not always fully sustained once the drug is stopped. Long-term use and heavy mucosal stimulation can induce neoplastic change and requires monitoring. Presently, the drug is expensive and is not easily available.

7.11.1 Transplantation

The child with IF is a prime candidate for intestinal transplantation to restore enteral autonomy and remove the risks from long-term parenteral nutrition and central venous catheters. Transplantation requires a suitable donor, complex surgery, and skilled post-operative care. Donor organ availability can be an issue, as also is the size discrepancy between the child's smaller abdominal domain and adult bowel or liver-bowel grafts. Lifelong immunosuppression is essential to avoid acute graft rejection and graft versus host reaction (GVH). Post-transplant immunoproliferative disease (PTLD) is a constant threat that often recedes when immunosuppression is stopped, which then threatens graft function and survival. Constant monitoring is advisable because of the risk of sepsis and neoplasia. Chronic rejection is 'difficult' to treat and is a major concern that leads to loss of bowel function. Spontaneous graft tolerance not requiring immunosuppression is a rare phenomenon, and the induction of tolerance is not a consistent option.

There is a general agreement that transplantation should not be the first line of management for a child with intestinal failure but should be considered when there has been a loss of central venous access, irreversible liver injury, or poor-quality life after autologous bowel reconstruction. Appropriate early management of the IF patient attempts to avoid transplantation by establishing safe parenteral nutrition that avoids liver injury, careful central venous catheter management and preservation of central access portals, and judicious surgery for maximal preservation of autologous bowel for expansion and reconstruction (AGIR). Better enteral absorption from autologous bowel and reduced parenteral nutrition are compatible with a life of acceptable quality and are a lesser-risk alternative to transplantation.

At the present time, post-transplant patient survival is 76–92% at 1 year following bowel and liver-bowel transplantation, 60–65% at 5 years with a lesser figure, 57% for graft survival, and around 50% at 10 years. While the intestinal transplant is functional, patients benefit from not requiring parenteral nutrition but must often contended with episodes of acute rejection that require intricate management and detract from the quality of post-transplant life. Insidious chronic graft failure remains a major concern at 5–10 years post-transplant, which requires graft removal and a return to parenteral nutrition, with an option for re-transplantation. The issues surrounding transplantation, which are constantly updating, will not be discussed further [16]. It is, however, relevant to note that despite the morbidity and mortality, for those with no other options, transplantation is a potentially life-enhancing management [17, 18].

7.12 Conclusion

Over the last 50 years, the management of IF has been transformed [19] with refinements in parenteral nutrition, absorption and adaptation enhancing drugs, autologous gastrointestinal reconstruction, improvement in immunosuppression, and transplantation. However, even present techniques have grave limitations; indeed, 'the transplant donor must die for the recipient to live'!

The future lies in avoiding intestinal failure by better management as for S-NEC; further understanding of stem cell technology; restructured gene transfer to replace abnormal gene mutants, as in cystic fibrosis; less toxic immunosuppression; and induction of tolerance following transplantation. The urge to 'do more with autologous bowel' must remain the ultimate solution and a potent driver towards innovative AGIR techniques for bowel elongation and for growing new functional autologous tissue towards enteral autonomy.

In writing this chapter and in proposing the unconventional, I have attempted to stimulate the reader's imagination, and I have dared to hope that there will come a day when the patient with intestinal failure can look confidently to enteral autonomy and a normal life *on his own reconstructed bowel.* The ingenuity of great men, research, and a modicum of prayer promise a better future, transforming the despair of intestinal failure into the sumptuous reality of a 'gourmet meal and a glass of vintage wine'!

References

1. Pironi L, Arends J, Baxter J, Bozzetti F, Pelaez RB, Cuerda C, et al. ESPEN endorsed recommendations. Definition and classification of intestinal failure in adults. Clin Nutr. 2015;34:171–80. https://doi.org/10.1016/j.clnu.2014.08.017.
2. Bell MJ, Ternberg JL, Feigin RD, Keating JP, Marshall R, Barton L, et al. Neonatal necrotizing enterocolitis: therapeutic decisions based upon clinical staging. Ann Surg. 1978;187(1):1–7. https://doi.org/10.1097/00000658-197801000-00001.
3. Epelman M, Daneman A, Navarro OM, Morag I, Moore AM, Kim JH, et al. Necrotizing enterocolitis: review of state-of the art imaging finding with pathologic correlation. Radiographics. 2007;27:285–305. https://doi.org/10.1148/rg.272055098.
4. Bianchi A, Dickson AP. Elective delayed reduction and no anesthesia: minimal intervention management for gastroschisis. J Pediatr Surg. 1998;33(9):1338–40. https://doi.org/10.1016/S0022-3468(98)90002-1.
5. Bianchi A, Dickson AP, Alizai NK. Elective delayed midgut reduction—no anaesthesia for gastroschisis: selection and conversion criteria. J Pediatric Surg. 2002;37(9):1334–6. https://doi.org/10.1053/jpsu.2002.35003.
6. Touloukian RJ, Walker Smith GJ. Normal intestinal length in preterm infants. J Pediatr Surg. 1983;18(6):720–3. https://doi.org/10.1016/S0022-3468(83)80011-6.
7. Bianchi A. Intestinal loop lengthening—a technique for increasing small intestinal length. J Pediatr Surg. 1980;15(5):145–51. https://doi.org/10.1016/S0022-3468(80)80005-4.
8. Boeckman CR, Traylor R. Bowel lengthening for short gut syndrome. J Pediatr Surg. 1981;16(6):996–7. https://doi.org/10.1016/s0022-3468(81)80863-9.
9. Kim HB, Fauza D, Garza J, Oh J-T, Nurko S, Jaksic T. Serial transverse enteroplasty (STEP): a novel bowel lengthening procedure. J Pediatr Surg. 2003;38(3):425–9. https://doi.org/10.1053/jpsu.2003.50073.
10. Piper H, Modi BP, Kim HB, Fauza D, Glickman J, Jaksic T. The second STEP: the feasibility of repeat serial transverse enteroplasty. J Pediatr Surg. 2006;41(12):1951–6. https://doi.org/10.1016/j.jpedsurg.2006.08.015.
11. Cserni T, Varga G, Erces D, Kaszaki J, Boros M, Laszlo A, et al. Spiral intestinal lengthening and tailoring—first in vivo study. J Pediatr Surg. 2013;48(9):1907–13. https://doi.org/10.1016/j.jpedsurg.2013.01.048.
12. Pigot F, Messing B, Chaussade S, Pfeiffer A, Pouliquen X, Jian R. Severe short bowel syndrome with a surgically reversed small bowel segment. Dig Dis Sci. 1990;35(1):137–44.
13. Panis Y, Messing B, Rivet P, Coffin B, Hautefeuille P, Matuchansky C. Segmental reversal of the small bowel as an alternative to intestinal transplantation in patients with short bowel syndrome. Ann Surg. 1997;225:401–7.
14. Bianchi A. From the cradle to enteral autonomy: the role of autologous gastrointestinal reconstruction. Gastroenterology. 2006;130(2):S138–46. https://doi.org/10.1053/j.gastro.2005.09.070.
15. Greig CJ, Oh PS, Gross ER, Robert A, Cowles RA. Retracing our STEPs: four decades of progress in intestinal lengthening procedures for short bowel syndrome. American Journal of Surgery. 2019;217(4):772–82. https://doi.org/10.1016/j.amjsurg.2018.11.025.
16. Baradwaj S, Tandon P, Gohel TD, Brown J, Steiger E, Kirby DF, et al. Current status of intestinal and multivisceral transplantation. Gastroenterol Rep. 2017;5(1):20–8.
17. Abu-Elmagd KM, Armanyous SR, Fujiki M, Parekh NR, Osman M, Scalish M, et al. Management of 500 patients with gut failure at a single centre: surgical innovation versus transplantation with a novel predictive model. Ann Surg. 2019;270(4):656–74.
18. Abu-Elmagd KM, Kosmach-Park B, Costa G, Zenati M, Martin L, Koritsky DA, et al. Long-term survival, nutritional autonomy, and quality of life after intestinal and multivisceral transplantation. Ann Surg. 2012;256(3):494–508.
19. Jeppesen PB. The long road to the development of effective therapies for the short gut syndrome: a personal perspective. Dig Dis Sci. 2019;64(10):2717–35. https://doi.org/10.1007/s10620-019-05779-0.

Children with Obesity

8

Susann Weihrauch-Blüher, Oliver Mann,
Georg Singer, and Holger Till

8.1 Introduction

The pandemic of childhood obesity has continuously increased during the past decades, and especially morbid obesity in our youngsters still increases [1]. As in adults, the excess adipose tissue triggers multiple immunological and metabolic pathways, resulting in serious cardiometabolic comorbidities such as disturbed glucose metabolism leading to prediabetes or type 2 diabetes (T2DM), nonalcoholic fatty liver disease (NAFLD), hyperlipidemia, and hyperuricemia [2–4]. Importantly, many adolescents with severe obesity remain obese into adulthood and develop major cardiovascular morbidities in early adulthood [5]. Recent data, for instance, suggest that obesity that has already started in childhood is associated with a significantly higher risk of developing certain malignancies later in life [6, 7].

Obesity in childhood or adolescence is defined—as in adults—by the body mass index (BMI). However, percentiles are applied to define the degree of obesity. In pediatrics, overweight is classified as BMI ≥90th and <97th percentile, obesity as BMI ≥97th and <99.5th percentile, and extreme (morbid) obesity as BMI ≥99.5th percentile. Age- and sex-specific percentile curves are available for different nations and countries, and in Germany, percentiles by Kromeyer-Hauschild et al. are applied [8].

The therapy for childhood obesity is complex, and conservative lifestyle intervention programs remain the first line of treatment, representing the "gold standard" for therapy. However, the long-term success of lifestyle intervention programs for reducing weight remains disputed. A recent study has revealed that despite having multiple improvements in health measures, such as a reduction in sweet drink intake, BMI standard deviation score (SDS) reduction at 12 months was lost at 24 months in 121 participants (60% of participants at baseline) [9]. Moreover, a meta-analysis including 11 randomized controlled clinical trials indicated that long-term school-based interventions on physical activity and dietary habits received by children aged 6–12 years seem to have no effect on BMI [10].

As far as drug therapy in childhood obesity is concerned, the only available medication in

S. Weihrauch-Blüher
Clinic for Pediatrics I, Pediatric Endocrinology, University Hospital Halle (Saale), Halle, Germany
e-mail: susann.weihrauch-blueher@uk-halle.de

O. Mann
Department of General, Visceral and Thoracic Surgery, Medical Center Hamburg-Eppendorf (UKE), Hamburg, Germany
e-mail: omann@uke.de

G. Singer · H. Till (✉)
Department of Pediatric and Adolescent Surgery, Medical University of Graz, Graz, Austria
e-mail: georg.singer@medunigraz.at; holger.till@medunigraz.at

M. Lima, M. C. Mondardini (eds.), *Frailty in Children*,
https://doi.org/10.1007/978-3-031-24307-3_8

Europe so far includes metformin, which is licensed for children ≥12 years with already manifest T2DM and glucagon-like peptide-1 receptor agonists, representing the only medication in Europe licensed by the European Medicines Agency (EMA) in early 2021 for the treatment of pediatric obesity.

In addition to the abovementioned lifestyle intervention programs and drug therapies, metabolic-bariatric surgery (MBS) is a treatment option for morbidly obese adolescents following strict inclusion and exclusion criteria (see below) [3, 11, 12]. The current international recommendations and guidelines for MBS in adolescence are presented and discussed in the following chapter.

8.2 Indication for Bariatric Surgery in Children and Adolescents

MBS for adolescents was first reported in the 1980s but has only gained importance since around 2000. The American Society for Metabolic and Bariatric Surgery (ASMBS) Pediatric Committee has recently updated its guidelines [3] and has suggested that adolescents with class II obesity and a diagnosed comorbidity or with class III obesity should be considered for MBS [13]. A thorough preoperative evaluation including metabolic profiling should be performed by an interdisciplinary team. Moreover, sufficient education must be provided explaining the surgical interventions and the necessary postoperative lifestyle changes [13].

Indications for MBS in morbidly obese adolescents vary between countries within Europe. However, the European Association for the Study of Obesity and the European Chapter of the International Federation for the Surgery of Obesity agreed on interdisciplinary European guidelines on MBS in adolescents in 2013 [14]. According to these guidelines, bariatric surgery can be considered in adolescents

1. With a BMI >40 kg/m^2 and at least one confirmed comorbidity (see below)
2. Following at least 6 months of structured conservative therapy in a specialized center
3. Showing skeletal and developmental maturity (Tanner stage IV)
4. Capable of committing to comprehensive medical and psychological evaluation before and after surgery
5. Willing to participate in a postoperative multidisciplinary treatment program
6. Able to access surgery in a unit with specialist pediatric support (nursing, anesthesia, psychology, postoperative care)

Moreover, bariatric surgery can even be considered in genetic syndromes, such as Prader–Willi syndrome, but only after careful consideration by an expert medical, pediatric, and surgical team [14].

The German guideline published by the German Society for General and Visceral Surgery describes a BMI ≥35 kg/m^2 and at least one diagnosed somatic and/or psychosocial comorbidity as indications for bariatric surgery in children and adolescents. In patients with a BMI ≥50 kg/m^2, surgery can be considered even without any comorbidity. However, 95% of the predicted final height or Tanner stage IV should have been reached, and at least 6 months of unsuccessful conservative interdisciplinary lifestyle intervention should have been performed [15].

Exclusion criteria for bariatric surgery in adolescents include the following

- Severe psychiatric disorders (unstable psychosis, borderline personality, severe depression, and personality disorders) and diagnosed eating disorders
- Alcohol and/or drug abuse
- Pregnancy (present or planned within 18 months after surgery)
- Inability of the patient to participate in long-term interdisciplinary follow-up at the obesity center

Most multidisciplinary MBS programs recommend a protein-rich liquid diet to induce weight loss and decrease the liver size, which should be started already preoperatively. Such conditioning improves surgical safety, operative times, and intraoperative blood loss [12]. Before MBS, a comprehensive medical examination for existing metabolic and/or cardiovascular comorbidities and a psychosocial evaluation should be performed.

Surgery should be performed in a specialized facility, and treatment should be interdisciplinary, including a pediatric surgeon or bariatric surgeon with many years of experience in obesity and metabolic surgery (including in adolescents), a pediatrician, a dietitian, a psychologist, and a sports medicine specialist. In the first postoperative year, in particular, a standardized follow-up in a specialized obesity center with regular medical examinations, nutritional advice, and psychological care, as well as a supportive family environment, is essential.

8.3 MBS in Adolescents: Operative Procedures

According to present guidelines, MBS should be performed in high-volume centers specialized in the medical and surgical treatment of morbid obesity at any age. Thus, it seems highly advisable for pediatric surgeons to join a high-volume center for adult bariatric surgery. In the United States, the Metabolic and Bariatric Surgery Accreditation and Quality Improvement Program (MBSAQIP) requires for adolescent bariatric surgery that a children's hospital conducting fewer than 25 stapling cases per year invites an MBSAQIP-verified bariatric surgeon on each case [13].

Pathophysiologically, a fundamental distinction is made between the so-called restrictive versus malabsorptive procedures. Restrictive procedures "simply" tighten the stomach, for example, by placing an adjustable band around a small portion of the fundus [laparoscopic adjustable gastric banding (LAGB)]. This maneuver creates a pouch and a small channel into the remaining stomach. The volume of food passing through the band may be adjusted by changing the diameter of the band. The continuity of the gastrointestinal tract remains intact.

The Roux-en-Y gastric bypass (RYGB) remains the "gold standard" of all malabsorptive procedures. Technically, the stomach is resected close to the gastroesophageal junction, leaving only a small pouch of approximately 20 mL. A loop of the small bowel is anastomosed to this gastric pouch (alimentary loop), while the rest of the stomach, the duodenum, and the adjoining proximal small intestinal loops are initially excluded from the food route (biliodigestive loop). Further distal (100–170 cm), both loops are joined (common channel), allowing for the absorption of food.

Sleeve gastrectomy [laparoscopic sleeve gastrectomy (LSG)] serves both principles. Basically, the stomach is resected longitudinally, leaving a "restricted" volume of approx. 50–100 mL. This procedure was first recommended by the authors as a "stand-alone" technique for young adolescents in 2008 [16]. Metabolically, it is assumed that the resection of the gastric fundus also removes large parts of ghrelin production. Since ghrelin induces feelings of hunger in the central nervous system (arcuate nucleus), the removal of ghrelin-producing cells induced changes in eating behavior [17–19]. Valid studies have shown that it is almost as effective as RYGB for weight loss and improving comorbidities [20]. Thus, LSG has gained general acceptance and has become the most commonly performed MBS procedure in adolescents [3].

8.4 Results of MBS in Adolescents

8.4.1 Effects on Weight Status

Data for comparing clinical and metabolic outcomes for RYGB and LSG are available from the American Teen-LABS Consortium. These show a sustainable weight reduction of 27% in 242 adolescents (161 RYGB, 67 LSG, and 14 LAGB) after 3 years. There were no significant differences between RYGB and LSG (mean weight loss: RYGB 28% and LSG 26%). The adjustable gastric band (LAGB) performed worst (8%) [20].

Previous studies support these findings. A systematic review article and a meta-analysis on weight loss after bariatric surgery in adolescence have shown that the mean BMI difference between the initial examination at the time of the operation and the examination after 1 year was 13.5 kg/m^2 (95% confidence interval −14.1 to 11.9 kg/m^2). Weight loss was greatest after RYGB and least after treatment with an adjustable gastric band (AGB) [21].

However, these findings should be interpreted and discussed with caution since long-term data are not yet available for adults, and studies in adults with obesity who have undergone MBS have shown that many patients gain weight again after 3–10 years, regardless of the surgical method used [22].

8.4.2 Effects on Preexisting Comorbidities

In adulthood, LSG and LAGB have revealed similar efficacy at 1-year and 3-year follow-ups with regard to weight loss and the improvement of comorbidities [18]. In adolescents with obesity, initial results revealed a significant improvement in the preexisting T2DM, obstructive sleep apnea syndrome, bronchial asthma, NAFLD and dyslipidemia [23, 24]. More specifically, the preexisting T2DM has improved or even resolved in 90%, dyslipidemia in 66%, arterial hypertension in 74%, and impaired kidney function in 86% of affected adolescents, as shown in the Teen LABS study [20]. Ryder et al. demonstrated that in adolescents with severe obesity who are undergoing MBS, the risk of cardiovascular endpoints later in life has significantly improved [5]. These findings are comparable to long-term outcome data in adults after MBS [25–28].

In addition, an improvement in insulin sensitivity and glucose homeostasis, decrease in serum-free fatty acid levels, increase in the adiponectin/leptin ratio, and decrease in interleukin-6 and C-reactive protein have been reported in adolescents following MBS [29–32].

8.4.3 Complications

MBS is a high-risk operation and may induce distinct surgical complications. Basically, there are more "technical" complications with LAGB. In up to 30% of all cases, dislocations of the band or erosions into the stomach may be encountered, requiring revisional surgery. Paulus et al. have compiled the complication rate in bariatric surgery in adolescence in their current systematic review: complications occurred in around 11% of patients who received AGB, including dislodgement of the band and port revisions [33]. Due to the high rate of long-term revisional surgery, in adults, AGB has become a very rare procedure in the past years.

In malabsorptive techniques, the "principle may become a problem," meaning that malnutrition, vitamin deficiencies, or electrolyte imbalances may occur long-term. The most important and most frequent long-term complication in adolescents after bariatric surgery, however, are deficiency symptoms of vitamins or trace elements, which occur after all three surgical procedures. Deficiency symptoms should therefore be recognized and corrected before the operation. The most common vitamin deficiency symptoms following RYGB are vitamin B12 deficiency, thiamine deficiency, and vitamin D deficiency [34].

Vitamin deficiency remains an issue after MBS: as shown in the Teen-LABS study, 37% of adolescent patients had a vitamin D deficiency preoperatively, which persisted in 43% of the patients 3 years after RYGB and SG. A preexisting vitamin B12 deficiency worsened significantly 3 years postoperatively. Furthermore, 5% of the patients had an iron deficiency preoperatively, and 3 years postoperatively, this rate increased to 57% [20]. A lifelong vitamin substitution after bariatric surgery is therefore recommended and should be followed up during regular visits.

8.5 Discussion

MBS for the treatment of adolescents with morbid obesity has evolved from being a controversial issue to becoming a distinct recommendation within the past 20 years. Overall, laparoscopic Roux-en-Y gastric bypass (LRYGB) has been the most commonly used method to date in extremely obese adolescents [35–43]. Historically, the laparoscopically adjustable gastric band (LAGB) had also been used frequently [36]. LSG has gained general acceptance and has become the most common operation performed in morbidly obese adolescents [3].

Independent of the procedure applied, surgery should only be performed in high-volume treatment centers, and management should involve an interdisciplinary team experienced in the treatment and handling of adolescents with obesity, including postoperative care. An indication for MBS in adolescents requires strict international recommendations and guidelines, and the American Society for Metabolic and Bariatric Surgery (ASMBS) Pediatric Committee recommends that MBS should not be withheld from adolescents with severe comorbidities.

According to available data from adults, MBS can improve insulin resistance and secretion independently of weight loss by influencing gastrointestinal hormones. In some patients, a complete remission of T2DM occurred just a few days after bariatric surgery and thus before significant weight loss was recorded [44, 45], suggesting that MBS directly influences the hormonal control of the glucose balance [46]. However, additional factors, such as adherence to diet recommendations and genetic predisposition, seem to play a role as well [47, 48]. The highest remission rates in type 2 diabetes have been achieved after RYGB and after biliopancreatic diversion with duodenal switch (BPD/DS). Remission rates ranging between 40 and 100% have been described for the different surgical procedures, with gastric bypass appearing to have higher remission rates than the purely restrictive procedures [44, 46, 49]. BPD and BPD/DS can completely normalize diabetic metabolism in most patients [50]. The remission rates in type 2 diabetes reached an average of 76.8%; 38% after gastric banding, 84% after RYGB, and 98% after BPD with or without duodenal switch [51]. Procedures like BPD with or without duodenal switch are reserved for a minority of (very sick) patients, mainly due to their potential long-term complications—and in children and adolescents, only extremely limited data exist [45, 52, 53].

Available data and, especially, results from the Teen-LABS Consortium suggest that MBS may improve preexisting impaired glucose metabolism and other cardiometabolic comorbidities even in this age group of adolescent patients and can be even more effective than in adults [54–56]. However, data were to date mostly obtained from retrospective studies—with the exception of the Teens-LAB study. Long-term data on adolescents who have undergone MBS are still pending. There are still no definitive therapy recommendations, in particular on the bariatric methods suitable for children and adolescents. The implementation of randomized controlled clinical trials is therefore essential, and metabolic surgery as well as follow-up examinations should thus only be performed by specialized centers, which offer a long-term interdisciplinary treatment approach.

References

1. World Health Organization. Fact sheet on obesity and overweight. https://www.who.int/news-room/fact-sheets/detail/obesity-and-overweight. Accessed 29 Oct 2021.
2. Oberbach A, Neuhaus J, Inge T, Kirsch K, Schlichting N, Bluher S, et al. Bariatric surgery in severely obese adolescents improves major comorbidities including hyperuricemia. Metabolism. 2014;63(2):242–9. https://doi.org/10.1016/j.metabol.2013.11.012.
3. Pratt JSA, Browne A, Browne NT, Bruzoni M, Cohen M, Desai A, et al. ASMBS pediatric metabolic and bariatric surgery guidelines, 2018. Surg Obes Relat

Dis. 2018;14(7):882–901. https://doi.org/10.1016/j.soard.2018.03.019.

4. Lautenbach A, Wienecke JW, Stoll F, Riedel N, Mann O, Huber TB, et al. Bariatric surgery is protective against renal function decline in severely obese patients in the long-term. Obes Surg. 2021;31(3):1038–45. https://doi.org/10.1007/s11695-020-05096-w.
5. Ryder JR, Xu P, Inge TH, Xie C, Jenkins TM, Hur C, et al. Thirty-year risk of cardiovascular disease events in adolescents with severe obesity. Obesity (Silver Spring). 2020;28(3):616–23. https://doi.org/10.1002/oby.22725.
6. Llewellyn A, Simmonds M, Owen CG, Woolacott N. Childhood obesity as a predictor of morbidity in adulthood: a systematic review and meta-analysis. Obes Rev. 2016;17(1):56–67. https://doi.org/10.1111/obr.12316.
7. Weihrauch-Bluher S, Schwarz P, Klusmann JH. Childhood obesity: increased risk for cardiometabolic disease and cancer in adulthood. Metabolism. 2019;92:147–52. https://doi.org/10.1016/j.metabol.2018.12.001.
8. Kromeyer-Hauschild K, Wabitsch M, Kunze D, Geller F, Geiß HC, Hesse V, et al. Perzentile für den body-mass-index für das Kindes- und Jugendalter unter Heranziehung verschiedener deutscher Stichproben. Monatsschr Kinderheilkd. 2001;149(8):807–18. https://doi.org/10.1007/s001120170107.
9. Anderson YC, Wynter LE, O'Sullivan NA, Wild CEK, Grant CC, Cave TL, et al. Two-year outcomes of Whanau Pakari, a multi-disciplinary assessment and intervention for children and adolescents with weight issues: a randomized clinical trial. Pediatr Obes. 2021;16(1):e12693. https://doi.org/10.1111/ijpo.12693.
10. Cerrato-Carretero P, Roncero-Martin R, Pedrera-Zamorano JD, Lopez-Espuela F, Puerto-Parejo LM, Sanchez-Fernandez A, et al. Long-term dietary and physical activity interventions in the school setting and their effects on BMI in children aged 6–12 years: meta-analysis of randomized controlled clinical trials. Healthcare (Basel). 2021;9(4):396. https://doi.org/10.3390/healthcare9040396.
11. Pedroso FE, Angriman F, Endo A, Dasenbrock H, Storino A, Castillo R, et al. Weight loss after bariatric surgery in obese adolescents: a systematic review and meta-analysis. Surg Obes Relat Dis. 2018;14(3):413–22. https://doi.org/10.1016/j.soard.2017.10.003.
12. Thenappan A, Nadler E. Bariatric surgery in children: indications, types, and outcomes. Curr Gastroenterol Rep. 2019;21(6):24. https://doi.org/10.1007/s11894-019-0691-8.
13. Pratt JSA, Roque SS, Valera R, Czepiel KS, Tsao DD, Stanford FC. Preoperative considerations for the pediatric patient undergoing metabolic and bariatric surgery. Semin Pediatr Surg. 2020;29(1):150890. https://doi.org/10.1016/j.sempedsurg.2020.150890.
14. Fried M, Yumuk V, Oppert JM, Scopinaro N, Torres AJ, Weiner R, et al. Interdisciplinary European guidelines on metabolic and bariatric surgery. Obes Facts. 2013;6(5):449–68. https://doi.org/10.1159/000355480.
15. AWMF-Leitlinie Chirurgie der Adipositas und metabolischer Erkrankungen, Registernummer 088-001, Entwicklungsstufe S3, Version 2.3, 2/2018. https://www.awmf.org/uploads/tx_szleitlinien/088-0011_S3_Chirurgie-Adipositas-metabolische-Erkrankugen_2018-02.pdf. Accessed 29 Oct 2021.
16. Till H, Bluher S, Hirsch W, Kiess W. Efficacy of laparoscopic sleeve gastrectomy (LSG) as a stand-alone technique for children with morbid obesity. Obes Surg. 2008;18(8):1047–9. https://doi.org/10.1007/s11695-008-9543-6.
17. Kiriakopoulos A, Varounis C, Tsakayannis D, Linos D. Laparoscopic sleeve gastrectomy in morbidly obese patients. Technique and short term results. Hormones (Athens). 2009;8(2):138–43. https://doi.org/10.14310/horm.2002.1230.
18. Shi X, Karmali S, Sharma AM, Birch DW. A review of laparoscopic sleeve gastrectomy for morbid obesity. Obes Surg. 2010;20(8):1171–7. https://doi.org/10.1007/s11695-010-0145-8.
19. Till HK, Muensterer O, Keller A, Korner A, Blueher S, Merkle R, et al. Laparoscopic sleeve gastrectomy achieves substantial weight loss in an adolescent girl with morbid obesity. Eur J Pediatr Surg. 2008;18(1):47–9. https://doi.org/10.1055/s-2008-1038356.
20. Inge TH, Courcoulas AP, Jenkins TM, Michalsky MP, Helmrath MA, Brandt ML, et al. Weight loss and health status 3 years after bariatric surgery in adolescents. N Engl J Med. 2016;374(2):113–23. https://doi.org/10.1056/NEJMoa1506699.
21. Black JA, White B, Viner RM, Simmons RK. Bariatric surgery for obese children and adolescents: a systematic review and meta-analysis. Obes Rev. 2013;14(8):634–44. https://doi.org/10.1111/obr.12037.
22. Odom J, Zalesin KC, Washington TL, Miller WW, Hakmeh B, Zaremba DL, et al. Behavioral predictors of weight regain after bariatric surgery. Obes Surg. 2010;20(3):349–56. https://doi.org/10.1007/s11695-009-9895-6.
23. Messiah SE, Lopez-Mitnik G, Winegar D, Sherif B, Arheart KL, Reichard KW, et al. Changes in weight and co-morbidities among adolescents undergoing bariatric surgery: 1-year results from the bariatric outcomes longitudinal database. Surg Obes Relat Dis. 2013;9(4):503–13. https://doi.org/10.1016/j.soard.2012.03.007.
24. Alqahtani AR, Elahmedi MO, Al Qahtani A. Co-morbidity resolution in morbidly obese children and adolescents undergoing sleeve gastrectomy. Surg Obes Relat Dis. 2014;10(5):842–50. https://doi.org/10.1016/j.soard.2014.01.020.
25. Aminian A, Zajichek A, Arterburn DE, Wolski KE, Brethauer SA, Schauer PR, et al. Association of metabolic surgery with major adverse cardiovascular outcomes in patients with type 2 diabetes and obesity. JAMA. 2019;322(13):1271–82. https://doi.org/10.1001/jama.2019.14231.

26. Benotti PN, Wood GC, Carey DJ, Mehra VC, Mirshahi T, Lent MR, et al. Gastric bypass surgery produces a durable reduction in cardiovascular disease risk factors and reduces the long-term risks of congestive heart failure. J Am Heart Assoc. 2017;6(5):e005126. https://doi.org/10.1161/JAHA.116.005126.
27. Romeo S, Maglio C, Burza MA, Pirazzi C, Sjoholm K, Jacobson P, et al. Cardiovascular events after bariatric surgery in obese subjects with type 2 diabetes. Diabetes Care. 2012;35(12):2613–7. https://doi.org/10.2337/dc12-0193.
28. Sjostrom L, Peltonen M, Jacobson P, Sjostrom CD, Karason K, Wedel H, et al. Bariatric surgery and long-term cardiovascular events. JAMA. 2012;307(1):56–65. https://doi.org/10.1001/jama.2011.1914.
29. Schauer PR, Burguera B, Ikramuddin S, Cottam D, Gourash W, Hamad G, et al. Effect of laparoscopic Roux-en Y gastric bypass on type 2 diabetes mellitus. Ann Surg. 2003;238(4):467–84. https://doi.org/10.1097/01.sla.0000089851.41115.1b.
30. Min T, Prior SL, Dunseath G, Churm R, Barry JD, Stephens JW. Temporal effects of bariatric surgery on adipokines, inflammation and oxidative stress in subjects with impaired glucose homeostasis at 4 years of follow-up. Obes Surg. 2020;30(5):1712–8. https://doi.org/10.1007/s11695-019-04377-3.
31. Unamuno X, Izaguirre M, Gomez-Ambrosi J, Rodriguez A, Ramirez B, Becerril S, et al. Increase of the adiponectin/leptin ratio in patients with obesity and type 2 diabetes after Roux-en-Y gastric bypass. Nutrients. 2019;11(9):92069. https://doi.org/10.3390/nu11092069.
32. Wijayatunga NN, Sams VG, Dawson JA, Mancini ML, Mancini GJ, Moustaid-Moussa N. Roux-en-Y gastric bypass surgery alters serum metabolites and fatty acids in patients with morbid obesity. Diabetes Metab Res Rev. 2018;34(8):e3045. https://doi.org/10.1002/dmrr.3045.
33. Paulus GF, de Vaan LE, Verdam FJ, Bouvy ND, Ambergen TA, van Heurn LW. Bariatric surgery in morbidly obese adolescents: a systematic review and meta-analysis. Obes Surg. 2015;25(5):860–78. https://doi.org/10.1007/s11695-015-1581-2.
34. Saltzman E, Karl JP. Nutrient deficiencies after gastric bypass surgery. Annu Rev Nutr. 2013;33:183–203. https://doi.org/10.1146/annurev-nutr-071812-161225.
35. Pratt JS, Lenders CM, Dionne EA, Hoppin AG, Hsu GL, Inge TH, et al. Best practice updates for pediatric/adolescent weight loss surgery. Obesity (Silver Spring). 2009;17(5):901–10. https://doi.org/10.1038/oby.2008.577.
36. Jen HC, Rickard DG, Shew SB, Maggard MA, Slusser WM, Dutson EP, et al. Trends and outcomes of adolescent bariatric surgery in California, 2005–2007. Pediatrics. 2010;126(4):e746–53. https://doi.org/10.1542/peds.2010-0412.
37. Livingston EH. Surgical treatment of obesity in adolescence. JAMA. 2010;303(6):559–60. https://doi.org/10.1001/jama.2010.99.
38. Treadwell JR, Sun F, Schoelles K. Systematic review and meta-analysis of bariatric surgery for pediatric obesity. Ann Surg. 2008;248(5):763–76. https://doi.org/10.1097/SLA.0b013e31818702f4.
39. O'Brien PE, Sawyer SM, Laurie C, Brown WA, Skinner S, Veit F, et al. Laparoscopic adjustable gastric banding in severely obese adolescents: a randomized trial. JAMA. 2010;303(6):519–26. https://doi.org/10.1001/jama.2010.81.
40. Korenkov M, Sauerland S. Clinical update: bariatric surgery. Lancet. 2007;370(9604):1988–90. https://doi.org/10.1016/S0140-6736(07)61844-3.
41. Lawson ML, Kirk S, Mitchell T, Chen MK, Loux TJ, Daniels SR, et al. One-year outcomes of Roux-en-Y gastric bypass for morbidly obese adolescents: a multicenter study from the Pediatric Bariatric Study Group. J Pediatr Surg. 2006;41(1):137–43. https://doi.org/10.1016/j.jpedsurg.2005.10.017.
42. Sugerman HJ, Wolfe LG, Sica DA, Clore JN. Diabetes and hypertension in severe obesity and effects of gastric bypass-induced weight loss. Ann Surg. 2003;237(6):751–6. https://doi.org/10.1097/01.SLA.0000071560.76194.11.
43. Lanthaler M, Sieb M, Strasser S, Weiss H, Aigner F, Nehoda H. Disappointing mid-term results after laparoscopic gastric banding in young patients. Surg Obes Relat Dis. 2009;5(2):218–23. https://doi.org/10.1016/j.soard.2008.08.007.
44. Blackburn GL, Wollner SB, Jones DB. Bariatric surgery as treatment for type 2 diabetes. Curr Diab Rep. 2010;10(4):261–3. https://doi.org/10.1007/s11892-010-0118-2.
45. Schauer PR, Bhatt DL, Kirwan JP, Wolski K, Aminian A, Brethauer SA, et al. Bariatric surgery versus intensive medical therapy for diabetes—5-year outcomes. N Engl J Med. 2017;376(7):641–51. https://doi.org/10.1056/NEJMoa1600869.
46. Spanakis E, Gragnoli C. Bariatric surgery, safety and type 2 diabetes. Obes Surg. 2009;19(3):363–8. https://doi.org/10.1007/s11695-008-9687-4.
47. Anguita-Ruiz A, Bustos-Aibar M, Plaza-Díaz J, Mendez-Gutierrez A, Alcalá-Fdez J, Aguilera CM, et al. Omics approaches in adipose tissue and skeletal muscle addressing the role of extracellular matrix in obesity and metabolic dysfunction. Int J Mol Sci. 2021;22(5):2756. https://doi.org/10.3390/ijms22052756.
48. Krause C, Geissler C, Tackenberg H, El Gammal AT, Wolter S, Spranger J, et al. Multi-layered epigenetic regulation of IRS2 expression in the liver of obese individuals with type 2 diabetes. Diabetologia. 2020;63(10):2182–93. https://doi.org/10.1007/s00125-020-05212-6.
49. Maggard MA, Shugarman LR, Suttorp M, Maglione M, Sugerman HJ, Livingston EH, et al. Meta-analysis: surgical treatment of obesity. Ann Intern Med. 2005;142(7):547–59. https://doi.org/10.7326/0003-4819-142-7-200504050-00013.
50. Dixon JB, O'Brien PE, Playfair J, Chapman L, Schachter LM, Skinner S, et al. Adjustable gas-

tric banding and conventional therapy for type 2 diabetes: a randomized controlled trial. JAMA. 2008;299(3):316–23. https://doi.org/10.1001/jama.299.3.316.

51. Buchwald H, Williams SE. Bariatric surgery worldwide 2003. Obes Surg. 2004;14(9):1157–64. https://doi.org/10.1381/0960892042387057.
52. Hedberg J, Sundstrom J, Sundbom M. Duodenal switch versus Roux-en-Y gastric bypass for morbid obesity: systematic review and meta-analysis of weight results, diabetes resolution and early complications in single-centre comparisons. Obes Rev. 2014;15(7):555–63. https://doi.org/10.1111/obr.12169.
53. Yu J, Zhou X, Li L, Li S, Tan J, Li Y, et al. The long-term effects of bariatric surgery for type 2 diabetes: systematic review and meta-analysis of randomized and non-randomized evidence. Obes Surg. 2015;25(1):143–58. https://doi.org/10.1007/s11695-014-1460-2.
54. Inge TH, Prigeon RL, Elder DA, Jenkins TM, Cohen RM, Xanthakos SA, et al. Insulin sensitivity and beta-cell function improve after gastric bypass in severely obese adolescents. J Pediatr. 2015;167(5):1042–8 e1. https://doi.org/10.1016/j.jpeds.2015.08.020.
55. Inge TH, Zeller MH, Jenkins TM, Helmrath M, Brandt ML, Michalsky MP, et al. Perioperative outcomes of adolescents undergoing bariatric surgery: the teen-longitudinal assessment of bariatric surgery (Teen-LABS) study. JAMA Pediatr. 2014;168(1):47–53. https://doi.org/10.1001/jamapediatrics.2013.4296.
56. Brandt ML, Harmon CM, Helmrath MA, Inge TH, McKay SV, Michalsky MP. Morbid obesity in pediatric diabetes mellitus: surgical options and outcomes. Nat Rev Endocrinol. 2010;6(11):637–45. https://doi.org/10.1038/nrendo.2010.167.

9 Frailty in Children with Oncological Disease

Andrea Pession and Laura Ronchini

Children with an oncological disease are at a major risk of frailty from the moment of diagnosis; this risk increases during the treatment process and remains elevated in the follow-up period and over. Thanks to the progress in the treatment of childhood malignancies, the prevalence of childhood cancer survivors increases over the years, but consequently, also the prevalence of frailty increases [1, 2]. It is estimated that 1 in 600 young adults in western countries is a survivor of childhood cancer [3].

The prevalence of frailty among childhood cancer survivors has been estimated by Ness et al. in a report from the St. Jude Lifetime Cohort Study [1]. Using the criteria proposed by Fried et al. [4] (see below), the prevalence of frailty reported among 1922 childhood cancer survivors, with a mean age of 33.6 ± 8.1 years, was 13.1% among women and 2.7% among men, with rates increasing with age [1]. These rates are similar to those described among older individuals (age ≥65 years) [1, 5, 6]. These data highlights that frailty is a phenotype typical of ageing, which prematurely occurs in young adult survivors of childhood cancer [1, 5].

Frailty among childhood cancer survivors consists of a phenotype characterized by reduced physical, cognitive and psychological reserve and function. This condition implies vulnerability, increased susceptibility to developing chronic conditions, more frequent hospitalization, and reduced quality of life [5].

Frailty is the result of physical and cognitive impairment, consequent to the oncologic disease status, medications and procedures for the treatment of cancer, such as chemotherapy, radiotherapy and surgery.

At the diagnosis of neoplasia, frailty is a consequence of the disease, which confers an increased risk of other illnesses (infection, coagulopathy and other conditions depending on the site of cancer) and mortality.

Frailty increases during treatment; cancer therapies have a lot of side effects, like nausea and vomiting, loss of weight, alopecia, muscle weakness and acute illness, with an increased risk of organ damage, the onset of chronic conditions and mortality.

Cranial radiotherapy has a major effect on central nervous system structures, such as the hypothalamic–pituitary axis, resulting in an increased risk of frailty related to the relevant impact of these structures on development and physical and cognitive functions [5]. However,

A. Pession
Paediatric Unit, IRCCS Azienda Ospedaliero-Universitaria di Bologna, Bologna, BO, Italy
e-mail: andrea.pession@unibo.it

L. Ronchini (✉)
Paediatric Unit, IRCCS Azienda Ospedaliero-Universitaria di Bologna, Bologna, BO, Italy

Specialty School of Paediatrics, University of Bologna, Bologna, BO, Italy
e-mail: laura.ronchini@studio.unibo.it

M. Lima, M. C. Mondardini (eds.), *Frailty in Children*,
https://doi.org/10.1007/978-3-031-24307-3_9

not only children exposed to cranial radiation are at increased risk of frailty; every cytotoxic therapy may have a significant impact on vital organs and may have consequences on physical and cognitive functions over a lifetime, resulting in an increased risk of frailty [5].

The psychological aspect is also important because a child, who, until the day before, went to school, played with friends and stayed well at home with family without worries, suddenly finds himself having to face hospitalization, chemotherapy and surgery and no longer being able to go to school, play with friends and go about the daily activities.

However, the phase during which frailty becomes more prominent and represents a central problem in patients' life is during follow-up. Indeed, during this phase, the effects of therapies and the insults received during the active disease and treatment come to the surface, and the risk of incidence of chronic disease, disability and reduction of the quality of life becomes more evident.

Both neoplasia and cytotoxic therapies create an environment characterized by inflammation, oxidative stress, deoxyribonucleic acid (DNA) damage, telomere shortening and mitochondrial dysfunction [5, 7]. These biological effects result in the premature ageing of the cells and tissues, leading to an increased risk of the onset of chronic diseases, disability and mortality [5, 7].

The prevalence of frailty increases with age and is affected by an incorrect lifestyle. Sedentary life, a diet rich in fat, smoking, drinking alcohol and other bad habits contribute to cell ageing, increase the prevalence of frailty and, as a consequence, increase the incidence of chronic illnesses, hospitalization, poor fitness and mortality [5, 8].

It is important to monitor childhood cancer survivors with a specific screening program to early identify the subjects with signs of prefrailty or frailty, who are at major risk of developing chronic diseases and disabilities.

The definition of frailty phenotype proposed by Fried et al. [4] is composed of five indicators of reduced physiological reserve: (1) sarcopenia (low muscle mass), (2) weakness (decreased muscle strength), (3) poor endurance (self-reported exhaustion), (4) slowness (slow walking speed) and (5) low activity (poor physical activity) [4] (Table 9.1). By evaluating these conditions, we can define prefrail patients as subjects with two of these indicators and frail patients as subjects with three or more of these indicators [4, 5] (Table 9.1).

Table 9.1 Definition of prefrailty and frailty phenotypes, proposed by Fried et al.

(1) Sarcopenia (low muscle mass)	Prefrailty: the presence of 2 indicators
(2) Weakness (decreased muscle strength)	Frailty: the presence of 3 or more indicators
(3) Poor endurance (self-reported exhaustion)	
(4) Slowness (slow walking speed)	
(5) Low activity (poor physical activity)	

Prefrailty, a milder phenotype that precedes frailty, has a higher prevalence among survivors of childhood cancer [1]. The prevalence of prefrailty reported by Ness et al. was 31.5% among women and 12.9% among men [1]. These data suggest that a significant proportion of young adult survivors of childhood cancer lose physiologic reserve and are prefrail or frail; specifically, nearly 8% are frail and 22.2% are prefrail, with a higher prevalence of both phenotypes in women than men [7].

By identifying these high-risk patients, it is possible to adopt tailored strategies to prevent physical and/or psychological decline [5]. For example, neuromuscular involvement is one of the first signs of frailty, manifesting with a deficit in neuromuscular control, decline in muscle strength, weakness and low muscle mass [5]. Patients with one or more of these signs should be referred for tailored intervention with physical exercise and an active lifestyle [5]. The screening program has to be structured to identify these early dysfunctions and also chronic diseases (for example endocrinological, cardiological, pneumological, neurocognitive) to get an early diagnosis and implement correct treatment [5].

Also, adequate psychological support is useful to prevent the incidence of mental disorders, such as depression or anxiety [5].

Finally, the screening program has to guide patients in adopting a healthy lifestyle [5].

The consequences of cancer treatment, for which frail childhood cancer survivors are at a major risk, involve different organs and systems: the musculoskeletal system, cardiovascular system, respiratory system, endocrine system, and neurocognitive and psychological functions.

9.1 Musculoskeletal System

Muscle weakness, exhaustion, reduced exercise tolerance and sarcopenia are some of the first signs of frailty [1, 4, 5]. Reduced muscle mass and strength are typical of the frailty phenotype and have important implications on the quality of life. Muscle weakness in young adults results in reduced physical performance, with, consequently, limitations of daily activities, reduced exercise tolerance and a sense of frustration.

Reduced skeletal muscle mass is part of the alterations of body composition consequent to cancer treatment, characterized by a loss of lean body mass and sarcopenic obesity [9]. This phenotype is more frequent among young adults treated for childhood acute lymphoblastic leukaemia because of the high-dose glucocorticosteroid therapy [9]. The loss of muscle mass implies changes in muscle composition, leading to reduced muscle strength [9].

It is important that all children treated for cancer are offered tailored exercise programs to enhance muscle strength and prevent physical decline. It is also important, as mentioned above, to guide children and their families to adopt an active lifestyle during follow-up.

A deficit in bone mineral density is a common late effect of treatment for childhood acute lymphoblastic leukaemia [10]. The mainly responsible factors for a deficit in bone mineral density are glucocorticoids, alkylating agents and methotrexate [10]. Also, cranial and gonadal radiation therapy contributes to the impairment of bone mineral density, through the adverse impact on the hypothalamic–pituitary axis and gonadal function [10, 11]. Indeed, hormonal deficiency, in particular sex hormone and growth hormone deficiency, contributes to low bone mineral density [10, 11]. An adequate screening program is mandatory to ensure the early detection of hormonal deficiency and a prompt start of hormone replacement therapy, when necessary, to improve bone mineral density and prevent complications. Indeed, low bone mineral density leads to an increased risk of fracture, impairment in mobility, physical limitation, and pain [10]. Additionally, a healthy lifestyle, avoiding smoking and drinking alcohol and promoting physical activity are important to improve clinical outcomes.

9.2 Cardiovascular System

Cardiovascular diseases are possible complications of cancer therapies, both during treatment and during follow-up, as late effects [12]. The frequency of cardiovascular complications increases during years after antineoplastic treatment, up to 30 years after cancer diagnosis [12].

Childhood cancer survivors are at major risk of different heart and vascular diseases: congestive heart failure, myocardial infarctions, valvular abnormalities and pericardial disease [12, 13]. Death from cardiovascular disease is the leading non-oncologic cause of mortality among adult survivors of childhood cancer, who have a significantly higher risk of cardiovascular illness and death from cardiac events compared with matched-age healthy subjects [12].

The effects of chemotherapy on the myocardium and vascular structures are various and might be serious. Anthracyclines are the most notorious among cytotoxic agents for being cardiotoxic. The use of anthracyclines, in particular after exposure to a cumulative dose of 250 mg/m^2 or more, is associated with the onset of dilated cardiomyopathy, a chronic condition that may be progressive, leading to congestive heart failure [12]. Dilated cardiomyopathy is characterized by the thinning of the ventricular wall and the decreasing of myocardial contractility due to progressive myocardial fibrosis as a consequence of the loss of myofibrillar content, which occurs after anthracycline exposure [13, 14]. Dilated cardiomyopathy may occur early, up to many years after treatment with anthracyclines, and it is dose dependent [13, 14]. Risk factors associated with the onset of anthracycline-related congestive heart failure are young age during treatment, female gender and exposure to heart radiation [13].

Other antineoplastic agents may be cardiotoxic, such as alkylating agents, anti-metabolites, vinca alkaloids and biological agents [12].

Also, chest radiotherapy is responsible for heart and vascular damage; the described late effects of radiation therapy are myocardial fibrosis, pericardial alterations, arrhythmia, valvulopathy, coronary artery disease and heart failure [12]. The risk of cardiac sequelae from radiation therapy is higher in patients who have received a cardiac radiation dose of more than 1500 cGy [12].

Moreover, a sedentary lifestyle with low physical activity and a diet rich in fat and smoking are deleterious for cardiovascular function and contribute to the progression of impairment in cardiac function and vessel wall integrity. Hence, low physical activity and loss of lean body mass, part of the frailty phenotype in childhood cancer survivors, contribute to cardiovascular impairment and increase early cardiac morbidity and mortality.

Tailored ongoing monitoring is very important in childhood cancer survivors to identify also late-onset cardiovascular consequences of cancer therapies. An accurate physical examination and anamnesis of daily activities and lifestyle have to be associated with non-invasive tests (such as electrocardiogram and echocardiogram) to early detect signs and symptoms of cardiovascular diseases or an incorrect lifestyle and rapidly carry out interventions to prevent damage progression [13].

9.3 Respiratory System

The adverse effects of cancer treatment on the lung may consist of diminished pulmonary function, lung fibrosis, interstitial lung disease, restrictive and obstructive pulmonary disease, and pleurisy.

The respiratory complications of cancer therapies can be categorized into acute (during treatment), early (months after treatment) and late (years after treatment) effects [3].

Therapies responsible for pulmonary damage are chest radiation, busulfan, bleomycin, cyclophosphamide, nitrosoureas and chest surgery [15, 16], with a higher risk of pulmonary sequelae in patients undergoing a combination of pulmotoxic treatments [17]. The effects of these treatments add to other unfavourable conditions, such as infections or other organ impairment, and all these factors are responsible for an adverse pulmonary outcome [3].

The respiratory symptoms of lung impairment are chronic cough, shortness of breath, dyspnoea, reduced exercise tolerance, recurrent respiratory tract infections and need for supplementary oxygen [15]. Based on the severity of symptoms, pulmonary complications can be classified, grading from mild to life-threatening conditions, to implement appropriate treatments [3].

The occurrence of pulmonary injury is particularly evident as a consequence of chest radiation [3]. The adverse effects of radiation on the lung can be divided into three phases: an immediate effect is induced by oxidative stress, which causes DNA damage and cell apoptosis and creates an inflammatory environment; an inflammatory response conduce to a repair process, during which tissue remodelling occurs, and this results in fibrosis; the onset of a vicious circle of cell injury, inflammation and repair creates a hypoxic environment that enhances pulmonary injury and fibrosis, leading to chronic lung damage and chronic lung disease [3]. In the subacute phase (within months after radiotherapy), radiation injury may manifest as radiation pneumonitis, an inflammatory disease characterized by mild to severe dyspnoea and cough [3]. In the chronic phase (years after radiotherapy), lung fibrosis may occur; patients may be asymptomatic for many years and progressively develop symptoms (dyspnoea, hypoxemia, shortness of breath), which become more severe during years till the onset of a chronic respiratory failure, pulmonary hypertension and heart failure [3]. Pulmonary damage induced by radiation therapy is dose dependent [3].

Particular pulmonary complications, which deserve a separate discussion, are late effects of allogeneic haematopoietic stem cell transplantation (HSCT), which are caused by an immune-mediated mechanism, Graft versus Host Disease (GvHD) [3]. Idiopathic Pneumonia Syndrome and Bronchiolitis Obliterans Syndrome are immune-mediated lung diseases typical of the allogeneic HSCT setting [3].

Idiopathic Pneumonia Syndrome (IPS) occurs within weeks to months after HSCT and is characterized by alveolar damage with significant alterations at chest radiograph; patients present with cough, progressive dyspnoea and need for supplementary oxygen, without identification of an infectious aetiology [3]. Treatment is steroid based and the prognosis is poor [3].

Bronchiolitis Obliterans Syndrome (BOS) is a chronic obstructive lung disease, occurring months after HSCT with impairment in pulmonary function, an obstructive pattern, and alterations at high-resolution chest computed tomography (air trapping and ground-glass opacity); patients clinically present with cough, wheezing, exercise-induced shortness of breath and dyspnoea and reduced exercise tolerance [3]. Treatment is based on immunosuppressive agents [3].

During the conditioning regimen, pulmotoxic agents are used, in particular busulfan and cyclophosphamide; so the effects of lung injury secondary to treatment and immune-mediated pulmonary complications are often difficult to discriminate [3]. Additionally, in the HSCT setting, pulmonary infections (bacterial, fungal and viral infections) may contribute to lung injury and pulmonary dysfunction, thus, lung disease may be the consequence of all these multiple factors [3].

Overall, pulmonary late-effects of cancer therapies result in a reduced quality of life in survivors of childhood cancer, who may become limited in daily activities, with increased morbidity and mortality [15].

These patients have to be aware of the adverse effects of smoking and exposure to occupational agents on pulmonary functions and need to be monitored in a follow-up program to identify the onset of new respiratory symptoms, considering that the effects of cancer therapies may occur after many years and lung diseases, such as lung fibrosis, may remain asymptomatic for a long time and become symptomatic after years from the end of treatment [15].

Therapy-based screening programs, including complete medical assessment with lung function tests, to detect also asymptomatic pulmonary sequelae, should be adopted for a tailored follow-up of treatment-related complications [3]. A long-term follow-up is recommended for all childhood cancer survivors, who were exposed to pneumotoxic therapies, providing regular visits and pulmonary function tests at scheduled time points and whenever it proves necessary [3]. Identification of pre-symptomatic lung disease is important to implement a correct treatment and prevent the progression of respiratory dysfunction and the onset of symptoms [3].

9.4 Endocrine System

Hormone deficiency and metabolic disorders are possible late effects of cancer treatment, in particular after chemotherapy and cranial and gonadal radiation.

Female survivors of childhood cancer are at increased risk of premature ovarian failure (POF), especially survivors exposed to pelvic radiation and alkylating agents, with the highest risk in patients exposed to both these treatments, because of the synergistic deleterious effect between radiation and alkylating agents on gonads [18].

POF is a primary ovarian condition, which consists in premature depletion of ovarian follicles and compromises endocrine and reproductive ovarian function, before the age of 40 years [18, 19]. POF may manifest with absent puberty (primary amenorrhea) or interrupted puberty (secondary amenorrhea), according to the age and stage of puberty during cancer treatment [18]. POF may occur during cancer treatment or promptly after the end of therapy, but most frequently POF occurs years after treatment, during follow-up [18].

The laboratory signs of POF are decreased levels of gonadal hormones and increased levels of gonadotropins [19]; levels of anti-mullerian hormone (AMH), an indicator of the follicular reserve, are typically low and inhibin B, a predictor of follicular depletion, may lower before the rise of gonadotropins [19].

Clinically, patients with POF present with pubertal delay (absent menarche, absent development of secondary sexual characters and reduced growth velocity), if they were pre-pubertal children at the time of exposure to gonadotoxic therapies; whereas, the post-pubertal onset of POF is characterized by the disappearance of menstrual cycles [19].

POF results in impaired fertility and hormonal and metabolic imbalance (abdominal obesity, dyslipidaemia, impaired glucose tolerance and hypertension), which increases the risk of cardiovascular disease and reduced bone mineral density [18, 20, 21]. Moreover, POF is associated with the frailty phenotype [18].

Sex hormone replacement therapy to induce puberty and replace gonadal hormones' metabolic effects may be an option in the management of patients with POF [18, 19].

Growth hormone deficiency is another possible late effect of cancer treatment, especially after exposure to cranial radiation, as a result of the damaging effect of radiations on the hypothalamic–pituitary axis [13].

Growth hormone deficiency may result in short stature, altered body composition (reduced lean body mass and increased fat body mass), reduced bone mineral density and metabolic disorders, which increase the risk of cardiovascular disease [13, 22]. Indeed, childhood cancer survivors with growth hormone deficiency are at increased risk of obesity, hyperlipidaemia, hyperinsulinemia and hypertension, resulting in a higher risk of vascular alteration and cardiovascular events [13].

Obesity may be induced by growth hormone deficiency but this is not the only cause; obesity among childhood cancer survivors is the result of multiple factors: hormone deficiency, steroid therapy, physical inactivity and reduced energy expenditure, caused by low muscle mass, muscle weakness and reduced exercise tolerance [13].

Obesity and abnormal body composition are risk factors for insulin resistance and diabetes [13].

Other endocrine abnormalities may occur in childhood cancer survivors: thyroid dysfunction (both primary and secondary to TSH/TRH deficiency), adrenal insufficiency, hyperprolactinemia; endocrine disease secondary to impairment of anterior pituitary functions (growth hormone deficiency, TSH deficiency, ACTH deficiency, LH/FSH deficiency and gonadotropin-dependent precocious puberty) may occur especially in survivors of central nervous system tumours and in particular tumours involving the hypothalamic–pituitary region, as a result of the tumour mass effect, surgery and cranial radiation [22–25]. Childhood cancer survivors who were exposed to cranial radiotherapy to treat any type of tumour have been reported to be at increased risk to develop hypothalamic–pituitary disorders, as a result of irradiation involving the hypothalamic–pituitary area [26, 27].

In addition to hypothalamic–pituitary radiation, also chemotherapy with alkylating agents and intrathecal chemotherapy represent risk factors for the onset of hypothalamic–pituitary dysfunctions [22].

Growth hormone deficiency and LH/FSH deficiency are associated with frailty phenotypes, characterized by low muscle mass and poor exercise tolerance in survivors with growth hormone deficiency; slowness in survivors with LH/FSH deficiency and muscle weakness and low physical activity with low energy expenditure in survivors with growth hormone deficiency or LH/FSH deficiency [27]. Cognitive dysfunctions, in particular impairment of memory and processing speed, have been associated with growth hormone deficiency and TSH deficiency among childhood cancer survivors [22].

Hence, hypothalamic–pituitary disorders have been associated with physical and neurocognitive dysfunction in childhood cancer survivors; therefore, hormone replacement therapy may improve health outcomes and quality of life in this population [22].

Endocrine function testing and complete physical examination with particular attention to growth, body composition, body proportions and stage of puberty is an essential part of childhood cancer survivors' follow-up, in order to early detect endocrine system disorders and start an appropriate treatment if necessary.

9.5 Neurocognitive Function

Both neurological and cognitive adverse effects of cancer treatments have been reported in childhood cancer survivors.

Acute neurological complications may occur during treatment, such as vincristine-induced peripheral neuropathy, described in children during treatment for acute lymphoblastic leukaemia [13, 28]. This entity consists of painful distal polyneuropathy, involving both sensitive and motor nerve fibres [13]. Patients with peripheral neuropathy reduce physical activity and immobility contributes to muscle wasting, weakness and reduced mobility of the joints [13]. This condition was reported to be transient, but recovery may be delayed and in some cases incomplete; indeed, nerve injury may result in persistent deficits and long-term neuropathy [13, 29].

Acute neurotoxicity may be also consequent to intrathecal chemotherapy with methotrexate and cytarabine, leading to stroke-like syndromes, seizures, myelopathy and encephalopathy [13]. Systemic methotrexate contributes both to acute and long-term neurotoxicity of other central nervous system-directed therapies [13].

Long-term neurological impairment in childhood cancer survivors involves different functions: speech, balance and coordination, neurosensory functions, neuromuscular control and motor functions.

Speech may be compromised in survivors of posterior fossa tumours, as a result of surgical resection [23]. Cerebellar mutism, a phenomenon that may follow resection of cerebellar tumours is transient and is characterized by gradual recovery [23]. But neurological complications of posterior fossa tumours are not always transients; indeed, impairment in speech and reading may be persistent [23, 30]. Moreover, survivors of cerebellar tumours, who had not manifested cerebellar mutism, have been reported to exhibit ataxic dysarthria and slower speech, with increased incidence and exacerbation in patients exposed to cranial radiation [23].

Reading, walking, coordination and balance may be undermined in survivors of posterior fossa tumours because of the impairment of oculomotor function, as a result of the damage to essential structures involved in the coordination of eye movements [23, 31].

Visual impairment may occur in survivors of hypothalamic–pituitary tumours and the deficit may persist and deteriorate for years [23].

Also, hearing impairment may occur after treatment for childhood cancer; in particular platinum-based antineoplastic agents (cisplatin, carboplatin) may induce high-frequency hearing loss [23].

Additionally, survivors of brain tumours are at increased risk for late onset of epilepsy and migraine [23].

Cognitive functions may be impaired in childhood cancer survivors. In particular, memory, processing speed, executive function and attention may result compromised as a result of cancer treatment, especially in patients exposed to cranial radiotherapy, with a higher risk in patients who were exposed to radiation at a younger age, in particular younger than 6 years [13, 32]. After cranial radiotherapy, cognitive functions decline over time, suggesting accelerated ageing, which could increase the risk of early-onset dementia [32]. Histopathological effects of cranial radiation on central nervous system structures usually become evident months to years after radiation therapy and consist of subacute leukoencephalopathy and cortical atrophy [13]. White matter damage correlates with the severity of cognitive dysfunction [13].

Not only survivors treated with cranial radiation are at risk for neurocognitive impairment. Also, survivors of childhood cancer who were treated only with chemotherapy and not exposed to cranial radiotherapy are at increased risk for neurocognitive dysfunctions [13, 32].

Central nervous system tumours confer risk for cognitive impairment, which is affected by tumour size and location and surgical complications (e.g. vascular injury) [32].

Impairments of learning, memory and executive function have been reported in children with tumours of the supratentorial midline, also before radiation therapy [23].

Attention deficit is common among childhood brain tumour survivors, regardless of the type of received treatment [23]. Attention deficit disorder appears to worsen cognitive outcomes, exacerbating impairment of other neurocognitive functions, such as executive function and processing speed [23].

Neurocognitive impairment has an important impact on the quality of life of childhood cancer survivors, resulting in academic difficulties, lower educational achievement, difficulty in finding a job, marrying and independent living [13].

9.6 Psychological Function

A diagnosis of cancer is a cause of stress because turns life upside down and is associated with a fear of dying, therefore children and adolescents diagnosed with cancer are at risk for psychological disorders which may occur at the time of diagnosis but may also be late-onset and long-term.

Psychological experiences lived by the child and his family during the illness lead the patient into a parallel world, in which he is obliged to abandon all his habits and his daily life and where the protagonist isn't, often, himself anymore but his illness, and all the rest takes a second place. This is true, especially in adolescence, when the patient is fully aware of the gravity of the illness, the path of care that awaits him and the prognosis; in this case, illness often becomes fixed thinking in the patient's life. While cancer in childhood remains more confined and is lived more by the family than by children themselves because they maintain other interests, keep alive their desire for games, their curiosity, their cheerfulness and they don't allow the illness to become the protagonist of their life. One aspect to consider, though, is that cancer in childhood determines a completely different experience of childhood and occurring in a such crucial moment for the neurocognitive and character development of the child can have important consequences both from the emotional and the neuropsychiatric points of view. In addition, cytotoxic therapies and especially cranial radiotherapy can lead to consequences on neurocognitive development that are greater the younger the patient is.

A diagnosis of cancer is a traumatic event, so childhood cancer survivors may manifest posttraumatic stress symptoms and disorder, also many years after the end of treatments, during adulthood [33]. Reports documented that posttraumatic stress disorder occurs in 10–20% of childhood cancer survivors [33–35]. Young adult survivors of childhood cancer who develop posttraumatic stress disorder have a lower quality of life concerning their psychosocial well-being [33, 34]. Indeed, these patients experience emotional distress and psychological disorders, such as anxiety, depression, somatization, obsessive-compulsive behaviour, hostility, paranoid ideation and psychoticism [33]. Furthermore, survivors with posttraumatic stress disorder have more difficulties to achieve their life goals, such as attaining academic achievements, gaining employment and getting married and these dysfunctions may have a relevant impact on self-esteem and psychosocial health [33]. It has been reported that subjective perception of cancer disease severity, the intensity of treatments, late effects and their impact on quality of life is a determining factor in the occurrence of posttraumatic stress disorder, suggesting that subjective impressions have a more relevant psychological impact than the objective measures of the disease and treatment severity [34].

The psychological implications of a diagnosis of cancer during adolescence deserve a dedicated section. Adolescence is a vulnerable phase of development, during which children become more independent, establish a sense of self, and set their interests and future goals [36].

During this growing and developing phase, relationship with peers is crucial [36]. The diagnosis of cancer at this delicate stage leads to a disruption of daily life, isolation of the patient from friends and a return to dependence on parents, caused by the side effects of antineoplastic treatment, which make the patient weak and in need of constant support [36]. Moreover, the side effects of treatment, such as alopecia, diarrhoea, weight loss, nausea and vomiting, lead the patient to no longer recognize his or her own body and this situation increases stress and can cause anxiety and depression [36].

Also after completion of the therapeutic program, in adulthood, the survivor must face up the adverse effects of treatment, long-term complications, such as neurocognitive and endocrinological disorders, cardiopulmonary diseases and frailty phenotype and this can cause clinically relevant psychological disorders [36]. Another condition which represents a source of long-term stress is the so-called Damocles syndrome, characterized by the fear of a possible relapse of primary cancer or the onset of secondary malignancy [36].

Posttraumatic stress, depression and anxiety are common among young adult survivors of cancer diagnosed during adolescence [36]. Therefore, the effects of a cancer diagnosis on mental health don't limit to the diagnosis or treatment phases but they also persist in future, in adulthood and influence a patient's psychological development and mental health for a long time [36].

Particular attention to the onset of psychological disorders among adult survivors of cancer diagnosed during childhood and adolescence is mandatory during follow-up because psychological dysfunction as a result of a cancer diagnosis may occur also years after the completion of medical treatment and early psychological intervention is essential to ameliorate psychosocial outcome [36].

9.7 Secondary Malignancies

One of the most fearsome events in survivors of childhood cancer, along with the relapse of the first neoplasia, is the development of a secondary malignancy. Secondary malignancies in cancer survivors may occur from a couple of months to years after the end of treatments for first cancer. The vast majority of secondary malignancies occur years to decades after the completion of original cancer treatment, up to 30 years after the diagnosis of primary neoplasia, with higher rates within the first 10 years [37].

Risk factors associated with an increased risk for secondary malignancies in childhood cancer survivors are related both to possible genetic predisposition and adverse effects of cytotoxic therapies.

Therapy-related risk factors for secondary malignancies consist of exposure to chemotherapeutic agents and ionizing radiation.

Among cytotoxic drugs, alkylating agents and topoisomerase inhibitors are the main actors involved in secondary cancer predisposition [37]. Alkylating agents (e.g. cyclophosphamide, ifosfamide, busulfan, melphalan) are part of therapeutic regimens used to treat haematologic malignancies and solid tumours and for HSCT conditioning [37]. Treatment with alkylating agents increases the risk of secondary haematologic malignancies, specifically therapy-related acute myeloid leukaemia (t-AML); this entity typically occurs within 5–7 years after primary cancer treatment and in many cases is preceded by a myelodysplastic syndrome (MDS) [37]. The concurrent use of alkylating agents with epipodophyllotoxins may result in an even higher risk of t-AML [37].

The response to alkylating agents varies among individuals as a result of polymorphisms in genes encoding DNA repair proteins crucial for sensitivity to alkylating agents; therefore, further knowledge about this variability could result in the personalization of dosing regimen to minimize toxicity without compromising antineoplastic effect [37].

Also, topoisomerase II inhibitors, especially epipodophyllotoxins (such as etoposide), increase the risk of t-AML [37]. t-AML consequent to topoisomerase II inhibitors occurs with earlier onset compared to t-AML consequent to alkylating agents, typically within 2–3 years after treatment [37].

Exposure to etoposide is also associated with an increased risk of solid secondary malignancies in patients treated for bone tumours [37].

Radiation therapy is used to treat various types of solid and haematologic paediatric malignancies and may be part of the HSCT conditioning regimen in the form of total body irradiation (TBI). The increased risk of secondary malignancies in childhood cancer survivors treated with radiation is well documented [37, 38]. Secondary malignancies after radiotherapy generally occur after a long latency period (10–15 years after radiation therapy) [37]. Radiation-induced secondary malignancies typically consist of solid tumours which occur at the site of primary irradiation [37]. Breast and thyroid carcinoma, lung cancer, nonmelanoma skin cancer, bone and soft tissue sarcomas, and central nervous system tumours, such as meningiomas and gliomas, are some types of secondary neoplasms observed in survivors of childhood cancer treated with radiation therapy [37]. Considering the deleterious effects of radiation on organs and systems (endocrine system, cardiovascular system, respiratory system and neurocognitive function) and the high risk of secondary malignancies after radiotherapy, new therapeutic protocols to treat paediatric malignancies reduced radiation exposure and introduced innovative radiation techniques to minimize irradiation of healthy tissues, such as proton therapy [37].

A particular entity characteristic of patients undergoing HSCT is a post-transplant lymphoproliferative disease (PTLD), consequent to immunosuppression [37].

In paediatric oncology an aspect to consider is a genetic predisposition to cancer.

Germline mutations in cancer predisposition genes, responsible for childhood cancer predisposition syndromes, confer a high risk of malignancies. Children with cancer predisposition syndromes have an increased risk of developing cancer, multiple primary neoplasms may occur during their lifetime and also the risk of secondary malignancies, after primary cancer treatments, may be increased, as a result of increased susceptibility to the adverse effect of cytotoxic therapies.

Hereafter, some cancer predisposition syndromes are mentioned [39]

- Li–Fraumeni syndrome, caused by mutations in TP53 gene;
- Fanconi anaemia, caused by mutations in genes encoding proteins which are crucial in DNA repair;
- GATA2 deficiency, caused by mutations in GATA2 gene;
- Neurofibromatosis 1, caused by mutations in NF1 gene;
- Retinoblastoma predisposition, caused by mutations in RB1 gene;
- Noonan syndrome, caused by mutations in PTPN11 and other genes encoding proteins involved in the Ras/Raf/MAPK pathway;
- APC-associated polyposis conditions, caused by mutations in APC gene.
- Beckwith–Wiedemann syndrome, caused by alterations in the short arm of chromosome 15, in the region 11p15.
- DICER1 syndrome, caused by mutations in DICER1 gene;
- Down syndrome, caused by trisomy 21.

Jongmans et al. [40] proposed a selection tool to identify children with cancer with potential genetic predisposition for cancer [40]. This tool includes criteria involving five main items: family history of malignancies and/or consanguinity, type of childhood cancer, multiple neoplasms, congenital anomalies and/or signs and symptoms evocative of cancer predisposition syndromes, and increased treatment toxicity [40]. Children with cancer who meet one or more of these criteria deserve genetic counselling [40]. Recognition of cancer predisposition is essential to monitor patients and their families with a focused screening program [40].

Considering the high risk of secondary malignancies, which persists for many years after primary cancer treatment, all childhood cancer survivors have to be monitored over a prolonged follow-up period with tailored surveillance programs.

9.8 Conclusions

In summary, considering the advances achieved in the treatment of childhood cancer, there will always be more childhood cancer survivors and their life expectations will always be longer. But antineoplastic treatments aren't unfortunately without complications, which, as we have seen, can also last a long time with an impact on health and on life quality even after many years from the end of the therapeutic program. We understand, so, how important is an adequate risk stratification in paediatric oncology, to obtain an increasing personalized treatment, based on specific characteristics of neoplasia and of patient, to reach a satisfying antineoplastic efficacy with the least number of adverse effects, both immediate and long-term ones. It is also fundamental to understand, always better, the late effects of antineoplastic treatments and the frailty phenotype of childhood cancer survivors, to follow patients with an individualized program, early recognize problems and promptly act with the necessary support, to improve outcome.

References

1. Ness KK, Krull KR, Jones KE, Mulrooney DA, Armstrong GT, Green DM, et al. Physiologic frailty as a sign of accelerated aging among adult survivors of childhood cancer: a report from the St Jude lifetime cohort study. J Clin Oncol. 2013;31(36):4496–503.
2. Robison LL, Hudson MM. Survivors of childhood and adolescent cancer: life-long risks and responsibilities. Nat Rev Cancer. 2014;14:61–70.
3. Versluys AB, Bresters D. Pulmonary complications of childhood cancer treatment. Paediatr Respir Rev. 2016;17:63–70.
4. Fried LP, Tangen CM, Walston J, Newman AB, Hirsch C, Gottdiener J, et al. Frailty in older adults: evidence for a phenotype. J Gerontol. 2001;56(3):146–57.
5. Ness KK, Armstrong GT, Kundu M, Wilson CL. Frailty in childhood cancer survivors. Cancer. 2015;121(10):1540–7.
6. Collard RM, Boter H, Schoevers RA, Voshaar RCO. Prevalence of frailty in community-dwelling older persons: a systematic review. J Am Geriatr Soc. 2012;60:1487–92.
7. Ness KK, Kirkland JL, Gramatges MM, Wang Z, Kundu M, Mccastlain K, et al. Premature physiologic aging as a paradigm for understanding increased risk of adverse health across the lifespan of survivors of childhood cancer. J Clin Oncol. 2018;36(21):2206–15.
8. Delaney A, Howell CR, Krull KR, Brinkman TM, Armstrong GT, Chemaitilly W, Wilson CL, Mulrooney DA, Wang Z, Lanctot JQ, Johnson RE, Krull MR, Partin RE, Shelton KC, Srivastava DK, Robison LL, Hudson MM, Ness KK. Progression of frailty in survivors of childhood cancer: a St. Jude lifetime cohort report. J Natl Cancer Inst. 2021;113(10):1415–21.
9. Marriott CJC, Beaumont LF, Farncombe TH, Cranston AN. Body composition in long-term survivors of acute lymphoblastic leukemia diagnosed in childhood and adolescence: a focus on sarcopenic obesity. Cancer. 2018;124(6):1225–31.
10. Wilson CL, Chemaitilly W, Jones KE, Kaste SC, Srivastava DK, Ojha RP, et al. Modifiable factors associated with aging phenotypes among adult survivors of childhood acute lymphoblastic leukemia. J Clin Oncol. 2016;34(21):2509–15.
11. Gurney JG, Kaste SC, Liu W, Srivastava DK, Chemaitilly W, Ness KK, Lanctot JQ, Ojha RP, Nottage KA, Wilson CL, Li Z, Robison LL, Hudson MM. Bone mineral density among long-term survivors of childhood acute lymphoblastic leukemia: results from the St. Jude lifetime cohort study. Pediatr Blood Cancer. 2014;61(7):1270–6.
12. Mulrooney DA, Yeazel MW, Kawashima T, Mertens AC, Mitby P, Stovall M, Donaldson SS, Green DM, Sklar CA, Robison LLLW. Cardiac outcomes in a cohort of adult survivors of childhood and adolescent cancer: retrospective analysis of the childhood cancer survivor study cohort. BMJ. 2009;339:b4606.
13. Ness KK, Armenian SH, Kadan-Lottick NGJ. Adverse effects of treatment in childhood acute lymphoblastic leukemia: general overview and implications for long-term cardiac health. Expert Rev Hematol. 2011;4(2):185–97.
14. Adams MJ, Lipshultz SE. Pathophysiology of anthracycline- and radiation-associated cardiomyopathies: implications for screening and prevention. Pediatr Blood Cancer. 2005;44(7):600–6.
15. Mertens AC, Yasui Y, Liu Y, Stovall M, et al. Pulmonary complications in survivors of childhood and adolescent cancer. A report from the childhood cancer survivor study. Cancer. 2002;95(11):2431–41.
16. Visscher H, Otth M, Feijen EAML, Nathan PC, Kuehni CE. Cardiovascular and pulmonary challenges after treatment of childhood cancer. Pediatr Clin N Am. 2020;67(6):1155–70.
17. Mulder RL, Thönissen NM, van der Pal HJ, Bresser P, Hanselaar W, Koning CC, Oldenburger F, Heij HA, Caron HN, Kremer LC. Pulmonary function impairment measured by pulmonary function tests in long-term survivors of childhood cancer. Thorax. 2011;66(12):1065–71.
18. Chemaitilly W, Li Z, Krasin MJ, Brooke RJ, Wilson CL, Green DM, Klosky JL, Barnes N, Clark KL, Farr JB, Fernandez-Pineda I, Bishop MW, Metzger M, Pui CH, Kaste SC, Ness KK, Srivastava DK, Robison LL, Hudson MM, Yasui YSC. Premature ovarian insufficiency in childhood cancer survivors: a report from the St. Jude lifetime cohort. J Clin Endocrinol Metab. 2017;102(7):2242–50.

19. Beck-Peccoz P, Persani L. Premature ovarian failure. Orphanet J Rare Dis. 2006;1(9):9.
20. Daan NM, Muka T, Koster MP, Roeters van Lennep JE, Lambalk CB, Laven JS, Fauser CG, Meun C, de Rijke YB, Boersma E, Franco OH, Kavousi MFB. Cardiovascular risk in women with premature ovarian insufficiency compared to premenopausal women at middle age. J Clin Endocrinol Metab. 2016;101(9):3306–15.
21. Popat VB, Calis KA, Vanderhoof VH, Cizza G, Reynolds JC, Sebring N, Troendle JFNL. Bone mineral density in estrogen-deficient young women. J Clin Endocrinol Metab. 2009;94(7):2277–83.
22. van Iersel L, Li Z, Srivastava DK, Brinkman TM, Bjornard KL, Wilson CL, Green DM, Merchant TE, Pui CH, Howell RM, Smith SA, Armstrong GT, Hudson MM, Robison LL, Ness KK, Gajjar A, Krull KR, Sklar CA, van Santen HMCW. Hypothalamic-pituitary disorders in childhood cancer survivors: prevalence, risk factors and long-term health outcomes. J Clin Endocrinol Metab. 2019;104(12):6101–15.
23. Janss AJ, Mazewski C, Patterson B. Guidelines for treatment and monitoring of adult survivors of pediatric brain tumors. Curr Treat Options Oncol. 2019;20(1):10.
24. van Iersel L, van Santen HM, Potter B, Zhang H, Chemaitilly W, Conklin HM, et al. Clinical impact of hypothalamic–pituitary disorders after conformal radiation therapy for pediatric low-grade glioma or ependymoma. Pediatr Blood Cancer. 2020;67(12):e28723.
25. Zhou Z, Zhang S, Hu F. Endocrine disorder in patients with craniopharyngioma. Front Neurol. 2021;12:737743.
26. Follin C, Erfurth EM. Long-term effect of cranial radiotherapy on pituitary–hypothalamus area in childhood acute lymphoblastic leukemia survivors. Curr Treat Options Oncol. 2016;17(9):50.
27. Chemaitilly W, Li Z, Huang S, Ness KK, Clark KL, Green DM, et al. Anterior hypopituitarism in adult survivors of childhood cancers treated with cranial radiotherapy: a report from the St Jude Lifetime Cohort Study. J Clin Oncol. 2015;33(5):492.
28. Gomber S, Dewan P, Chhonker D. Vincristine induced neurotoxicity in cancer patients. Indian J Pediatr. 2010;77(1):97–100.
29. Ramchandren S, Leonard M, Mody RJ, Donohue JE, Moyer J, Hutchinson RGJ. Peripheral neuropathy in survivors of childhood acute lymphoblastic leukemia. J Peripher Nerv Syst. 2009;14(3):184–9.
30. Huber JF, Bradley K, Spiegler BJ, Dennis M. Long-term effects of transient cerebellar mutism after cerebellar astrocytoma or medulloblastoma tumor resection in childhood. Childs Nerv Syst. 2006;22(2):132–8.
31. Peeler CE. A review of visual and oculomotor outcomes in children with posterior fossa tumors. Semin Pediatr Neurol. 2017;24(2):100–3.
32. Krull KR, Hardy KK, Kahalley LS, Schuitema I, Kesler SR. Neurocognitive outcomes and interventions in long-term survivors of childhood cancer. J Clin Oncol. 2018;36(21):2181–9.
33. Meeske KA, Ruccione K, Globe DR, Stuber ML. Posttraumatic stress, quality of life, and psychological distress in young adult survivors of childhood cancer. Oncol Nurs Forum. 2001;28(3):481–9.
34. Rourke MT, Hobbie WL, Schwartz L, Kazak AE. Posttraumatic stress disorder (PTSD) in young adult survivors of childhood cancer. Pediatr Blood Cancer. 2007;49:177–82.
35. Lee Y, Judge S. Posttraumatic stress in long-term young adult survivors of childhood cancer: a questionnaire survey. Int J Nurs Stud. 2007;44:1406–17.
36. Seitz DCM, Besier T, Debatin K, Grabow D, Dieluweit U, Hinz A, et al. Posttraumatic stress, depression and anxiety among adult long-term survivors of cancer in adolescence. Eur J Cancer. 2010;46(9):1596–606. https://doi.org/10.1016/j.ejca.2010.03.001.
37. Choi DK, Helenowski I, Hijiya N. Secondary malignancies in pediatric cancer survivors: perspectives and review of the literature. Int J Cancer. 2014;135:1764–73.
38. Friedman DL, Whitton J, Leisenring W, Mertens AC, Hammond S, Stovall M, et al. Subsequent neoplasms in 5-year survivors of childhood cancer: the childhood cancer survivor study. J Natl Cancer Inst. 2010;102:1083–95.
39. Ripperger T, Bielack SS, Borkhardt A, Brecht IB, Burkhardt B, Calaminus G, et al. Childhood cancer predisposition syndromes—a concise review and recommendations by the Cancer Predisposition Working Group of the Society for Pediatric Oncology and Hematology. Am J Med Genet. 2017;173:1017–37.
40. Jongmans MC, Loeffen JL, Waanders E, Hoogerbrugge PM, Ligtenberg MJ, Kuiper RPHN. Recognition of genetic predisposition in pediatric cancer patients: an easy-to-use selection tool. Eur J Med Genet. 2016;59(3):116–25.

Part IV

Operational Improvement Strategies

Operational Improvements in Neonatal Surgery

10

Olivier Reinberg

10.1 Introduction

Frailty has been introduced as a common geriatric syndrome that embodies an elevated risk of decline in health and function among the elderly. Patients with frailty have a higher risk for postoperative complications and mortality, even after minor surgical procedures. As the population ages, geriatricians and public health practitioners try to understand and, if possible, beneficially intervene in factors and processes that put elders at such risk, especially the increased vulnerability of such group to stressors (e.g., heat and cold, infection, injury) [1, 2]. Despite the identification of frailty as a significant predictor of poor health outcomes in adults, there is currently no consensus on how to define, measure, and diagnose this syndrome. Several tools and scores to quantify physiologic stress for surgical procedures and predict outcomes have been suggested, but the ideal tool for use in a clinical setting is still missing.

The concept of frailty is new in children. Frailty in children and adolescents suffering cardiac [3] or neurosurgical [4] diseases or cancers [5] has, however, been studied due to the related increased risk of morbidity and mortality. On the other hand, neonates and infants, who bear particular risks of adverse outcomes, have scarcely been the subject of systematic investigation.

Frailty in neonates can be due to different conditions, with consequent different behaviors. Frailty may be innate to the neonate himself (i.e., preterm, small for gestational age), be linked to the particular conditions of the neonate (i.e., infections, malformations), or result from the impact of a surgical procedure (i.e., bowel resection and anastomose). Understanding the role of frailty in the neonate's diagnosis is further compounded by great differences associated with gestational ages (GAs) and birth weights.

Therefore, we are dealing with a heterogeneous group of patients sharing solely the common thread of frailty while presenting different surgical problems, various conditions, and a broad range of GAs and weights (see Table 10.1 for definitions [6]). The pediatric surgeon has to anticipate a multitude of potential complications, associated with either the original disorder or its prescribed medical and surgical treatment.

The purpose of this chapter is to give pediatric surgeons tools to evaluate the frailty of surgical neonates in order to minimize stress induced by the proposed surgery and ultimately improve its outcome.

O. Reinberg (✉)
Lausanne, Switzerland

M. Lima, M. C. Mondardini (eds.), *Frailty in Children*,
https://doi.org/10.1007/978-3-031-24307-3_10

Table 10.1 Definitions based on Ref. [6]

In this chapter, neonates will be defined as pre-, term, and postterm babies up to 1 month of life
A premature (preterm) infant is defined as a baby born before completing 37 weeks of gestation age (WGA)
A term infant is defined as a baby born after completing 37 weeks of gestation. A postmature (postterm) infant is one who has completed more than 42 weeks of gestation
A baby is designated to be small for gestational age (SGA) if he is under the tenth percentile for weight for gestational age
The normal birth weight for a term infant is defined as 2500 g
Low birth weight (LBW) is defined as an infant weighing between 1500 and 2500 g
An infant is designated as having very low birth weight (VLBW) if he is between 1000 and 1500 g
Extremely low birth weight (ELBW) is defined as a birth weight of less than 1000 g

10.2 What Is Neonatal Surgery?

Neonatal surgery is performed shortly immediately after birth or in the following days or weeks. Neonatal surgery is highly complex and, often, a risky procedure that involves a multidisciplinary team of specialists, including obstetricians, pediatric anesthetists, neonatologists, the neonatal intensive care unit (NICU) team, and pediatric surgeons. In some circumstances and if possible, a member of the ethical committee should be present (see below).

The operation must be the result of a joint team decision. While some procedures are, undoubtedly, lifesaving, the question is what quality of life is to be expected for the patient in both the short and long terms. The team must debate why the risk to operate on such frail neonate is deemed acceptable, in lieu of opting to postpone a surgical procedure to a later time when the infant becomes stronger. Alternatively, partial or incomplete surgery can be suggested to mitigate inherent surgical risks, for instance in the case of esophageal atresia (EA), in a very frail neonate. In such a case, we suggest a tracheo-esophageal fistula ligation alone without esophageal anastomosis to protect his airways until a total correction could be done. Petrosyan et al. have shown that staged repair in very low birth weight neonates may have a good outcome, with a significantly lower rate of anastomotic complications and overall morbidity [7]. Patients at the highest risk for necrotizing enterocolitis (NEC) are preterm low birth weight (LBW) infants. A certain number of these neonates suffer NEC and will require surgery. Due to a prevailing very severe infection, the conditions of these extremely fragile children are poor, and the mortality rate may reach 30–40% [8]. An option is to perform a stoma proximal to the first necrosis/peroration and a postponed anastomosis.

The concept of emergency procedures has evolved. Decades ago, EA or congenital diaphragmatic hernias (CDH) were operated upon at birth. Today, proper stabilization of the neonate in a NICU, dedicated investigations, and a consensual decision to operate are the rules, an approach that changed dramatically the prognosis. We do not operate anymore on a hypothermic baby with metabolic imbalances and with poor knowledge of his conditions due to incomplete preoperative workup.

10.3 A Very Special Population

Preterm birth accounts for 11% of all live births worldwide and is increasing in most countries [9]. In recent years, survival rates of even the most immature preterm infants have improved significantly, enabling pediatric surgeons to participate in the management of patients with very immature and unique physiology. Nonetheless, these infants are still at risk for neurologic sequelae that extend beyond the neonatal period [10]. About one fourth of survivors of extremely preterm birth suffer from relevant neurological impairment [11].

It is not surprising that pediatric surgeons have to deal with many preterm and LBW neonates since congenital anomalies and syndromes are associated with premature labor. In fact, many abnormal fetuses are spontaneously aborted early in pregnancy [12, 13]. Of those who are carried beyond the first half of pregnancy, more than half are delivered preterm [14, 15] and may have restricted intrauterine growth [16–18]. The strongest effect was seen for chromosome anomalies and central nervous system malformations, including neural tube defects [17] and also, for instance, in abdominal wall defects.

Major concerns are related to the risk of bleeding in the brain. Any condition that raises intracranial blood pressure (i.e., high-pressure ventilation, high pressure in the superior vena cava due to pneumothorax insufflation) may cause bleeding. Disruption of the coagulating factors related to surgical bleeding may impair an already poor coagulation.

Low birth weight (LBW) and *ipso facto* very low birth weight (VLBW) children bear a risk of poor growth and neurodevelopmental development *per se* [19]. Extremely low birth weight (ELBW) infants without anomalies are at significantly increased risk for neonatal morbidities, such as bronchopulmonary dysplasia and NEC, which compromise their ability to achieve adequate nutrition for growth [20]. The incidence of such neonatal comorbidities in ELBW infants with severe, life-threatening congenital anomalies is unknown. Children with ELBW born with major anomalies have nearly double the risk for neurodevelopmental impairment, a higher risk of poor growth, and about three times greater risk of rehospitalization when compared with ELBW infants without major anomalies. The extreme frailty of these ELBW infants had to be added to their pathologies, and their relatively poor outcomes need to be explained. There is evidence that these infants remain medically fragile after discharge from the NICU: 30% of infants with major anomalies were rehospitalized four or more times in the first year of life [19].

Continuous monitoring of neonatal brain activity using amplitude-integrated electroencephalography (aEEG) has become more and more widespread in recent years [21]. A field of clinical use of aEEG is the prediction of cerebral outcome after birth asphyxia in term infants. It has also been used before, during, and after neonatal surgery in pre- and full-term babies [22]. During anesthesia, depression of brain activity was seen, with background patterns ranging from flat trace to discontinuous normal voltage. After cessation of anesthesia, recovery to preoperative brain activity occurred within 24 h in 86% of the preterm and 96% of the term infants, respectively. This reduction was related to GA and the dose of sevoflurane.

10.4 Does Prenatal Diagnosis Modify Neonatal Treatment and Early Outcome of Frail Surgical Neonates?

Recent advances in imaging techniques, such as three-dimensional (3D) and four-dimensional (4D) ultrasound, fetal magnetic resonance imaging, noninvasive serum analyses screening, and molecular genetics, have all significantly improved the knowledge and management of the structural anomalies of the fetus in the prenatal period.

Prenatal diagnosis, which must be completed through a multidisciplinary meeting, shall be used to optimize fetal, perinatal, and postnatal management to define the best timing for birth and to assist in a cost/benefit analysis of an early delivery. Should the risk of premature labor exist, even if in an unexpected urgent scenario, prenatal diagnosis allows the team time to give medical treatment (steroids) to accelerate lung maturation.

Very few studies have been able to show the benefits of the prenatal diagnosis of congenital malformations for live-born infants. Quartermain et al. [23], and some other pediatric cardiac surgeons using the Society of Thoracic Surgeons Congenital Heart Surgery database, demonstrated the benefits of prenatal diagnosis in children with congenital heart disease, associated with significantly lower rates of preoperative risk factors for cardiac surgery. Garabedian et al. have studied the impact of prenatal diagnosis on outcomes based on a study of 469 babies born with different types of EA between 2008 and 2010 in France [24]. In their study, prenatal diagnosis did not interfere with the delay between birth and first intervention and with the neonatal treatment and 1-year outcome. Cases with antenatal detection had a higher morbidity rate, possibly related to the EA type, type I and/or long gap being more frequently diagnosed antenatally. The benefits of prenatal diagnosis were related to both antenatal parental counseling and the more frequent in utero transfer, thus minimizing the risk for the baby when transfer takes place in an incubator.

Garne et al. report an analysis of 14 registries within a sample of 1047 live-born infants bearing one or more gastrointestinal malformations (EA, duodenal atresia, omphalocele, gastroschisis, and diaphragmatic hernia) from the European Registration of Congenital Anomalies and Twins (EUROCAT, European registries of congenital malformations) database. Median GA at birth was lower in prenatally diagnosed cases for all five malformations, although not statistically significant for gastroschisis. The difference in GA at birth between prenatally and postnatally diagnosed infants with gastrointestinal malformations is sufficient to increase the risk of mortality for the prenatally diagnosed infants. They conclude that clinicians need to balance the risks of early delivery against the benefits of clinical convenience when making case management decisions after prenatal diagnosis. This may be because the benefits of prenatal diagnosis are outweighed by the problems arising from a lower GA at birth [25].

10.5 Neonates Undergoing Surgery are at Risk *Per Se*

Several studies demonstrated that neonates undergoing surgery have higher morbidity and mortality compared to older children and adults [26, 27]. A project of the American College of Surgeons National Surgical Quality Improvement Program Pediatric (ACSNSQIP-P) Participant Use File (PUF) aimed to compare risk-adjusted outcomes of neonates versus other pediatric surgical patients. The overall 30-day mortality rate for preterm neonates, term neonates, and nonneonates was, respectively, 4.9%, 2.0%, and 0.1%, and morbidity was 27.0%, 17.0%, and 6.4%. The study demonstrated that preterm neonates have a significantly increased risk of morbidity and mortality compared to nonneonates. There was no significant difference, however, between the outcomes of preterm neonates compared to term neonates [28]. The procedures with the most morbidity in the data set included enterectomy with anastomosis or enterostomy, CDH repair, gastroschisis repair, and ventriculoperitoneal shunt placement. The morbidity rate for these procedures ranged from 37 to 53%. Overall, the 20 most morbid procedures made up only 4% of the entire NSQIP-P PUF study cohort, though they accounted for 44% of the mortality and 11% of the composite morbidity of the cohort [28]. Different conclusions come from another study encompassing 18,437 infants less than 30 days old undergoing noncardiac surgical procedures. In-hospital mortality for premature infants was 10.5%, compared with 2.0% for full-term neonates. In addition to the risk category, the clinical variables improving the prediction of in-hospital deaths were prematurity, serious respiratory conditions, NEC, neonatal sepsis, and congenital heart disease [29]. Thus, it is not clear whether prematurity is a significant risk factor for mortality for neonates undergoing surgery or not.

Why is there such frailty in surgical neonates? The reason is that besides specific problems related to surgery and anesthesiology, the physiology of the neonate differs from children. The transition from intrauterine to extrauterine life requires major cardiovascular, respiratory, and immunologic changes and does not allow neonates to appropriately respond to the stress of a surgical insult [28, 29].

10.6 Identified Preventable Risk Factors

The frailty of surgical neonates can be evaluated preoperatively through cumulative risk factors related to pathology and the child's condition. The following factors must be considered risk factors for the potential occurrence of postoperative complications: vital organ impairment, thoracic or abdominal surgeries, preterm birth, low postconceptual age, and perioperative hemodynamic instability (defined by pre- and peroperative fluid bolus or inotropic agent use) [30,

31]. Michelet et al. studied the major nonsurgical postoperative complications following neonatal surgery [32]. They identified four factors as independent predictors of postoperative complications: postconceptual age of less than 40 weeks, a history of cardiac malformations, hyaline membrane disease or NEC, preoperative NICU stay at the time of surgery, and intraoperative fluid bolus administration. Interestingly, the type of surgery (including major surgeries or thoracic surgeries) and the duration of anesthesia (correlated with the duration of surgery, the invasiveness and complexity of patient preparation: central line placement) were not found to be predictive of nonsurgical postoperative complications in multivariate analysis. However, being aware of these factors may be helpful in perioperative preventive strategies.

Metabolic-functional frailty of the neonate can be impaired by an infected lung, pneumonia, and/or empyema [33]. These conditions can adversely affect a surgical procedure or may require a thoracic procedure per se. The causes of pneumonia in the neonatal period are mainly due to *Streptococcus agalactiae* (group B streptococcus), *Escherichia coli*, *Cytomegalovirus*, and *Listeria monocytogenes* [34]. The cornerstones of treatment are supportive care (analgesia, oxygen, fluid balance control) and adequate antibiotics [33, 34]. Pneumonia complicated by pulmonary necrosis, lung abscess, parapneumonic effusion, and empyema may need invasive treatment, including interventional radiology and surgical procedures. A balance of interests must be done between the risk taken during anesthesia and surgery under such conditions or the risk taken while waiting for improvement with time. Surgery on an infected lung can induce or aggravate, for instance, parapneumonic effusion, pleural empyema, or pulmonary necrosis, thus reducing the lung's ampliation, raising pulmonary pressure and leading to congestive heart failure. Infectious processes of the abdominal cavity can extend to the pleural cavity because of the presence of unclosed openings between the pleura and peritoneum in neonates.

However, the long-term outcome for children being operated on in spite of a lung infection is generally good, although recovery is usually more complicated and prolonged when compared with children without [33].

The spectrum of congenital lung diseases requiring surgery includes congenital pulmonary airway malformations (CPAM), intra- and extrapulmonary sequestrations, and symptomatic congenital lobar emphysema. Early surgery for prenatally diagnosed pulmonary malformations is indicated if symptoms such as respiratory or hemodynamic effects are present. In asymptomatic children, early resection was advocated to prevent pulmonary infections. The risk of infection until 3 months appears low. Stanton et al. [35] opined that asymptomatic antenatally detected infants developed symptoms later, at a median age of 6.9 months (range: 2–10 months). Pelizzo et al. [36] reported chronic inflammation in 50% of asymptomatic CPAM resected at 3 months of age. Therefore, thoracoscopic lobectomy or segmentectomy during the neonatal period remains desirable for asymptomatic cases but not as an early procedure. It may be safer by 2–3 months even in slightly symptomatic cases with mediastinal deviation, as long as the symptoms are mild enough to wait.

Pulmonary infections are favored by aspirations, not because of possibly infected gastric liquid in a nonfed baby but due to its irritative acid component on immature lungs, which may impair the child's ventilatory conditions. Thus, it is important to prevent aspirations, with efficient gastric aspirations before surgery, especially in ventilated neonates. In the case of a nonpatent esophagus, the tube must be placed in the upper pouch.

Infections play a major role in the frailty of neonates. Nosocomial risk exists, as demonstrated in French maternity departments (3% in postnatal beds). The incidence rates are 7.5–12.7% or 1.3–8.5 per 1000 days in neonatal care units and 14.2% or 11.7 per 1000 days in neonatal intensive care units (NICUs). Gram-positive cocci bloodstream infections are the most common nosocomial infections in the NICU, but viral gastroenteritis is more frequent in neonatal care units. Risk factors include low birth weight, small GA and intravascular catheter in the NICU, and, for viral nosocomial infections, visits and winter outbreaks [37]. Thus, patients entering the NICU can already be colonized. Therefore, antimicrobials are the most commonly prescribed drugs in the NICU but are, unfortunately, quite often used inappropriately with various short- and long-term effects, namely, the creation of multidrug-resistant pathogens. Neonatal infections from multidrug-resistant strains are associated with increased mortality, excessive cost, prolonged hospitalization, and therapeutic challenges [38]. Additionally, the colonization of newborns with these pathogens makes them a potential source of nosocomial outbreaks [39]. For all the above reasons, the rational use of antimicrobials in NICUs is imperative, and structured antimicrobial stewardship interventions should be in place.

The concept that the newborn infant emerges from a sterile environment is obsolete. In utero colonization may have major impacts on the developing mammal in terms of developing immunity and metabolism, which, with epigenetic modifications, will lead to diseases in later life. The personal microbial profile that develops during and after birth depends on the mode of delivery, the type of feeding (human milk vs formula), and various other environmental factors to which the newborn is exposed. During the last decade, published data suggest long-term effects of the overuse of antimicrobials during the neonatal period, through their effect on the intestinal microbiome, including the development of atopic diseases, colic, and NEC [40], and it also impairs the development of normal microbiota in the neonatal lung [41].

Preinfected children are predisposed to surgical site infections and increased morbidity and mortality. Few studies are exclusively dedicated to surgical infections in the NICU. A Canadian study reports on surgical site infections occurring within 30 days in a series of 724 infants who underwent 1039 surgical interventions between 2004 and 2009 [42]. The overall surgical site infection rate was 4.3 per 100 interventions, up to 19 per 100 dirty interventions. Very low birth weight infants were overrepresented as children with gastroschisis compared to other neonates.

Catania et al. conducted a meta-analysis on the same subject, including 48 studies (16,442 neonates, 946 surgical site infections; 5.7%) [43]. It shows that predictive factors for surgical site infection development were GA, birth weight, age at surgery, length of surgical procedure, number of procedures per patient, length of preoperative hospital stay, and preoperative sepsis. Conversely, preoperative antibiotic use was not significantly associated with the development of surgical site infections.

10.7 Where to Operate?

Neonates in need of surgery are traditionally transferred from the NICU to the main operation room (OR). The transportation of critical patients could worsen their clinical condition and increase the complication rate by up to 70% [44, 45]. This is mainly due to hypothermia, changes in variations in the heart rate and blood pressure, and accidental displacements of vascular accesses or endotracheal tubes. If transportation is unavoidable, we strongly advocate for the use of specially dedicated devices for neonatal transportation. If not available, cotton roll/aluminum foils/woolen cap and socks cover over the head and limbs should be used.

Since the 1980s, many teams have promoted surgeries performed inside the NICU, i.e., bedside surgery, to avoid adverse events during transportation and to provide continuity of care with the same intensive care team. Bedside surgery must achieve similar results to those done in the main OR. The benefits and risks of performing surgery on critically ill newborns in the NICU compared to those of conducting surgery outside the NICU have been widely reported in the literature. The first official survey from the Italian Society of Pediatric Surgery (ISPS) was dedicated to bedside surgery in neonatal intensive care units (NICUs) in Italy. Bedside surgeries were done in 34 Italian NICUs in 2020 [46]. Most of these neonates requiring surgery in the NICU are premature or LBW, may be on prolonged ventilator support, and/or suffer cardiorespiratory instability. The most frequently selected indications for surgery were pneumothorax, pleural effusion, pericardial effusion, central venous catheter positioning, intestinal perforation, patent ductus arteriosus ligation, and CDH.

Major surgeries, such as abdominal laparotomy drainage for NEC, are reported starting in 1977 [47], ligation of patent ductus arteriosus since 1982 [48], and cure of CDH since 1999 [49], even in VLBWI (<1000 g and/or <28 WGA) [50].

Besides common facilities (ventilator, oxygen, suction, monitoring), additional requirements for surgery in the NICU are needed, including instruments for major surgery brought from the main OR, sealing devices, radiant warmer, appropriate light, and sufficient space around the bed to ensure sterility.

Bedside surgery is not part of the guidelines of the British Association of Perinatal Medicine (Standards for Hospitals Providing Neonatal Intensive and High Dependency Care and Categories of Babies Requiring Neonatal Care). Nevertheless, the feasibility, safety, and cost-effectiveness of surgeries performed in the NICU have been proven and should be considered to minimize risks associated with transportation in frail neonates.

10.8 Surgery on Neonates

From a technical point of view, there are fewer differences between full-term and premature patients than between neonates and infants. Without entering into questions of specific techniques, we should point out that surgeries on neonates must be minimally invasive, even if not minimal invasive surgery (MIS) (laparoscopy, thoracoscopy, and closed surgeries through a visualization system): appropriate small instruments, binoculars, or microscopes are mandatory, i.e., "no touch handling."

Neonates are susceptible to heat loss because of their proportionally large surface area, low body-fat-to-body-weight ratio, and limited heat sink capacity due to their small size. They have poorly developed thermoregulatory mechanisms to adjust their body temperature to variations within the OR environment. Hypothermia during neonatal surgery may affect vital organs' circulation, such as cerebral, myocardial, and renal, and these organs are more sensitive to subsequent ischemia. In addition, poorer blood circulation requires an extra supply of calories, which, in turn, prompts the necessity of placing the neonate in a neutral (thermoneutral) environment, i.e., in a range of ambient temperatures suitable for an infant, at a minimal metabolic rate, to maintain a constant normal body temperature by vasomotor control. The core temperature must be monitored. In full-term neonates, the critical temperature ranges between 32 and 34 °C; in LBW infants, this critical range goes up to between 34 and 35 °C.

Factors contributing to hypothermia in the OR are the type and duration of surgery and the OR temperature before and during surgery. The operating room air conditioner must be off. The OR must be preheated, and frequent opening of the doors prior to and during surgery must be avoided. Different setups can be used to prevent hypothermia during neonatal surgery, including, for example, resorting to an automatic warming system, such as the use of a Bair-Hugger®. During open surgery, any exposed intestine or lung should be frequently irrigated with warm saline and wrapped in towels.

10.9 Minimal Invasive Surgery (MIS) on Neonates

Most congenital anomalies have been reported to be feasible and safe under MIS. The advantages of MIS have been widely reported: minimal surgical stress, better view, shorter stay in the NICU, less pain, and improved cosmetics. Nevertheless, neonatal MIS faces the surgeon with hemodynamic alterations generated by the insufflation of CO_2 to create a working space. These changes differ in neonates from older children and result in tissue oxygen delivery [51]. The data collected regarding alterations in cerebral oxygenation during laparoscopic procedures in children have been limited and nonhomogeneous [52, 53]. The use of near-infrared spectroscopy measuring perioperative brain oxygenation [regional cerebral oxygen saturation ($rScO_2$)] has significantly improved our understanding. For example, Tytgat et al. have studied the impact of neonatal thoracoscopic repair of EA with the insufflation of CO_2 at 5 mmHg. Intrathoracic CO_2 insufflation caused a reversible decrease in SaO_2 and pH and an increase in $paCO_2$. The $rScO_2$ was higher at anesthesia induction but remained stable, and within normal limits, during and after the CO_2 pneumothorax, which suggests no hampering of cerebral oxygenation by the thoracoscopic intervention resulting from changes in the ventilation [53]. It proves the importance of the rapid recognition of low cerebral perfusion and its prompt correction, with the main goal of avoiding negative postoperative neurodevelopmental outcomes following pediatric surgical procedures.

Our French-speaking group of MIS conducted a multicentric study based on the experience of eight pediatric surgery centers [54] to evaluate the safety, as well as the complication rate, of laparoscopy and thoracoscopy during the first month of life.

The observed complications and the surgical recommendations to prevent them are listed in Table 10.2. Significant risk factors for complications due to insufflation include the young age of the patient, low body temperature, thoracic insufflation, high insufflation pressure and flow, and the length of the surgery.

Table 10.2 Risk factors for neonatal MIS and prevention strategies [54]

Identified risk factor	Strategy for prevention
Patient's age	Careful evaluation in premature and VLBW
Low t° at the beginning of surgery	Prevent hypothermia during transportation
	Automatic warming system (Bair Hugger®)
High insufflation pressure	Low-pressure insufflation
Duration of insufflation	Low-flow and intermittent insufflation
Length of surgery >100 min	Preset length of surgery in agreement with anesthetists
	Monitoring of t°, PaO_2, and $ETCo_2$

A major point emerging from this study is that the neonate has a high and specific sensitivity to the insufflation of CO_2. Respiratory (hypercapnia, hypoxemia), hemodynamic, and thermic balances were altered in 12% of cases. It was possible to compensate for these imbalances through ventilatory adjustments, vascular expansion, and external warming. A pressure of 8 mmHg appeared to be the limit, beyond which the risk for poor tolerance to insufflation increased. At the beginning of our MIS practice in neonates, we were lacking working space and resorted to more insufflation than today. With experience and better port placements, we have proven that using intermittent low-flow and low-pressure insufflation avoids a rise in CO_2 and hypothermia.

10.9.1 Hypercapnia

A significant amount of CO_2 is absorbed through the distended peritoneal surface, resulting in frequent and potentially marked hypercapnia [55]. Due to the ratio surface/weight in neonates, the peritoneal and pleural absorption surface per unit of weight is high in neonates, resulting in hypercapnia. There are options to reduce hypercapnia using alternative insufflation gases such as helium, argon, nitrogen, or even air, but, alas, none of them dissolve as rapidly as CO_2, creating a potential risk of embolism. In addition, none are as cheap as CO_2.

Hypercapnia produces acidosis (7.4–6.9): $PaCO_2$ rises to a plateau in 15 min, and then pH falls with an associated decreased cerebral perfusion in the neonates (≈20%) [56]. Hypercapnia increases with pressure: at 5 mmHg insufflation, no effect is observed, while at 10 mmHg, hemodynamic instability and a decrease in cerebral perfusion/oxygenation are detected on piglets [56].

End-tidal CO_2 ($EtCO_2$) monitoring and subsequent compensation by appropriate ventilation is mandatory because it is correlated with high CO_2 arterial pressure ($PaCO_2$) and low pH and, consequently, may expose the infant to per-operative acidosis and the alteration of cerebral circulation. Cyanotic congenital heart diseases increase this risk.

10.9.2 Hypoxemia

Hypoxemia is the other secondary effect induced by MIS. It is observed more frequently with thoracoscopy than with laparoscopy due to the restriction on ventilation. Continuous monitoring of O_2 saturation, a high inspiratory fraction of O_2, and the use of minimal intermittent insufflation pressure prevent hypoxemia. With experience, we have limited ventilatory restrictions. For instance, when we did the first cure of EA (2000), single-lung ventilation via mainstem intubation and blockage using a Fogarty catheter was needed to improve visualization. Nowadays, with appropriate port placements, prone position, and intermittent low-pressure pneumothorax insufflation, we can dispense single-lung ventilation, and patients are conventionally intubated in the trachea and better ventilated on both lungs. Other teams experienced the same evolution with the same benefits; i.e., the changes observed in $PaCO_2$ and pH in the neonates undergoing thoracoscopic repair of EA/TEF were not significant [57]. Another concern is the risk of intracranial bleeding and correlated brain damage. The youngest the neonate is, the higher is the risk. A rise of pressure in the thorax, for instance, due to high-pressure pneumothorax, compromises venous return in the superior vena cava, thus inducing intracranial hypertension with a risk of bleeding. This is why we must carefully evaluate this risk with premature and VLBW children.

10.9.3 Hypothermia

MISs are closed procedures and, therefore, should prevent tissues from drying and cooling. However, they require gas (CO_2) insufflation from a bottle. Liquid gas, when expanded through the insufflator, comes dry and cold, contributing to cooling the child. Consequent hypothermia from insufflation is directly correlated with operating time in neonatal MIS. It was observed that a cutoff above 100 min triples the risk of adverse events [54]. Attempts have been made to heat and humidify the CO_2. A meta-analysis (Cochrane), including 22 studies, compared heated (with or without humidification) with cold gas insufflation in adult and adolescent populations undergoing laparoscopic abdominal procedures. Despite the small increase in core body temperature (of 0.31 °C) with heated CO_2 compared to the cold CO_2 group, the difference is unlikely to be of clinical significance and does not account for improved patient outcomes. Therefore, there is no apparent and clear evidence of a benefit in the use of heated gas insufflation, with or without humidification, when compared to cold gas insufflation. It should be noted, however, that because no neonate was included, we are lacking conclusive information [58].

10.10 Postoperative Care

10.10.1 Where Should the Surgical Neonates Be Nursed Postoperatively?

In 1999, the Surgical Services for the Newborn of Royal College of Surgeons strongly recommended that surgical neonates be concentrated in specialist pediatric surgical units that are adequately staffed with trained pediatric surgeons and medical and nursing personnel and fitted with the right equipment to care for these infants. In the case of preterm infants and those with complex congenital malformations, it recommended a multidisciplinary approach especially involving neonatologists and specialists in perinatal medicine/obstetricians [59]. But in 2008, a survey of neonatal surgical units in the UK revealed that surgical neonates were not following this recommendation and were managed in a variety of wards—medical NICUs, pediatric intensive care units, stand-alone neonatal surgical units, and pediatric medical/surgical wards [60].

This is not surprising as only a few surgical departments worldwide have enough cases to support a dedicated unit throughout the year, enough staff to devote sufficient time to medical care in addition to their surgical activities, and appropriate equipment to care for these infants. In most places, therefore, it is difficult to envisage dedicated neonatal surgical units being managed exclusively by pediatric surgeons.

The question raised by Ramji et al. is that since most of the preoperative and postoperative care of surgical neonates is similar to the medical needs of sick neonates, why not manage them in medical NICUs, with support from the surgeons? It is true that many of such physiological needs are similar to those of most medical NICUs. However, among all births with certain specialized needs, the medical and nursing staffs in medical NICUs have insufficient training and exposure to surgical neonates. Additionally, placing surgical neonates in nonsurgical units would dilute the pediatric surgeons' training and experience in managing these uncommon patients [61].

We believe that surgical neonates should be admitted to a NICU since the best-trained specialist to manage all types of neonates (LBW and VLBW, preterm and term babies) is the neonatologist [61]. Such a recommendation does not preempt the contribution of a minimum daily multidisciplinary staff. Neonatal surgical care modules and curricula must be developed, both for the trainees as well as for the nurses, to improve their expertise in the care of surgical neonates. Additionally, pediatric surgical nurses should be admitted to such a unit and ought to participate in the training of the nonsurgical team.

10.10.2 Early Refeeding

In neonatal surgical patients, proper nutrition must be delivered to meet their proportionately large energy requirements. It is important to continue providing developmental care during the postoperative period, as well as to offer positive oral stimulation for neonates who will not be able to feed enterally for some period after surgery.

Traditionally, enteral nutrition following abdominal surgery in children has been delayed to prevent complications. The use of *nil per os* (NPO) for extended periods of time, in particular on neonates with long-gap EA, gastroschisis, and congenital heart disease, should be abandoned. Parenteral nutrition prevents the development of malnutrition but increases the risks of sepsis and metabolic complications, and its high cost makes it a less desirable method for delivering calories when the gastrointestinal tract can be used [62].

Early enteral refeeding has been proven beneficial and is one of the recommendations of both the European (ESPGHAN) and the North American Society for Pediatric Gastroenterology, Hepatology, and Nutrition (NASPGHAN). We should not wait anymore for bowel movements to restart oral or enteral feeding after surgery, often on day 1.

In 2010, the Committee on Nutrition of the ESPGHAN published the following statements and recommendations [63]. Enteral nutrition support involves the delivery of nutrients via feeding tubes, as well as specialized oral nutritional supplements. Enteral nutrition support is recommended in a patient with at least a partially functioning digestive tract when oral intake is inadequate or the ingestion of normal food is inappropriate to meet the patient's needs. Enteral nutrition delivery may be gastric or postpyloric. Whenever possible, intragastric is preferred to postpyloric delivery of nutrients, and intermittent rather than continuous feeding, considering it is more physiological. However, continuous feeding has the advantage of providing more energy and better weight gain in selected groups of patients. Postpyloric access is indicated only in clinical conditions in which aspiration, gastroparesis, gastric outlet obstruction, or previous gastric surgery precludes gastric feeding or when early postoperative feeding after major abdominal surgery is considered. It should be noted, though, that transpyloric feeding offers no protection against aspiration, vomiting, diarrhea, or abdominal distention [64–66].

If and when available, a mother's breast milk or bank human milk should always be preferred to formula [65, 66]. The beneficial effects of breast milk have been demonstrated for term, near-term, and even LBW neonates [67], including improved cognitive skills, improved behavior ratings, and decreased rates of infection. In 1997 and 2005, the American Academy of

Pediatrics (AAP) published position statements recommending breast milk for premature and other high-risk infants by breastfeeding and/or using the mother's own expressed milk. We must empower mothers to continue providing human milk for their surgical neonate as human milk is often the key to enteral success after surgery. If not available, bank human milk should be used [65–69].

10.10.3 Enhanced Recovery After Surgery (ERAS®)

Guidelines by the ERAS® Society integrate evidence-based practices into multimodal care pathways, which have improved outcomes in multiple adult surgical specialties. A multidisciplinary pediatric ERAS group created in 2020 has recommended guidelines for perioperative care in neonates undergoing intestinal resection surgery [70]. Limited applications of ERAS in children have demonstrated reduced surgical infections, readmissions, reoperations, LOS, and cost [71–73].

The ERAS recommendations are summarized in Table 10.3 [70]. More recently, the benefits of ERAS protocols have been extended to the management of intubated neonates in the NICU. Wakimoto et al. compared 58 neonates intubated for a surgical procedure, of which 28 were extubated immediately and 30 were extubated in a delayed fashion. The delayed extubation group showed a higher overall incidence of adverse respiratory events, which led them to recommend extubation as early as possible after neonatal surgery [74].

Table 10.3 Enhanced Recovery After Surgery (ERASO) Society recommendations: guidelines for enhanced perioperative care in neonatal intestinal surgery [70]

Item	Recommendation	Quality	Strength
Surgical practices	Perform primary anastomosis as the first choice in patients with uncomplicated intestinal atresia	Very low	Weak
Antimicrobial prophylaxis	Administer appropriate preoperative antibiotic prophylaxis within 60 min prior to skin incision	Low	Weak
	Discontinue postoperative antibiotics within 24 h of surgery, unless ongoing treatment is required	Low	Weak
Preventing intraoperative hypothermia	Continuously monitor intraoperative core temperature and take pre-emptive measures to prevent hypothermia (<36.5 °C) and maintain normothermia	Low	Strong
Perioperative fluid management	Use perioperative fluid management to maintain tissue perfusion and prevent hypovolemia, fluid overload, hyponatremia, and hyperglycemia	Moderate	Weak
Perioperative analgesia	Unless contraindicated, administer acetaminophen regularly during the early postoperative period (not on an "as needed" basis) to minimize opioid use	High	Strong
	Use an opioid-limiting strategy is recommended in the postoperative period. Manage breakthrough pain with the lowest effective dose of opioid with continuous monitoring	Moderate	Strong
	Use regional anesthesia and acetaminophen perioperatively in combination with general anesthesia. Multimodal strategies including regional techniques should be continued postoperatively	High	Strong
	Provide lingual sucrose/dextrose to reduce pain during naso/orogastric tube placement and other minor painful procedures	High	Strong
Optimal hemoglobin	Restrict transfusions to maintaining HgB ≥90 (9 g/dL for a term neonate with no oxygen requirement. Term neonates within the first week of life, intubated or with an oxygen requirement should be transfused to maintain a HgB ≥110 (11 g/dL)	Low	Weak

(continued)

Table 10.3 (continued)

Item	Recommendation	Quality	Strength
	Use written transfusion guidelines and take into account not only a target hemoglobin threshold, but also the clinical status of the neonate and local practices	Low	Weak
Perioperative communication	Implement perioperative multidisciplinary team communication with a structured process and protocol ("pre- and postoperative huddle") utilizing established checklists	Moderate	Strong
Parental involvement	Facilitate hands on care and purposeful practice by parents that is individualized to meet the unique needs of parents early during the admission. Sustain these to build the knowledge and skills of parents to take on a leading role as caregivers and facilitate their readiness for discharge	High	Strong
Postoperative nutritional care	Start early enteral feeds within 24–48 h after surgery when possible. Do not wait for formal return of bowel function	High	Weak
	Use breast milk as the first choice for nutrition	High	Strong
	Monitor urinary sodium in all neonates with a stoma. Target urinary sodium should be greater than 30 mmol/L and exceed the level of urinary potassium	Low	Weak
Mucous fistula refeeding	Use mucous fistula refeeding in neonates with enterostomy to improve growth	Moderate	Weak

10.11 Complications

The Clavien-Dindo classification, applied to identify the presence of surgical complications within 30 days in neonates, showed a 23% incidence of at least one serious complication. The authors identified four independent risk factors for severe postoperative complications: reoperation, operation for CDH, preterm (<32 WGA), and abdominal surgery [75].

De Bruin et al. studied postoperative deaths after neonatal surgery in their institution during a 7-year period, including children of any age up to 18. Among 45,182 procedures, the all-cause 24-h hospital mortality was 13 per 10,000 anesthetics, while the all-cause 30-day in-hospital mortality was 42 per 10,000 anesthetics. In total, the passing of five patients was partially assigned to anesthesia, and in four patients, surgery was the partially contributing factor. Mortality was higher in neonates (38%) and infants (21%), in children with American Society of Anesthesiologists (ASA) physical status III and IV, and in emergency- and cardiothoracic surgery [75].

10.12 Long-Term Follow-Up of Frail-Operated Neonates

Concerns about favorable outcomes after neonatal surgery are not enough. Increasing interest has been raised regarding the incidence of neurodevelopmental delay in children with noncardiac congenital anomalies (NCCA) requiring neonatal surgery. In 2015, Stolwijk et al. undertook a systematic meta-search to determine the incidence of and potential risk factors for such outcomes [76]. The meta-analysis showed a cognitive score of 0.5 SD below the population average and delayed motor development in 25% of cases. Several of these studies report risk factors for psychomotor delay, including LBW, a higher number of congenital anomalies, the duration of hospital admission, and repeated surgery.

In a retrospective cohort analysis performed on 5920 extremely LBW neonates surviving beyond 12 h of life at 19 neonatal network centers between 1998 and 2001, those with significant anomalies were more likely to die before 18–22 months' corrected age. ELBW born with major anomalies have nearly twice the risk for neurodevelopmental impairment, an increased risk of poor growth, and more than three times greater risk of rehospitalization when compared with ELBW infants without major anomalies [19].

10.13 Surgery on Frail Neonates in Developing Countries

The World Health Organization (WHO) estimates that, globally, 150 million children suffer from some type of disability, most of whom reside in low- and middle-income countries (LMICs) with limited access to medical care [77, 78]. Great disparities exist in the accessibility to and the quality of pediatric surgical services between high-income countries (HICs) and LMICs. The incidence of congenital anomalies in LMICs seems to be between 3.9 and 11.8 per 1000 live births [79, 80]. Unfortunately, efforts to estimate the burden of pediatric surgical diseases in LMICs are limited by the rarity of population-based data. Subsequently, there is limited evidence on the incidence and predictors of neonatal mortality at the national level and on frailty in neonatal surgery.

According to a recent review aiming to determine the pattern of neonatal surgical conditions in Ghana [81], it appears that congenital anomalies are the fifth leading cause of under-five mortality. The overall mortality in the study was 13.5%, but congenital anomalies involving the digestive system including gastroschisis having the highest mortality rate (88%). Omphalocele (23.4%), gastroschisis (14.9%), and imperforate anus (n = 6, 12.8%) contributed to the most deaths. Birth weight was the most significant predictor of mortality. Neonates who were categorized as LBW (<2500 g) had three times the odds of dying when compared to those categorized as having normal birth weight. No EA and no CDH have been reported. However, there is a great disparity in the number of patients with treated EA, their number ranging from one to more than 80 patients per year in various neonatal surgical units in Africa [82]. According to Abdul-Mumin, "delayed access to care resulting in poor clinical condition on arrival, together with lack of neonatal surgical and anesthetic capacity, may have contributed to the higher mortality rates amongst neonates with digestive systems congenital anomalies." Misdiagnosis, delayed presentation of neonates with pneumonia, dehydration, and failure to feed are the rule in Africa [82].

A study has been done in Ethiopia, one of the countries with the highest neonatal mortality in Africa, that concerns neonates at large, not only those requiring surgery. Shorter birth interval (<18 months), small and large size at birth, no antenatal care visit, male sex, and twin births were significant predictors of neonatal mortality [83].

A Tunisian study (41 neonates, 2010–2017) recorded 24% of deaths during hospitalization. The highest rate of mortality was observed for CDH. Predictive variables of mortality were prematurity, LBW, the necessity of preoperative intubation, and duration of surgery of more than 2 h [84].

In a meta-analysis of publications on neonatal surgery in Africa (51 studies from 11 countries in the 1995–2014 period), the authors pointed out major documented challenges, such as delayed presentation and inadequate facilities in 39 studies (76.5%), lack of trained care team in 32 (63%), and the absence of NICU in 29 (57%) [85]. In spite of this demanding environment, they stated that improvements have been achieved in the outcomes of neonatal surgery in the past two decades [85].

Key reasons for the heightened mortality rates stem from a complex combination of social, cultural, economic, and geographic factors. In LMICs, many births occur at home, either with no attendants or with traditional birth attendants; pejorative cultural beliefs or ignorance about possible cures for defects may prevent families from seeking treatment. The local meaning of a disease or malformation differs according to cultural references. In many of them, it is not a personal concern that prevails but a collective one, and its management is multimodal [86]. If families do seek care, they must often travel great distances to reach medical facilities. Hypothermia following unsupervised transport over long distances is common. Delays in diagnosis for non-visible anomalies are the rule and are associated with misdiagnosed infectious diseases. Even neonates who are delivered in the hospitals are referred late to specialist centers, often not well resuscitated and transported in suboptimal conditions from far locations, on bad roads. These babies usually are hypothermic, septic, and hemodynamically unstable and frail on arrival at the referral centers.

These massive challenges are further exacerbated by the paucity of specialized care providers in LMICs. Most NICU units—if they exist—are not equipped for ventilation or parenteral nutrition for neonates or suffer incessant electricity outages [82].

Among the factors related to the children's condition, infection and prematurity play a major role in the poor outcome of neonatal surgery.

Neonatal sepsis, defined as a systemic infection in the first 28 days of life, encompasses bloodstream infections, meningitis, and pneumonia. It is the third most common cause of death among neonates, accounting for 225,000 deaths globally every year [87]. This seems to be a major concern in South Asia and sub-Saharan Africa, which have the highest burden of neonatal sepsis in the world, i.e., four to ten times higher than that in developed countries. Unlike high-income countries (HICs) with a predominance of group B *Streptococci*, Gram-negative germs predominate, possibly indicating the transmission of infections from the environment and healthcare providers. In addition, antimicrobial resistance has worsened in the last decade, with most antibiotics becoming ineffective. About 50–88% of common isolates from health facilities are resistant to first-line antibiotics—ampicillin and gentamicin [87, 88].

We have seen above how an infected lung can adversely affect a surgical procedure. Pneumonia represents the leading cause of mortality (more than two million deaths per year) in children less than 5 years of age worldwide [89]. Most cases of pneumonia occur in LMIC countries [90], where the problem of infection is a major concern, affecting the results of neonatal surgery. Sankar et al. call for urgent action to improve the quality of care at birth and implement antimicrobial stewardship in health facilities in South Asia, with the objective of reducing neonatal deaths from sepsis [88]. Among the proposals that directly involve pediatric surgeons, rational use of antibiotics is mandatory, i.e., avoiding unnecessary antibiotics, improving microbiology lab capacity, and obtaining blood cultures before the first dose [88].

Frailty is worsened by prematurity and low birth weight. Neonatal care in resource-limited LMICs differs significantly from the one afforded in HMIC settings. Therefore, it is not reasonable to extrapolate data from units in highly equipped countries. According to data collected in South Africa, results are surprisingly better than expected for children who survive the first hours/days, and birth weight or GA was not predictive of poor neurodevelopmental outcomes [91]. In fact, the results may reflect the low survival of babies with low birth weights: ventilatory support was not offered to infants with a birth weight lower than 900 g due to a very low survival percentage of infants with lower birth weights in these countries. The authors are silent on whether these LBW babies needed surgery, but results suggest no difference with highly equipped countries for those who survive long enough prior to entering an operating room.

It is an economic and moral imperative that global partners invest in pediatric surgery as a vital component for reducing the burden of diseases and malformations as a means to improve public health in LMICs. Healthy children are the single most important foundation and are the future of any society.

10.14 Teaching/Learning Surgery on the Frail Neonate

We have seen that the operating duration is correlated with adverse issues in neonates. Thus, the intervention timing and the skills of the surgeon play an important role. Consequently, the training of pediatric surgeons is part of the problem (or part of its solution?).

In 1989, the British National Confidential Enquiry into Perioperative Deaths (NCEPOD) in a report on perioperative pediatric deaths [92] recommended that "surgeons and anesthetists should not undertake occasional pediatric practice." This was also a statement of the European Union of Medical Specialists (EUMS) in 1995: "Surgeons taking care of children should have adequate training in a pediatric surgical unit. They should also continue to have regular exposure to this type of patients." Neonatal surgery should only be carried out by surgeons and anesthetists whose pediatric workload is of adequate volume to maintain a high level of surgical competence and allow the training of residents. Congenital birth defects complicate 3–6% of pregnancies, leading to live birth. As an example of structural birth defects associated with significant mortality/morbidity, CDH is among the most common anomalies, occurring in about one per 2000–3000 live births. Consequently, the opportunity of training—and keeping a desirable level of expertise—on CDH is low. Added to these facts, the combination of a shortened training period and the "new deal" on junior doctors about the accumulated number of hours has serious implications for training.

Nowadays, it is unacceptable to train on real frail patients. Advanced technologies, namely MIS and simulators, have been of great help in using simulation technology to reduce risks to both students and patients by allowing training, practice, and testing in a safe environment prior to real-world exposure. This is further supported by interest in the quality of care, restrictions on the use of animal models, limitations on the number of cases, medico-legal pressures, and cost-effective performance. Many models are available. The usefulness of mechanical simulators with faithful models has been proven efficient, for example, in EA [93, 94] or CDH [95]. They have facilitated shifting to realistic interactive models. Computerized modern technology with electronically assisted devices and virtual reality environments has provided new tools for mechanical simulation. Presently, there are tools to evaluate cognitive/clinical, technical, and social/interactive skills, which we have seen to be quite important in neonatal surgery. Surgical simulators (mechanical, computerized, virtual) and models (animals and interactive) are the right tools to learn, train, assess surgical skills, and keep the surgeon's expertise despite the small number of cases.

All this means that neonatal malformations need to be concentrated in centers to allow a sufficient caseload. There are arguments in favor of and against such large regional specialist pediatric centers. The benefits of centralization include the concentration of expertise, better-trained consultants on call, and more appropriate development of support services. The disadvantages include the burden of having children and their families far from their homes and the loss of expertise at a local level. The benefits of centralization, though, far outweigh the adverse effects of having to move children to a regional pediatric intensive care center [96].

Pediatric surgeons must ask their supervisory authorities to provide them with modern tools in order to avoid training on real babies. Although this is undoubtedly expensive, quoting Bok Derek from the Harvard Law School, "If you think education is expensive, try ignorance!" The major challenge faced by the new generation of pediatric surgeons is how to promote collaboration between pediatric surgical units and, in addition, how to create networks to expand the publication of multicenter prospective studies with adequate sample sizes.

10.15 Ethical Concerns

It is hard to conclude such a chapter without some ethical considerations. A couple of problems are involved: one, the relation between the surgeon, the parents or their representative, and members of the caregiver team and, the other, the way to handle new techniques.

Neonates are inherently unable to express their choice toward surgical procedures, and their parents or representatives are supposed to make such decisions based on the best interest of the child. Today, most discussions between the surgeon and the parents about an "unborn patient" take place before birth, during an antenatal consultation, usually in the presence of members of the caregiver team. The role of the surgeon is to explain the diagnosis, alternatives for treatment with their possible outcomes, potential complications, and long-term outcome.

For most pregnant women, receiving a prenatal diagnosis of any anomaly is frequently associated with intense feelings of shock and grief. The parents become frail themselves as this information ruins their expectation of a perfectly healthy child. During this time of crisis, parents are often faced with very, perhaps most, important choices about the pregnancy. They experience much stress and can quickly reach an information load saturation level that often translates into a need for multiple discussions. Levels of understanding, the cultural environment, and experience of professional support throughout this period of uncertainty, or even shock, can definitely impact decisions to be made and how they are subsequently perceived. If the "bad news" occurs once the child is born, this process is shortened by the urgent decision to be made, usually in the stressful environment of the NICU. Giving birth to a child with a life-limiting condition and deciding the possible termination of pregnancy for fetal anomaly are emotionally traumatic life events, both associated with psychological morbidity demanding appropriate support. In all cases, according to Nwomeh and Caniano [97], the following four elements must be a part of a fully informed process: (a) the physician to provide comprehensive information on which the decision to be made is supported; (b) a legal proxy is given to a person delegated to make decisions; (c) the named person demonstrates a full understanding of the intervention, including the indications, risks, and possible alternatives; and (d) written voluntary consent to the proposed intervention is agreed upon. In this process, good knowledge of frailty in neonates is mandatory to properly assess any increased risk of complications or poor issues.

When explaining proposed surgical procedures, we must consider that we are using new techniques rarely backed by randomized controlled trials. Broad evidence-based support for many of our interventions is missing due to the small number of patients and the lack of multicenter trials, especially if the results are affected by the variable frail conditions. Hall and Pierro have tried summarizing the evidence-based medicine (EBM) randomized controlled trial (RCT) (level I evidence) of some of the most common neonatal procedures. Their review highlights the fact that a quality evidence base supporting many of these interventions is lacking. Only a few randomized controlled trials have been done in neonatal diseases such as CDH, NEC, pyloric stenosis, and inguinal hernia. All of these trials have resulted from collaborations between pediatric surgical units firmly convinced of the importance of networks to promote multicenter prospective studies [98]. So how can we conduct an informed process if several parameters are lacking? We must refrain from saying "Everything will be fine"—a lie that will ruin parents' confidence. We must just be honest, tell the truth, and share what we know and what we ignore.

In the elderly, despite efforts over the past three decades and many suggested scales, an agreement on a standard instrument to identify frailty has not yet been achieved. Similar tools are still lacking for neonates, and we must keep working to develop them.

Acknowledgements My grateful thanks to Bernardo Fernandes for his help in reviewing the manuscript and for his wise comments and suggestions.

References

1. Hoogendijk EO, Jonathan Afilalo J, Ensrud KE, et al. Frailty: implications for clinical practice and public health. Lancet. 2019;394:1365–75.
2. Richards SJG, Frizelle FA, Geddes JA, et al. Frailty in surgical patients. Int J Color Dis. 2018;33(12):1657–66.
3. Panchangam C, White DA, Goudar S, et al. Translation of the frailty paradigm from older adults to children with cardiac disease. Pediatr Cardiol. 2020;41(5):1031–41.
4. Sherrod BA, Johnston JM, Rocque BG. Risk factors for unplanned readmission within 30 days after pediatric neurosurgery: a nationwide analysis of 9799 procedures from the American College of Surgeons National Surgical Quality Improvement Program. J Neurosurg Pediatr. 2016;18(3):350–62.

5. Ness KK, Armstrong GT, Kundu M, et al. Frailty in childhood cancer survivors. Cancer. 2015;121(10):1540–7.
6. Loretto G, Kelly M, Austin KM. Care of the surgical neonate. Oakbrook Terrace: American Pediatric Surgical Association; 2020. www.pedsurglibrary.com/apsa/view/Pediatric-Surgery-NaT/829030/all/view/Pediatric-Surgery-NaT/829030/all/Care_of_the_Surgical_Neonate
7. Petrosyan M, Estrada J, Hunter C, et al. Esophageal atresia/tracheoesophageal fistula in very low-birth-weight neonates: improved outcomes with staged repair. J Pediatr Surg. 2009;44(12):2278–81.
8. Raval MV, Hall NJ, Pierro A, Moss RL. Evidence-based prevention and surgical treatment of necrotizing enterocolitis-a review of randomized controlled trials. Semin Pediatr Surg. 2013;22(2):117–21.
9. Blencowe H, Cousens S, Oestergaard MZ, et al. National, regional, and worldwide estimates of preterm birth rates in the year 2010 with time trends since 1990 for selected countries: a systematic analysis and implications. Lancet. 2012;379:2162–72.
10. Saigal S, Doyle LW. An overview of mortality and sequelae of preterm birth from infancy to adulthood. Lancet. 2008;371:261–9.
11. Doyle LW. Neonatal intensive care at borderline viability— is it worth it? Early Hum Dev. 2004;80: 103–13.
12. Boué J, Boué A, Lazar P. Retrospective and prospective epidemiological studies of 1500 karyotyped spontaneous human abortions. Birth Defects Res A Clin Mol Teratol. 2013;97(7):471–86.
13. Creasy RK, Resnik R. Maternal-fetal medicine: principles and practice. 5th ed. Philadelphia: WB Saunders; 2004.
14. Holmes LB. Current concepts in genetics: congenital malformations. N Engl J Med. 1976;295(4):204–7.
15. Nelson T, Oakley GP, Shephard TH. Collection of human embryos and fetuses. In: Hook EB, Janerich DT, Porter IH, editors. Monitoring birth defects and environment: the problem of surveillance. New York: Academic Press; 1971.
16. Lindahl E, Michelsson K. Neurodevelopmental significance of minor and major congenital anomalies in neonatal high-risk children. Neuropediatrics. 1986;17:86–93.
17. Nikkilä A, Källén B, Marsál K. Fetal growth and congenital malformations. Ultrasound Obstet Gynecol. 2007;29(3):289–95.
18. Puccio G, Giuffré M, Piccione M, et al. Intrauterine growth restriction and congenital malformations: a retrospective epidemiological study. Ital J Pediatr. 2013;11(39):23–30.
19. Walden RV, Taylor SC, Hansen NI, National Institute of Child Health and Human Development Neonatal Research Network, et al. Major congenital anomalies place extremely low birth weight infants at higher risk for poor growth and developmental outcomes. Pediatrics. 2007;120(6):e1512–9.
20. Ehrenkranz RA, Younes N, Lemons JA, et al. Longitudinal growth of hospitalized very low birth weight infants. Pediatrics. 1999;104:280–9.
21. Rosen I. The physiological basis for continuous electroencephalogram monitoring in the neonate. Clin Perinatol. 2006;33:593–611.
22. Stolwijk LJ, Weeke LC, de Vries LS, et al. Effect of general anesthesia on neonatal aEEG—a cohort study of patients with non-cardiac congenital anomalies. PLoS One. 2017;12(8):e0183581.
23. Quartermain MD, Hill KD, Goldberg DJ, et al. Prenatal diagnosis influences preoperative status in neonates with congenital heart disease: an analysis of the Society of Thoracic Surgeons Congenital Heart Surgery Database. Pediatr Cardiol. 2019;40(3):489–96.
24. Garabedian C, Sfeir R, Langlois C, et al. Does prenatal diagnosis modify neonatal treatment and early outcome of children with esophageal atresia? Am J Obstet Gynecol. 2015;212(3):340.e1–7.
25. Garne E, Loane M, Dolk H, EUROCAT Working Group. Gastrointestinal malformations: impact of prenatal diagnosis on gestational age at birth. Paediatr Perinat Epidemiol. 2007;21(4):370–5.
26. Langham MR Jr, Walter A, Boswell TC, et al. Identifying children at risk of death within 30 days of surgery at an NSQIP pediatric hospital. Surgery. 2015;158(6):1481–91.
27. Saito JM, Chen LE, Hall BL, et al. Risk-adjusted hospital outcomes for children's surgery. Pediatrics. 2013;132:e677–88.
28. Bucher BT, Duggan EM, Grubb PH, et al. Does the American College of Surgeons National Surgical Quality Improvement Program pediatric provide actionable quality improvement data for surgical neonates? J Pediatr Surg. 2016;51(9):1440–4.
29. Lillehei CW, Gauvreau K, Jenkins KJ. Risk adjustment for neonatal surgery: a method for comparison of in-hospital mortality. Pediatrics. 2012;130:e568–74.
30. Stey AM, Kenney BD, Moss RL, et al. A risk calculator predicting postoperative adverse events in neonates undergoing major abdominal or thoracic surgery. J Pediatr Surg. 2015;50:987–91.
31. Catré D, Lopes MF, Madrigal A, et al. Predictors of major postoperative complications in neonatal surgery. Rev Col Bras Cir. 2013;40:363–9.
32. Michelet D, Brasher C, Ben Kaddour H, et al. Postoperative complications following neonatal and infant surgery: common events and predictive factors. Anaesth Crit Care Pain Med. 2017;36(3):163–9.
33. Loizzi M, De Palma A, Pagliarulo V, et al. Pulmonary infections of surgical interest in childhood. Thorac Surg Clin. 2012;22(3):387–401.
34. Thomas MF, Spencer DA. Management and complications of pneumonia. Pediatr Child Health. 2011;21(5):207–12.
35. Stanton M, Njere I, Ade-Ajayi N, et al. Systematic review and meta-analysis of the postnatal management of congenital cystic lung lesions. J Pediatr Surg. 2009;44:1027–33.

36. Pelizzo G, Barbi E, Codrich D, et al. Chronic inflammation in congenital cystic adenomatoid malformations. An underestimated risk factor? J Pediatr Surg. 2009;44:616–9.
37. Lachassinne E, Letamendia-Richard E, Gaudelus J. Epidémiologie des infections nosocomiales en néonatalogie [Epidemiology of nosocomial infections in neonates]. Arch Pediatr. 2004;11(3):229–33.
38. Stone PW, Gupta A, Loughrey M, et al. Attributable costs and length of stay of an extended-spectrum beta-lactamase-producing *Klebsiella pneumoniae* outbreak in a neonatal intensive care unit. Infect Control Hosp Epidemiol. 2003;24(8):601–6.
39. Gupta A, Della-Latta P, Todd B, et al. Outbreak of extended-spectrum beta-lactamase-producing *Klebsiella pneumoniae* in a neonatal intensive care unit linked to artificial nails. Infect Control Hosp Epidemiol. 2004;25(3):210–5.
40. Penders J, Kummeling I, Thijs C. Infant antibiotic use and wheeze and asthma risk: a systematic review and meta-analysis. Eur Respir J. 2011;38(2):295–302.
41. Gollwitzer ES, Saglani S, Trompette A, et al. Lung microbiota promotes tolerance to allergens in neonates via PD-L1. Nat Med. 2014;20(6):642–7.
42. Segal I, Kang C, Albersheim SG, et al. Surgical site infections in infants admitted to the neonatal intensive care unit. J Pediatr Surg. 2014;49(3):381–4.
43. Catania VD, Boscarelli A, Lauriti G, et al. Risk factors for surgical site infection in neonates: a systematic review of the literature and meta-analysis. Front Pediatr. 2019;29(7):101–11.
44. Vieira AL, dos Santos AM, Okuyama MK, et al. Factors associated with clinical complications during intrahospital transports in a neonatal unit in Brazil. J Trop Pediatr. 2011;57:368–74.
45. Schwebel C, Clec'h C, Magne S, et al. Safety of intrahospital transport in ventilated critically ill patients: a multicenter cohort study. Crit Care Med. 2013;41:1919–28.
46. Pelizzo G, Bagolan P, Morini F, et al. Bedside surgery in the newborn infants: survey of the Italian society of pediatric surgery. Ital J Pediatr. 2020;46(1):134–42.
47. Ein SH, Marshall DG, Girvan D. Peritoneal drainage under local anesthesia for perforations from necrotizing enterocolitis. J Pediatr Surg. 1977;12(6):963–7.
48. Eggert LD, Jung AJ, McGough EC, et al. Surgical treatment of patent ductus arteriosus in preterm infants—4 year experience with ligation in the newborn intensive care unit. Pediatr Cardiol. 1982;2:15–8.
49. Lago P, Meneghini L, Chiandetti L, et al. Congenital diaphragmatic hernia: intensive care unit or operating room? Am J Perinatol. 2005;22(4):189–97.
50. Avsar MK, Demir T, Celiksular C, Zeybek C. Bedside PDA ligation in premature infants less than 28 weeks and 1000 g. J Cardiothorac Surg. 2016;11(1):146–51.
51. Pelizzo G, Carlini V, Iacob G, et al. Pediatric laparoscopy and adaptive oxygenation and hemodynamic changes. Pediatr Rep. 2017;9(7214):21–5.
52. Tytgat SH, Stolwijk LJ, Keunen K, et al. Brain oxygenation during laparoscopic correction of hypertrophic pyloric stenosis. J Laparoendosc Adv Surg Tech A. 2015;25(4):352–7.
53. Tytgat SH, van Herwaarden MY, Stolwijk LJ, et al. Neonatal brain oxygenation during thoracoscopic correction of esophageal atresia. Surg Endosc Surg Endosc. 2016;30:2811–7.
54. Kalfa N, Allal H, Raux O. Multicentric assessment of the safety of neonatal videosurgery. Surg Endosc. 2007;21(2):303–8.
55. Bannister CF, Brosius KK, Wulkan M. The effect of insufflation pressure on pulmonary mechanics in infants during laparoscopic surgical procedures. Paediatr Anaesth. 2003;13:785–9.
56. Stolwijk LJ, Tytgat SH, Keunen K, et al. The effects of CO_2-insufflation with 5 and 10 mmHg during thoracoscopy on cerebral oxygenation and hemodynamics in piglets: an animal experimental study. Surg Endosc. 2015;29(9):2781–8.
57. Pierro A. Hypercapnia and acidosis during the thoracoscopic repair of oesophageal atresia and congenital diaphragmatic hernia. J Pediatr Surg. 2015;50(2):247–9.
58. Birch DW, Dang JT, Switzer NJ, et al. Heated insufflation with or without humidification for laparoscopic abdominal surgery. Cochrane Database Syst Rev. 2016;10(10):CD007821.
59. Surgical Services for the Newborn Report of the Royal College of Surgeons of England. 1999. http://www.baps.org.uk.
60. BAPS/Department of Health Survey of Neonatal Surgical Facilities. 2008. http://www.baps.org.uk/documents/Survey_neonatal_facilities.
61. Ramji S, Kler N, Kaur A. Where should the surgical neonates be nursed? J Neonatal Surg. 2012;1(2):24–6.
62. Mantegazza C, Landy N, Zuccotti GV, Köglmeier J. Indications and complications of inpatient parenteral nutrition prescribed to children in a large tertiary referral hospital. Ital J Pediatr. 2018;44(1):66–78.
63. Braegger C, Decsi T, Dias JA, et al. ESPGHAN Committee on Nutrition: practical approach to paediatric enteral nutrition: a comment by the ESPGHAN committee on nutrition. J Pediatr Gastroenterol Nutr. 2010;51(1):110–22.
64. Meert KL, Daphtary KM, Metheny NA. Gastric vs small-bowel feeding in critically ill children receiving mechanical ventilation: a randomized controlled trial. Chest. 2004;126:872–8.
65. Suri S, Eradi B, Chowdhary SK, et al. Early postoperative feeding and outcome in neonates. Nutrition. 2002;18(5):380–2.
66. Greer D, Karunaratne YG, Karpelowsky J, Adams S. Early enteral feeding after pediatric abdominal surgery: a systematic review of the literature. J Pediatr Surg. 2020;55(7):1180–7.
67. Vohr BR, Poindexter BB, Dusick AM, et al. Beneficial effects of breast milk in the neonatal intensive care unit on the developmental outcome of extremely low birth weight infants at 18 months of age. Pediatrics. 2006;118(1):e115–23.

68. Edwards TM, Spatz DL. An innovative model for achieving breast-feeding success in infants with complex surgical anomalies. J Perinat Neonatal Nurs. 2010;24(3):246–53.
69. Hylander MA, Strobino DM, Dhanireddy R. Human milk feedings and infection among very low birth weight infants. Pediatrics. 1988;102(3):e38.
70. Brindle ME, McDiarmid C, Short K, et al. Consensus guidelines for perioperative care in neonatal intestinal surgery: enhanced recovery after surgery (ERAS®) society recommendations. World J Surg. 2020;44:2482–92.
71. Shinnick JK, Short HL, Heiss KF, et al. Enhancing recovery in pediatric surgery: a review of the literature. J Surg Res. 2016;202(1):165–76.
72. Pearson KL, Hall N. What is the role of enhanced recovery after surgery in children? A scoping review. Pediatr Surg Int. 2017;33(1):43–51.
73. Short HL, Heiss KF, Burch K, et al. Implementation of an enhanced recovery protocol in pediatric colorectal surgery. J Pediatr Surg. 2017;53(4):688–92.
74. Wakimoto Y, Burjonrappa S. Enhanced recovery after surgery (ERAS) protocols in neonates should focus on the respiratory tract. Pediatr Surg Int. 2019;35(6):635–42.
75. de Bruin L, Pasma W, van der Werff DB, et al. Perioperative hospital mortality at a tertiary paediatric institution. Br J Anaesth. 2015;115(4):608–15.
76. Stolwijk LJ, Lemmers PM, Harmsen M, et al. Neurodevelopmental outcomes after neonatal surgery for major noncardiac anomalies. Pediatrics. 2016;137(2):e20151728.
77. World Health Organization. Health statistics and health information systems: life tables for WHO member states. Geneva: World Health Organization; 2011.
78. Sitkin NA, Ozgediz D, Donkor P, et al. Congenital anomalies in low- and middle-income countries: the unborn child of global surgery. World J Surg. 2015;39:36–40.
79. Wu VK, Poenaru D. Burden of surgically correctable disabilities among children in the Dadaab Refugee Camp. World J Surg. 2013;37(7):1536–43.
80. Wu VK, Poenaru D, Poley MJ. Burden of surgical congenital anomalies in Kenya: a population-based study. J Trop Pediatr. 2013;59(3):195–202.
81. Abdul-Mumin A, Anyomih TTK, Owusu SA, et al. Burden of neonatal surgical conditions in Northern Ghana. World J Surg. 2020;44(1):3–11.
82. Chirdan LB, Ngiloi PJ, Elhalaby EA. Neonatal surgery in Africa. Semin Pediatr Surg. 2012;21(2):151–9.
83. Tessema ZT, Tesema GA. Incidence of neonatal mortality and its predictors among live births in Ethiopia: Gompertz gamma shared frailty model. Ital J Pediatr. 2020;46(1):138–48.
84. Ammar S, Sellami S, Sellami I, et al. Risk factors of early mortality after neonatal surgery in Tunisia. J Pediatr Surg. 2020;55(10):2233–7.
85. Ekenze SO, Ajuzieogu OV, Nwomeh BC. Neonatal surgery in Africa: a systematic review and meta-analysis of challenges of management and outcome. Lancet. 2015;385(Suppl 2):S35.
86. Reinberg O. Des Dieux et des Hommes: approches de la maladie en Afrique et en Europe [Of gods and men: crossed analysis on medicine in Europe and Africa]. E-Mem Acad Natl Chir. 2014;13(4):075–84.
87. GBD 2016 Causes of Death Collaborators. Global, regional, and national age-sex specific mortality for 264 causes of death, 1980–2016: a systematic analysis for the Global Burden of Disease Study 2016 [Erratum in: Lancet. 2017 390(10106):e38]. Lancet. 2017;390(10100):1151–210.
88. Chaurasia S, Sivanandan S, Agarwal R, et al. Neonatal sepsis in South Asia: huge burden and spiralling antimicrobial resistance. BMJ. 2019;364:k5314.
89. Wardlaw T, Salama P, Johansson EW, et al. Pneumonia: the leading killer of children. Lancet. 2006;368(9541):1048–50.
90. Colin AA. Pneumonia in the developed world. Pediatr Respir Rev. 2006;7(Suppl 1):S138–40.
91. Ballot DE, Potterton J, Chirwa T, et al. Developmental outcome of very low birth weight infants in a developing country. BMC Pediatr. 2012;12:11.
92. NCEPOD. The national confidential enquiry into perioperative deaths (NCEPOD). Health Serv Manag. 1990;86(5):203.
93. Maricic MA, Bailez MM, Rodriguez SP. Validation of an inanimate low cost model for training minimal invasive surgery (MIS) of esophageal atresia with tracheoesophageal fistula (AE/TEF) repair. J Pediatr Surg. 2016;51(9):1429–35.
94. Barsness KA, Rooney DM, Davis LM, et al. Validation of measures from a thoracoscopic esophageal atresia/tracheoesophageal fistula repair simulator. J Pediatr Surg. 2014;49(1):29–32.
95. Barsness KA, Rooney DM, Davis L. Collaboration in simulation: the development and evaluation of a novel thoracoscopic neonatal simulator. J Pediatr Surg 2013;48(6):1232–8.
96. Arul GS, Spicer RD. In where should paediatric surgery be performed? Arch Dis Child. 1998;79(1):65–70.
97. Nwomeh BC, Caniano DA. Ethical considerations in pediatric surgery. In: Puri P, Höllwarth M, editors. Pediatric surgery. Berlin: Springer; 2009. https://doi.org/10.1007/978-3-540-69560-8_11.
98. Hall NJ, Eaton S, Pierro A. The evidence base for neonatal surgery. Early Hum Dev. 2009;85:713–8.

11 Operational Improvement in Pediatric Surgery

Catarina Barroso and Jorge Correia-Pinto

Abbreviations

DNR	Do not resuscitate
ERAS	Enhanced recovery after surgery
MIS	Minimally invasive surgery
OR	Operating room

11.1 Introduction

The prevalence of pediatric chronic diseases has increased worldwide over the last years due to the advancements in medical diagnosis, developing technology, and treatments for different illnesses and comorbidities. Nowadays, frail children represent an increasing proportion of the population of healthcare utilization. In a tertiary care hospital of a developed country, children with complex special health care comprehend around 15% of operative cases, with around 90% of them being scheduled procedures [1]. Frailty in children creates a unique challenge for the pediatric surgeon. These children often have several medical problems that require careful attention before surgery. They are at increased risk for requiring acute surgical interventions for complications and needs from previous surgeries or related to implanted surgical hardware (central venous access, enterostomy tubes, or peritoneal dialysis catheter, etc.). On the other hand, they may be scheduled for elective procedures to address sequelae of disease such as malnutrition, gastroesophageal reflux disease or other conditions [2]. They may also need a surgical procedure for a common pediatric pathology, such as inguinal hernia, phimosis, or acute appendicitis, etc.

In these chapters, we intend to consider strategies to improve perioperative management of this special-needs population.

11.2 Frail Children—Specific Considerations

Any kind of hospital admission involves risk to this vulnerable population once it is a break from home routine medication and medical care, exposure to the hospital environment, rotating provid-

C. Barroso
Pediatric Surgery Department, Hospital de Braga, Braga, Portugal

Life and Health Sciences Research Institute (ICVS), School of Medicine, University of Minho, Braga, Portugal
e-mail: catarina.barroso@hb.min-saude.pt

J. Correia-Pinto (✉)
Pediatric Surgery Department, Hospital de Braga, Braga, Portugal

ICVS/3B's-PT Government Associate Laboratory, Braga/Guimarães, Portugal
e-mail: jcp@med.uminho.pt

M. Lima, M. C. Mondardini (eds.), *Frailty in Children*,
https://doi.org/10.1007/978-3-031-24307-3_11

ers not familiarized with the patient, and generation of stress and anxiety [2, 3]. Frail children are at higher risk for prolonged length of stay compared to the general population, as they have more postoperative complications such as slow return of bowel function, hemodynamic instability, and respiratory insufficiency. Also, they have higher rates of readmissions, medical errors, as well as in-hospital mortality [2, 3]. Heterogeneity among this population, specific medication requirements, different anatomy or physiology, uncertainty about the best treatment protocol for the underlying conditions, developmental needs can make perioperative management challenging. Anatomic abnormalities such as micrognathia, muscular contractures, excessive adipose tissue, can make common procedures difficult (airway management, vascular access, positioning of the patient, etc). Previous surgery history is associated with postoperative adhesions, which can hamper surgical approach. Malnutrition can delay wound healing. Past hospital admissions and infectious disease history increases the risk for antimicrobial resistance, raising concerns on deciding prophylactic antibiotics and dealing with possible postoperative infection. Baseline organ dysfunction can require modifications in treatment algorithms as the threshold for starting treatment may be lower. Developmental or behavioral disabilities can make communicating pain and other symptoms difficult [2]. Familial socioeconomical insufficiencies may hamper the best clinical contacts and treatment adherence. There will be frail children that, due to their physical or clinical condition, do not arouse compassion. Eventually, we come across the ethical question that some of these patients require a lot more of us than we could possibly give in return, either emotionally, materialistically, and professionally.

11.3 Operational Improvement

The spectrum of frailty in children extends through all ages, originating from congenital and acquired conditions, with a range of static, potentially resolving, and progressively declining trajectories. Such heterogeneity presents challenges for categorization, prediction modeling, research, bedside care, and support of families. Nonetheless we intend to establish some strategies in preoperative evaluation, coordination of care, postoperative planning, and expectation to respond to these special-needs children.

11.3.1 Referencing and Multidisciplinary Team

First of all, frail children should receive surgical care at institutions that offer multidisciplinary, pediatric-centered care, involving pediatric surgery, pediatrics, pediatric anesthesiology, physiatry, psychology and social service, making an extensive preoperative planning possible. The team should be trained for complex special health care, meaning they should have experienced specialists, continuing education of healthcare providers, and guidelines for the management of these children [4]. It is essential that effective communication exists between all involved specialists of the team in order to have an organized, high-quality plan that fulfills the child's needs. It is useful to have a central practitioner coordinating care, which is usually the child's general pediatrician or family physician. The role would be to make the bond between every specialist, and also the family, providing organized and updated data [5]. When there is a planned surgery, the involved in-hospital specialists should stay informed of each other's plans.

Families or primary care providers always play an important role as they can provide invaluable patient-specific details, including health summaries, interpretation of the symptoms, rare disease-specific expertise. Specialists and generalists must always involve families in decision making, preoperative planning, and postoperative management and should be educated on successful means of interaction and communication.

11.3.2 Surgical Indication and Conservatism

The principles upon which medical decisions are made for frail children are the same as for any other child: autonomy, beneficence justice, non-maleficence, veracity, and fidelity [6]. Toward a potentially surgical problem, the decision making is not always easy and should be part of a multidisciplinary consensus. Discussions can be improved by engaging the family and the primary care team as shared decision-making promotes co-operation, with ultimate goals of improved health and satisfaction [7]. When cognitively competent, children should also be involved in decisions about their care, on the basis of developmental age. This can help them understand the condition and treatments, reduce fear, enhance self-confidence and acceptance, and improve collaboration with treatment decisions [6].

Nevertheless, a surgical procedure is a physical aggression, and it is well known that frail children have increased risk of prolonged length of stay due to pre-procedural optimization, overnight respiratory optimization, general uncertainty of response to procedural stress, and possible postoperative complications. There is also a higher rate of medical errors and even in-hospital death. The anxiety around the surgery and disruption it causes to the family dynamics is also important to take into account. Surgical indication should be a decision made after careful consideration of risks and benefits, keeping in mind that good outcomes likely reflect a conservative approach [1]. The surgeon must consider the natural history, the risks of surgery for mortality and morbidity, namely, postoperative complications, and decide if there is an absolute need to perform surgery or if the child would be able to have an acceptable quality of life with conservative treatment.

For hopelessly ill children, or who have a progressive degenerative neurologic disease, it is important to understand what are the parents' expectations and determine precociously if parents want care to be limited. Patients in palliative care may obviously benefit from surgical procedures as long as it is to provide relief and/or prevention of pain and discomfort. If parents request do not resuscitate (DNR) status for their child, it should be documented in the medical record for clarity and legal protection of the team. This does not mean they are not eligible for surgical procedures. Some patients with DNR status may have significant benefit with a surgical intervention, even though the procedure may not change the natural history of the underlying disease. The surgeon plays an important role to discern if the procedure is important or a futility for the purpose of prolonging life. If there is a disagreement between parents and physicians' decision, a second opinion from another specialist is recommended [8].

11.3.3 Day-Case Surgery and Early Discharge

The longer the length of hospital stay, the higher the risk of nosocomial infections, medical errors, stress and anxiety. There should always be an attempt to keep the admission as soon as possible. Therefore whenever it is feasible, the procedure should be in a day-case basis. This will only be possible if the underlying condition is stabilized, time of surgery is not very long (<120 min), postoperative pain can presumably be controlled (regional anesthesia, use of minimally invasive techniques), and there is no high risk of postoperative bleeding or alimentary intolerance [9].

When the procedure is not suitable for a day-case surgery, efforts should be made to reduce the length of stay as much as possible. Enhanced recovery after surgery (ERAS) has been a hot theme for adult surgeons lately, as it have been found to decrease hospital length of stay and complications in diverse adult surgical populations. These interventions theoretically maintain physiological homeostasis and minimize surgical stress, thus facilitating a quicker return to baseline. There is a paucity of literature assessing enhanced recovery protocols in the pediatric population, let alone in frail children, although there have been numerous pediatric studies demonstrating improved outcomes with isolated elements of ERAS (perioperative counseling, limited perioperative fasting, non-routine bowel preparation, antibiotic prophylaxis, use of short-acting anesthetics, epidural anesthesia/analgesia, limited use of narcotics, nausea and vomiting prophylaxis, early enteral intake and mobilization, and nonroutine use of surgical drains and tubes) [10]. Some of them have included frail children as oncologic patients and transplant recipients [11]. The creation of ERAS protocols in these populations must be an area of research as it seems to have a lot of potential in minimizing stress, complications, and length of stay. In fact, some elements of ERAS will be mentioned beneath as strategies for operational improvement, such as perioperative counseling, minimally invasive techniques, avoiding prolonged fasting, and postoperative pain management.

11.3.4 Pre-operative Planning

11.3.4.1 Patient and Family Preparation

The preoperative evaluation of frail children should comprehend common concerns that may impact perioperative decision-making. The surgeon must anticipate the unique intraoperative and postoperative potential challenges.

Preparing the child and family to face the surgery is important on a basis of good communication methods and promptness to answer doubts and questions. Adaptation to the hospital environment is a basic condition for a smooth uneventful stay. Some non-pharmacological adjuvant interventions proved to have a positive role on pediatric patients' outcomes, such as hospital decorations, facilities to play and participation in team games, miniature cars for children to play with while waiting for surgery and to drive them to the operating room (OR). The presence of hospital clowns helps in reducing stress and anxiety in children during medical procedures, induction of anesthesia, and as part of routine care. It might contribute to improve the psychological well-being and emotional responses in frail children and adolescents [12]. Also, while contributing to reduce parents' stress and anxiety, they can contribute for their respite by providing some distraction and entertainment for their child. Music has also the potential to reduce pain, anxiety, and distress in children undergoing surgery [13]. If possible, it brings calmness to the child to make a preparatory visit to the actual OR, where all the stages of surgery are explained. Right before surgery, the presence of parents provides comfort and assurance.

For hopelessly ill children with a DNR order, after a decision to undergo surgery, the team should always have a discussion with the family on their options. Cardiopulmonary resuscitation in the OR carries a much better medical prognosis than when performed in other hospital scenarios (around 50–80% of patients resuscitated in the OR return to their former level of functioning). At the OR, the event is always witnessed allowing rapid and effective intervention. Also, the adjacent cause is usually known, often reversible effects of anesthesia or hemorrhage and not usually due to the patient's underlying disease. So the family should decide whether to suspend the DNR order during surgery and the perioperative period, maintaining the original DNR order, or modifying the DNR order [8].

11.3.4.2 Medical Optimization

Whenever possible, frail children should be brought to their individual optimum level of health before undergoing a surgical procedure. Malnourished children (or at risk of malnourishment) should have a nutrition plan prior to surgery, either by optimizing oral intakes or by tube feedings. Prolonged fasting should be avoided, so clear liquids should be emphasized until 1–2 h before surgery. Although with some limitations, serum albumin is generally considered a useful index of nutritional status and the target serum level should be 4 g/dL [14]. Dehydration is common and frequently underdiagnosed in malnourished children who are affected by several kinds of disability, so it should be considered and treated before surgery [15]. Children with chronic disorders or renal disease often have associated anemia with usual hemoglobin concentrations of 6–9 g/dL. Target preoperative hemoglobin values should be individualized to the type of procedure planned and pointed after a discussion with the anesthesiologist. Coagulopathies and electrolyte imbalances must be corrected before surgery. Patients receiving corticosteroids for extended periods may not be able to support a natural stress response because of chronic suppression of the hypothalamic–pituitary–adrenal axis, so they should receive perioperative supplementation. Patients taking antihypertensive drugs should not suspend it, but must be closely monitored for intraoperative hypotension. Other drugs that should be continued in the perioperative period include antiepileptics, drugs for asthma, and immunosuppressants. Drugs that should be discontinued before surgery include anticoagulants, anti-thrombotic, nonsteroidal anti-inflammatory drugs, and diuretics. Patients with chronic lung disease should be preoperatively asymptomatic and for that, pharmacologic, environmental, or dietary control may be necessary. Medications should not be suspended during perioperative period. In some difficult cases, such as in cystic fibrosis, the pneumologist's cooperation is essential to optimize the patient before surgery to minimize the surgical risk. In patients with chronic kidney disease, renal function and electrolyte monitoring is important in the preoperative period, and any acid–base imbalances and electrolyte disturbances must be corrected. Careful attention must be paid to the patient's intake and output. The fasting period should not be prolonged before surgery because they can become dehydrated quickly. In such patients, securing peripheral intravenous access is always sensible, even before surgery. When prescribing drugs that are metabolized and excreted by the kidney, monitoring of serum drug levels is essential. In patients with chronic liver disease, edema or ascites should be treated preoperatively with diuretics and sodium-restricted diet. Liver enzyme levels and coagulation should be accessed before surgery. If coagulopathy is present, vitamin K and fresh frozen plasma should be ensured in the preoperative period as well as during surgery. When prescribing drugs that are metabolized and excreted by the liver, monitoring of serum drug levels is essential. Patients with neurological disease and seizure disorder are often considered at high risk of seizures occurring during or shortly after the procedure. There should be an appropriate plan for continued use of antiepileptic drugs throughout pre- and immediate postoperative period. In patients with obesity, measures should be taken to prevent deep vein thrombosis and pulmonary embolism, such as postoperative enoxaparin, elastic compression stockings and/or intermittent compression devices. Also, additional measures to prevent surgical site infection should be considered.

11.3.4.3 Anesthesia Plan

Frail children should always be under observation by an anesthesiology specialist prior to an elective surgery. The pediatric surgeon must communicate to the pediatric anesthesiologist the surgical plan so that together they can anticipate problems or concerns, especially for complex or uncommon procedures. The anesthesia team should be aware if the patient has a history of complications with anesthetics, malignant hyperthermia, coagulation disorders, or if the patient has symptoms of an upper respiratory tract illness that increases the risk of postintubation laryngotracheal edema. Preoperatively, the anesthesia team must have a plan, according to the surgical intervention, for postoperative pain control as caudal injection, epidural catheter insertion, or peripheral nerve block.

11.3.5 The Surgery

11.3.5.1 Positioning and Surgical Approach

Planning a surgical approach anticipatedly is very important considering these patients may have altered anatomy or surgical implanted devices that restrict standard surgical steps. In patients with neurological or neuromuscular diseases, the body habitus may hamper surgical positioning and access. For instance, in a patient with severe lower extremity contractures, a laparoscopic operation may not be feasible if there is no adequate extracorporeal clearance of laparoscopic instrumentation, unless there is an alternative for port sites position. Surgical implanted devices such as ventriculoperitoneal shunts or venous catheters, digestive or urinary stomas, previous scars may limit surgical approach like surgical incision site. Every detail must be considered when deciding what technique to perform, if any modification will be required, and what to do in case of a difficulty or complication.

11.3.5.2 Minimally Invasive Surgery (MIS)

Minimally invasive surgery revolutionized pediatric surgery since it has been proven to be feasible in a great proportion of pediatric surgery procedures. Advantages of minimally invasive surgery are unquestionable and well known throughout the fields of abdominal, thoracic, and urologic conditions. Of interest in this population, MIS is associated with decreased risk of infection, decreased recovery time and length of stay, greater surgical visualization and precision [16]. If surgery is inevitably a physical aggression, MIS tends to minimize it, as it is possible to make smaller incisions and limited mobilization of structures when trying to achieve an adequate exposure. Greater visualization, magnification, and precision might prove to be an advantage in children who have altered anatomy. MIS should always be considered a first-line approach after disclosing any kind of cardiopulmonary contra-indication.

11.3.5.3 Pre-operative Simulation

Whenever there is a high-complexity surgical case, experience and competency are expected of the team. In pediatric surgery, and specifically in frail children, there are some conditions that are rare, and the team will not have experienced significant case volume. Even if there is considerable volume of similar cases, each case might have particularities in this population. Frail children will be frequently complex cases owing to their altered anatomy and physiology, increased risk of complications, and less tolerability to minor errors and distractions. That is why preoperative simulation can improve safety and effectiveness of surgical procedures. Significant advances in diagnostic imaging modalities and image processing software enable surgeons to obtain detailed anatomical information preoperatively for each patient and incorporate this data in surgical simulation. A surgical simulator based on radiological images from an individual patient using three-dimensional visualization techniques may greatly assist surgeons to preoperatively rehearse an operation and facilitate sharing of information among the operative team [17]. Surgeons should have the means to achieve the best preparation they possible may have once we must always offer the best of our knowledge and competence to treat a child.

11.3.6 Postoperative Management

Together with the anesthesia team, a plan must be accomplished to minimize postoperative pain and analgesics requirement, which can involve epidural anesthesia/analgesia or a peripheral nerve block. These can be performed prior or immediately after surgery. Nausea and vomits prophylaxis should also be considered according to each surgical procedure and in high-risk patients. Oral/enteral feedings and physical mobilization should be started as early as possible. Tubes and catheters should be avoided or removed precociously. Every effort should be made so the child can have a safe and early discharge. Family support should be guaranteed during the admission and after discharge, reassuring they will have response to all of their concerns.

11.4 Conclusion

Optimal treatment for frail children may be challenging and requires an experienced pediatric-centered multidisciplinary team. The surgeon, together with the rest of the team and family, must bear in mind associated disorders, possible altered anatomy and physiology, and potential complications that may occur. Whenever there is a potentially surgical condition, the surgical indication must be analyzed, considering the risks and benefits. After the decision has been made, the team should carefully plan the procedure and implement individual pre-, peri-, and postoperative care in the child's best interests.

References

1. Graham RJ, Wachendorf MT, Burns JP, Mancuso TJ. Successful and safe delivery of anesthesia and perioperative care for children with complex special health care needs. J Clin Anesth. 2009;21(3):165–72. https://doi.org/10.1016/j.jclinane.2008.06.033.
2. Murphy Salem S, Graham RJ. Chronic illness in pediatric critical care. Front Pediatr. 2021;9:686206. https://doi.org/10.3389/fped.2021.686206.
3. Sacchetti A, Sacchetti C, Carraccio C, Gerardi M. The potential for errors in children with special health care needs. Acad Emerg Med. 2000;7(11):1330–3.
4. McAteer JP, LaRiviere CA, Drugas GT, Abdullah F, Oldham KT, Goldin AB. Influence of surgeon experience, hospital volume, and specialty designation on outcomes in pediatric surgery. JAMA Pediatr. 2013;167(5):468–75. https://doi.org/10.1001/jamapediatrics.2013.25.
5. Hamonet-Torny J, Le Bellego D, Jasper E, Suc A-L, Fourcade L. Regional consensus on the health care pathway of disabled children in surgery. Ann Phys Rehabil Med. 2016;59:e47. https://doi.org/10.1016/j.rehab.2016.07.109.
6. Okun A. Children who have special health-care needs: ethical issues. Pediatr Rev. 2010;31(12):514–7. https://doi.org/10.1542/pir.31-12-514.
7. Adams RC, Levy SE. Shared decision-making and children with disabilities: pathways to consensus. Pediatrics. 2017;139(6):956. https://doi.org/10.1542/peds.2017-0956.
8. Calkins CM, Oldham KT. Surgical problems of children with physical disabilities. Pediatr Surg. 2020;34:541–58. https://doi.org/10.1007/978-3-662-43588-5_36.
9. De Luca U, Mangia G, Tesoro S, Martino A, Sammartino M, Calisti A. Guidelines on pediatric day surgery of the Italian Societies of Pediatric Surgery (SICP) and Pediatric Anesthesiology (SARNePI). Ital J Pediatr. 2018;44(1):1–10. https://doi.org/10.1186/s13052-018-0473-1.
10. Shinnick JK, Short HL, Heiss KF, Santore MT, Blakely ML, Raval MV. Enhancing recovery in pediatric surgery: a review of the literature. J Surg Res. 2016;202(1):165–76. https://doi.org/10.1016/j.jss.2015.12.051.
11. Reismann M, von Kampen M, Laupichler B, Suempelmann R, Schmidt AI, Ure BM. Fast-track surgery in infants and children. J Pediatr Surg. 2007;42(1):234–8. https://doi.org/10.1016/j.jpedsurg.2006.09.022.
12. Lopes-júnior LC, Bomfim E, Olson K, et al. Effectiveness of hospital clowns for symptom management in paediatrics: systematic review of randomised and non-randomised controlled trials. Br Med J. 2020;371:m4290. https://doi.org/10.1136/bmj.m4290.
13. Van Der Heijden MJE, Araghi SO, Van Dijk M, Jeekel J, Hunink MGM. The effects of perioperative music interventions in pediatric surgery: a systematic review and meta-analysis of randomized controlled trials. PLoS One. 2015;10(8):1–11. https://doi.org/10.1371/journal.pone.0133608.
14. Viani K, Trehan A, Manzoli B, Schoeman J. Assessment of nutritional status in children with cancer: a narrative review. Pediatr Blood Cancer. 2020;67(S3):1–9. https://doi.org/10.1002/pbc.28211.
15. Calcaterra V, Cena H, Ruggieri A, et al. Metabolically unhealthy phenotype: a key factor in determining "pediatric" frailty. Pediatr Rep. 2021;13(3):340–6. https://doi.org/10.3390/PEDIATRIC13030042.
16. Schukfeh N, Kuebler JF, Dingemann J, Ure BM. Thirty years of minimally invasive surgery in children: analysis of meta-analyses. Eur J Pediatr Surg. 2020;30(5):420–8. https://doi.org/10.1055/s-0039-1687901.
17. Endo K, Sata N, Ishiguro Y, et al. A patient-specific surgical simulator using preoperative imaging data: an interactive simulator using a three-dimensional tactile mouse. J Comput Surg. 2014;1(1):2–9. https://doi.org/10.1186/s40244-014-0010-5.

12 Operational Improvement in Pediatric Neurosurgery

Barbara Spacca, Davide Luglietto, Octavian Vatavu, Ludovico D'Incerti, Germana Tuccinardi, Desy Butti, Leonardo Bussolin, Federico Mussa, and Lorenzo Genitori

Abbreviations

1H-MRS	H-magnetic resonance spectroscopy
AA	Amino acids
AC	Arachnoid cysts
ADC	Apparent diffusion coefficient
ASL	Arterial spin labeling
bFFE	Balanced fast field-echo
BOLD	Blood oxygenation level-dependent
CBF	Cerebral blood flow
Cho	Choline
CNS	Central nervous system
Cr	Creatine
CSF	Cerebrospinal fluid
CT	Computed tomography
DIPG	Diffuse intrinsic pontine glioma
DMN	Default mode network
DTI	Diffusion tensor images
DWI	Diffusion-weighted images
EES	Endoscopic endonasal surgery
ESC	Endoscopic strip craniectomy
ETV	Endoscopic third ventriculocisternostomy
FA	Fractional anisotropy
FIESTA	Fast imaging employing steady-state acquisition
FLAIR	Fluid-Attenuated Inversion Recovery
fMRI	Functional MRI
GE	Gradient echo
Gli	Glutamate glutamine
HARDI	High-angular resolution diffusion imaging
HCP	Hydrocephalus
ICA	Independent component analysis
Lip	Lipids
LITT	Laser interstitial thermal therapy
MAP	Mean arterial pressure
mI	Myoinositol
MPRAGE	Magnetization prepared—rapid gradient echo
MRI	Magnetic resonance imaging
MRS	Proton MR spectroscopy
MTT	Mean transit time
NAA	*N*-Acetylaspartate
NDI	Neurite density index

B. Spacca · D. Luglietto · F. Mussa · L. Genitori (✉)
Pediatric Neurosurgery Unit, IRCCS, Florence, Italy
e-mail: barbara.spacca@meyer.it; federico.mussa@meyer.it; lorenzo.genitori@meyer.it

O. Vatavu
School of Medicine, Scuola Superiore Sant'Anna, Pisa, Italy
e-mail: octavian.vatavu@santannapisa.it

L. D'Incerti
Radiology Unit, IRCCS, Florence, Italy
e-mail: ludovico.dincerti@meyer.it

G. Tuccinardi · D. Butti · L. Bussolin
Pediatric Neuroanesthesia Unit, IRCCS, Florence, Italy
e-mail: germana.tuccinardi@meyer.it; desy.butti@meyer.it; leonardo.bussolin@meyer.it

M. Lima, M. C. Mondardini (eds.), *Frailty in Children*,
https://doi.org/10.1007/978-3-031-24307-3_12

ODI	Orientation dispersion index
PWI	Perfusion-weighted imaging
ROSA	Robotic operating surgical assistant
SE	Spin echo
SPGR	Spoiled gradient-recalled
SWI	Susceptibility-weighted images
T	Tesla
TrueFISP	Fast imaging with steady-state free precession

12.1 Introduction

12.1.1 Frailty and Neurosurgery

Frailty is a clinical condition characterized by excessive vulnerability to endogenous and exogenous stressors due to a reduction of homeostatic reserve. It is a state defined by diminished strength, endurance, and reduced physiologic function which leads to major vulnerability for developing increased dependency and/or death [1]. Principal elements that define pediatric frailty can be found in the previous chapters.

Frailty in neurosurgery has been analyzed especially in older patients to predict their post-surgical outcome as shown by Pazniokas et al. [2]. Most of the studies included in the review showed an association between "frail" phenotype and poorer outcomes in terms of complications or mortality. For example, higher frailty assessed with mFI index showed higher mortality and poorer outcome in patients with spontaneous intracerebral hemorrhage. Frailty assessment is about to become a proven item in clinical evaluation in neurosurgery, especially in neuro-oncology, as many authors showed that frailty may be used as a prognostic value particularly for short-term postoperative complications [2–4]. Today, there are no available studies about pediatric frailty in neurosurgery.

12.1.2 But Why is Frailty an Important Concept in Pediatric Neurosurgery?

Frailty is a concept that has been introduced recently in medicine and it has been extended also to pediatric patients because

(a) Children have some features that make them generally frailer to surgery (such as higher risk of hemodynamic instability).
(b) The number of frail patients has increased due to improvements of therapy.

In fact, decades ago, many neurosurgical pathologies had very poor outcomes with high rates of mortality and morbidity. Technological, therapeutical, and surgical innovations caused an improvement of prognosis of most of these pathologies. Cerebral tumors are an example of this phenomenon. These tumors are the second most prevalent tumors in children. In the past, cerebral tumors had very high mortality and morbidity related to retarded diagnosis and minor technical tolls during surgery, but survival rate increased progressively in the last 30 years. In Italy, a statistically significant reduction was observed during the entire period 1970–2002. Mortality for central nervous system (CNS) tumors in children increased from 1970 to 1977, and decreased constantly thereafter up to 2008, similarly in boys and girls. The estimated annual percentage change for the first period was estimated to be 4.6% and 6.3%, with borderline significance, in boys and girls, respectively. In the following period, 1977–2008, estimated annual percentage change of age-adjusted mortality rates were − 2.3% in boys and − 2.6% in girls, both highly significant. The calculated average mortality rate for CNS tumors of 8.3 per million/year, during the period 2000–2008, with 59 deaths occurring annually. CNS tumors were more common in boys than in girls, with a 24% higher mortality rate [5].

Pediatric neurosurgical patients are considered frail patients as they are exposed to long-term treatments [6]. In fact, frailty is caused by both the underlying cerebral pathology and the treatment itself, and consequently patients have an increased risk of complications and sequelae.

Better therapies caused longer survival rates but, at the same time, determined an increase of complex patients, thus justifying the interest toward the concept of frailty.

12.1.3 Improvements in Pediatric Neurosurgery

The principal objective of today's neurosurgical practice is the cure (or control) of the pathology and at the same time the maintenance of the best possible quality of life. Minimally invasive approaches, adequate anesthesiologic procedure and reduction of surgery duration are important elements.

The aim of minimally invasive surgery is to minimize trauma of surgery without losing therapeutical efficacy [7]. The concept of minimally invasive was born in other fields, such as general and gynecological surgery, and neurosurgeons have applied it to their field through different techniques that will be described in the next paragraphs such as neuroendoscopy, stereotactic surgery, microsurgery, and robotics. The advantages of minimally invasive surgery are increased precision, less tissue disruption, lower morbidity, and shorter hospital stays [7].

Moreover, an increased attention to patients' needs have developed so that the improvement in neurosurgery implies a multidisciplinary approach. An example of this new exigency derives from the alteration of self-perception after cranial surgeries due to complete hair shaving. Traditionally, all patients underwent a complete hair shaving before craniotomy to avoid post-operative infections with a strong psychological impact. After years of this practice, it is now well understood that hair does not increase infections risks so it is sufficient to shave only the surface needed for the craniotomy or, in some cases, do not shave at all [8, 9]. Some studies have showed that not only psychological benefits are present, but also that complete hair shaving may lead to an increase of bacterial proliferation [10]. Moreover, limited hair shaving causes an improvement of quality of life and allows faster recovery to normal everyday activities even after complex brain surgeries. This practice started in the last decades of the twentieth century, but it spread only in the 2000s, and today it is a common practice in all neurosurgical departments.

Similar elements have emphasized that neurosurgical improvements must be oriented to multiple aspects and consider all the patients' frailties. The aim of this chapter is to analyze the most important improvements in pediatric neurosurgery, their impact, and future perspectives.

12.2 Pediatric Neuro-Anesthesia

Innovative and advanced neurosurgical and anesthesiologic techniques have improved the outcome of newborns and children who undergo this type of surgery [11]. The complexity of the approach to the pediatric patient depends on the age-related differences of cerebrovascular physiology and cranial ossification. During surgeries, very young children show a higher risk of hemodynamic instability due to a different distribution of the cardiac output, directed for a higher percentage to the CNS. The autoregulation of the blood flow is guaranteed for mean arterial pressure (MAP) between 60 and 20 mmHg. It is imperative to achieve stable hemodynamics not to induce hypotension or hypertension, which may cause respectively cerebral ischemia and, especially in the newborn, intraventricular hemorrhage [12].

Newborns and infants have higher risk of mortality and morbidity compared to any other age group. Great part of the complications is related to respiratory and cardiac events. The preoperative evaluation is essential, but often it is not possible in emergency. The anesthesiologic evaluation should particularly focus on airway management due to high rates of craniofacial malformations. Almost all the pediatric neurosurgeries are done under general anesthesia. General anesthesia needs one or more venous accesses and a meticulous management of the airways, usually done by orotracheal or nasotracheal intubation. In the last years, only for minor surgeries, the intubation has been replaced with laryngeal mask, a supraglottic device which requires a less invasive procedure. The laryngeal mask allows the insertion of a nasogastric tube to prevent lung aspiration. The mask can also be used in emergency for difficult airways [13]. In major neurosurgery, femoral central line is the most used because it does not interfere with cerebral venous drainage such as jugular catheters and it has no pneumothorax risk as in subclavian lines.

12.2.1 Intraoperative Monitoring

ASA monitoring standards may need additional parameters such as invasive arterial pressure monitoring though arterial catheter to be able to detect sudden hemodynamic instability caused by hemorrhage, cranial nerve manipulation, herniation syndromes, and venous embolism. Moreover, the arterial catheter allows multiple gas analysis during the surgery [12].

12.2.2 Hypothermia Prevention

The pediatric patient loses heat faster than the adult. This phenomenon concerns all the children, but it is effectively more important in newborns because of their absence of subcutaneous fatty tissue, the higher ratio between body surface and weight and due to the absence of shiver as a compensatory mechanism. During surgery, the risk of hypothermia is even higher due to low temperature of the operating room, the lack of thermoregulatory response due to general anesthesia, the surgery itself, and mechanical ventilation. Consequently, it is imperative to minimize heat loss through warming table pads and warm fluids.

12.2.3 Prevention of Dehydration and Hypoglycemia

Prolonged fasting should be avoided in pediatric patients because excessive fluid restriction may lead rapidly to dehydration and hypovolemia due to fast metabolism of these patients. Excessive fasting may also induce hypotensive events, metabolic acidosis, and severe hypoglycemia. Today, the pediatric patient can have a solid meal 6 h before surgery, mother's milk 4 h before and clear liquids until 1 h before [14]. This timing is important to allow the reduction of gastric volume. Nevertheless, there are still cases of high risk of dehydration due to the patient's pathology, but also in toddlers and newborns especially, if premature. Dehydration is dangerous during the induction phase of anesthesia because it may lead to bradycardia. The consequences of bradycardia are worse in extremely young patients. It is imperative to adhere strictly to protocols and if the patient is not able to drink, it is possible to inject fluids IV [14].

12.2.4 Transfusion

Blood transfusions may be necessary for blood loss of 15% of total blood volume or in the case of Hb concentration below 7 g/dL. The need for transfusion can be stated by hematocrit values and through the evaluation of hemodynamic response to hemorrhage. It is crucial that the surgeon and the anesthesiologist work very closely, especially during intracerebral manipulation, to avoid any changes to the cerebral microcirculation. Often, the need of transfusion anticipate alteration of hematocrit. The blood should be injected at a 37 °C temperature to prevent hypothermia. Tumescent Local Anesthesia in the area covered by the skin incision, is extremely useful to reduce blood transfusions and the volume of blood transfused intraoperatively, especially in low weight patients. Tumescent Local Anesthesia uses low concentration lidocaine (0.1%), adrenaline, sodium bicarbonate diluted in a large volume of saline or lactate Ringer. The cutaneous and subcutaneous infiltration with this solution takes advantage of its long-term efficacy to reduce the use of pain killers. The reduction of hemorrhage is caused by the vasoconstrictive effect induced by the adrenaline (alfa1-receptors) and by hydrostatic compression, while infectious complications are minimized by the bacteriostatic activity of lidocaine [15].

12.2.5 Patient Positioning

Patient positioning is essential in neurosurgery for the neurosurgical approach, but also for the anesthetist who must deal with possible complications of different positions. Prone positioning may cause neck and head venous congestion, a reduction of pulmonary compliance, an increase in abdominal pression, and caval compression. Extreme head flexion may determinate cerebral compression in patients affected by posterior fossa diseases, while an excessive head rotation may prevent venous drainage by the jugular veins and affect cerebral perfusion. Anti-decubitus devices are imperative in all types of surgery [11, 12]. In our department, the sitting position is being avoided from decades.

12.2.6 Newborn

Newborns (term or pre-term) have higher risks of complication related to anesthesia than older children due to the peculiarity of cardiovascular and respiratory systems. In fact, the responses to hypocapnia and hypoxia are reduced. In patients born before the 34th week of gestation, spontaneous apneas are frequent due to prematurity. Newborns have anatomical particularities such as bigger epiglottis in a more anterior position. Other difficulties are the much more frequent collapse of superior respiratory airways and the disproportion between head and body. Moreover, the respiration is necessarily nasal. Protective ventilation is essential to avoid pulmonary damage. At the same time, hyperoxygenation may be harmful in preterm newborns due to higher risk of obliterative retinopathy and bronchopulmonary dysplasia.

12.2.7 Syndromic Patient

Today, the registered syndromes are more than 10,000 and they are still increasing. The syndromic diagnosis is not always immediate, so it is possible for the anesthetist to face unexpected difficulties. In front of a syndromic patient, it is imperative to obtain the anamnesis and to undergo a meticulous preoperative evaluation, looking for any possible complication caused by the syndrome itself. Being aware of the difficulties related to the syndrome helps the anesthetist to choose the specific anesthesiologic technique, especially in case of difficult airway management, congenital cardiopathy, or malignant hyperthermia risk.

12.3 Pediatric Neuroimaging

Brain imaging is of paramount importance in the diagnosis and follow up of the entire spectrum of disorders of central nervous system. Imaging techniques are brain echography, computed X-ray tomography (CT), and magnetic resonance imaging (MRI). MRI is the gold standard for pediatric brain imaging. With time, extensive employment of MRI in pediatric allowed recognition of specific morphological and functional features of malformative, degenerative, neoplastic (Fig. 12.1), and vascular disorders.

Technical improvement allows high spatial and contrast resolution images that are mandatory in order to maximize the information gained from imaging studies performed either on 1.5 and 3 T equipment [16].

With respect to 1.5 T, imaging at 3 T allows higher resolution and more favorable signal-to-noise ratio with similar time. The small size of the pediatric brain and its higher content of water make more suitable employment of a 3 T unit. A 1.5 T unit can be more suitable if body imaging in addition to brain studies are performed. However, a 1.5 T unit with a dedicated pediatric brain coil can provide adequate imaging in most clinical situation. Due to higher signal-to-noise ratio, 3 T is the optimal choice when highest spatial resolution is required, such as MRI angiogra-

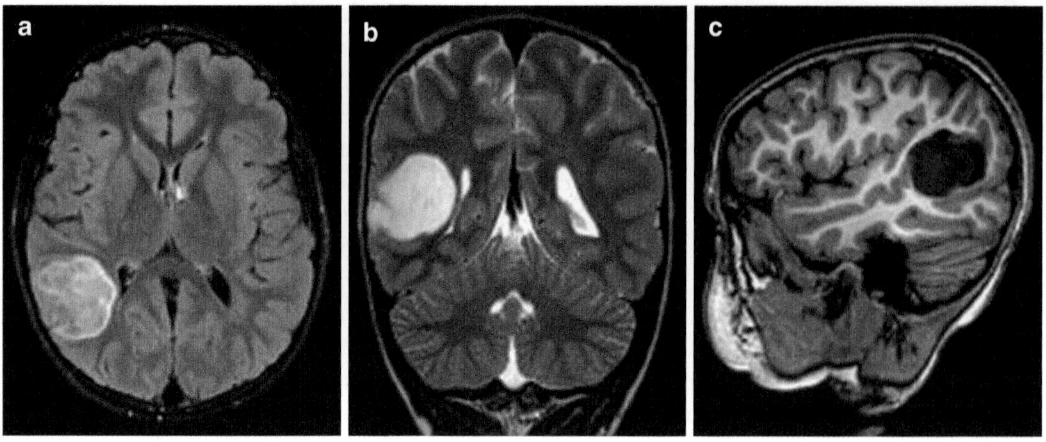

Fig. 12.1 (**a**) Axial FLAIR; (**b**) coronal T2-weighted image; (**c**) sagittal T1-weighted image demonstrating right posterior temporal and parietal nonenhancing lesion, with sharp margins, inhomogeneous hyperintensity on FLAIR and T2-weighted image consistent with DNET or ganglioglioma

phy, or in second-level MRI studies for small brain malformations. However, high signal-to-noise ratio also allow the best results when advanced MRI studies are performed [16].

Besides the strength of the magnetic field, hardware improvement, notable development of 32 channel phased-array head coils, and increase in the performance of the gradients allowed high spatial and contrast resolution, thus maximizing the advantages of high field strengths.

In pediatric patients, the clinical background and the chemical structure of the developing brain change over time, especially for neonates and young infants. Therefore, the MRI studies of the pediatric brain require imaging protocols specific for the different ages. Analogously, a specific training is required for neuroradiologists and MRI technicians involved in pediatric studies.

Careful review of patient history is always required prior to the MRI study, then careful checking of images and eventual protocol modification based on emerging findings must be performed in real time by the supervising neuroradiologist [16].

Whatever the field strength and the imaging protocol, motion artifacts are the main issue in pediatric neuroimaging. To overcome the problem, fast imaging techniques and specific modalities of sedation are employed [16]. Motion artifacts remain an issue for most studies of children younger than 8 years, for which sedation is almost always required.

Although sedation techniques are not discussed, it is important to remind that sedation of infants undergoing MRI studies requires MR compatible life support and monitoring equipment, and, above all, sedation must be performed by a specifically trained anesthesiologist, and that it is time consuming [17].

Sedation is not always necessary for MRI studies of neonates. They can undergo MRI if they are fed immediately prior to the study, kept warm, and earmuffs/earplugs are used to reduce the noise. Moreover, older children can avoid sedation if some MR-compatible audiovisual system is available, or if detailed explanation is provided by appropriately trained nurse or technician.

Noise reduction techniques have been developed by the main MRI vendors and are adopted in the more recent releases.

Fast MR techniques, called PROPELLER, BLADE, HASTE, depending on vendor, allow images of the entire brain without significant motion artifacts in less than 1 min, and are often adequate for diagnosis of hydrocephalus or acute infarcts, but do not provide complete evaluation of the brain, particularly in MRI studies for subtle malformations, metabolic disorders, or tumor progression [18].

The signal intensity and the contrast between grey and white matter change throughout the progression of the myelination, between birth, and 2 years of life. The changes of the MRI picture require careful evaluation of T1- and of heavily T2-weighted images. At birth and in the first 8 months of life, the white matter is incompletely myelinated and, due to its high content of water, it is hyperintense on T2-w.i. Therefore, the imaging parameters must be set in order to obtain the appropriate contrast between grey and white matter. In this period, the progression of the myelinating is better evaluated on T1-w.i. [16]. Between 6 and 8 months, the progression of myelination makes white matter isointense to the cortex. In this phase, the lack of contrast makes more difficult to detect signal abnormalities, and therefore to diagnose malformation of cortical development or small tumors, as well as to recognize the abnormal signal pattern of neurometabolic disorders [16].

FLAIR images have limited value in children younger than 1 year. After the signal intensity from the white matter reaches the normal value, FLAIR are complementary to T2-w.i. [19].

At 1.5 T, spin echo (SE) T1-weighted images usually provide adequate spatial and contrast resolution, and allow assessment of the overall anatomy of the brain.

At 3 T, differences in T1 relaxation times and magnetic susceptibility requires specific techniques and parameters. SE-T1-w.i. cannot be obtained. 3D-T1 volumetric sequence (SPGR, MPRAGE, 3D-FLASH, depending on vendor) must be performed, and, especially if a phased-array head coil and parallel imaging are available, they result in optimal demonstration of small anatomic detail. 0.7–1 mm isotropic voxel partitions and multiplanar reformations in the coronal and axial planes are usually employed in MRI studies' patients for developmental delay and for epilepsy, as they can demonstrate small cortical malformations, as well as reveal subtle areas of T1 shortening in injured brain, and for neuro-navigation.

High resolution volumetric 3D T2-w.i. (FIESTA, bFFE, TrueFISP, depending on vendor) are employed for demonstration of specific anatomic details of cranial nerves or orbits. For evaluation of the intraorbital tract of the optic nerves, fat suppression techniques or DIXON sequences are also available [16].

3D susceptibility-weighted images (SWI) and gradient echo (GE) T2-w.i. are highly sensitive in detecting hemosiderin and calcium deposits. While on GE images calcium and hemosiderin are almost indifferently hypointense, SWI raw phase images allow to distinguish the opposite phase of paramagnetic iron, as normally seen in nuclei pallidi, from diamagnetic calcium, as seen in choroid plexus [20].

Great care is required for administration of contrast medium in pediatric patients. There are indeed increasing concerns regarding cerebral deposition of gadolinium and about nephrogenic systemic fibrosis. Given the immaturity of the blood–brain barrier, children have to be considered at particular risk. Gadolinium administration should be recommended only in MRI studies for follow-up or suspected brain tumors, infective or inflammatory diseases, and absolutely avoided "just in case", or in absence of a definite indication [16].

12.3.1 Advanced MRI Techniques

Besides high contrast and spatial resolution sequences, advanced pediatric neuroimaging includes functional techniques that make more reliable and accurate the diagnosis in children with neurological diseases.

Advanced MRI sequences encompass diffusion-weighted- (DWI), diffusion-tensor (DTI) imaging, perfusion-weighted imaging (PWI), H-magnetic resonance spectroscopy (1H-MRS), and blood oxygenation level-dependent (BOLD) functional MRI (fMRI).

Advanced MRI techniques can deepen the understanding of the normal brain development. They are increasingly employed to obtain quantitative biomarkers in hypoxic–ischemic or traumatic brain injury, or for monitoring treatment of brain tumors, infective diseases, and neurometabolic disorders [21].

12.3.2 Diffusion-Weighted Imaging (DWI)

DWI is based on the magnitude of the random movement of water molecules between the different tissues of the brain.

The diffusion is therefore related to architectural factors. The diffusion rate of water molecules within the cerebrospinal fluid (CSF) is high, as it is not limited by cell membranes, with respect to gray or white matter, where it is limited by the cell membranes and tissue packing.

Specific MR sequences that are sensitive for diffusion, allow to translate different diffusion rates differences in MR signal, and to generate image contrast [21, 22].

Cellular membranes, axons, myelin, and tissue packing are the physiological barriers to water movement within the brain tissue, and therefore determinate the water diffusion in the brain.

Water molecules diffusion within the extracellular space can be described as decreased or "restricted" and increased or "facilitated." Diffusion is differentiated by means of qualitative evaluation and quantitative analysis of diffusion images (DWI images) and ADC maps and values.

On DWI images, decreased or restricted diffusion from limited water mobility within the brain tissues corresponds to bright signal and to dark appearance or low ADC values on ADC maps.

Restricted diffusion is mostly caused by abnormal intracellular accumulation of fluid, that results in cellular swelling, narrowing of the extracellular spaces, and reduced extracellular water mobility. Abnormal intracellular accumulation of fluid is usually referred to as cytotoxic edema. It is typically recognized in acute ischemia and traumatic brain injury. Decreased diffusion can also be detected in brain tumors with high cellularity and high nuclear-to-cytoplasmatic ratio. Moreover, diffusion is restricted in fluid with high viscosity, such as pus in an abscess.

Increased or "facilitated" diffusion is shown as dark or brain isointense signal on diffusion images and bright appearance or high ADC values on ADC maps. Increased diffusion is related to abnormal extracellular accumulation of fluid, "widened" extracellular spaces and therefore to increased extracellular water mobility. This kind of edema is referred to as vasogenic edema; it is caused by a vascular damage or injury to the blood–brain barrier, resulting in abnormal passage of fluid from the intravascular to the interstitial spaces. Vasogenic edema is observed in inflammatory and infective diseases and in chronic phase of stroke.

Furthermore, increased diffusion is seen in low-grade brain tumors, usually characterized by low cellularity, small nuclear area, and high amount of extracellular fluid [21].

12.3.3 Diffusion Tensor Imaging

Besides the magnitude of diffusion for each tissue voxel, diffusion tensor imaging (DTI) samples the principal direction and the three dimensional shape of diffusion [23]. In white matter tracts, diffusion is predominantly parallel to the long axis, and limited in the direction perpendicular to the tract. This directional diffusion can be represented as an ellipsoid, and is known as anisotropic diffusion. A minimum of six directions of diffusion is required to assess water molecular motion in a tissue using the diffusion tensor, in addition to one with no diffusion weighting. When the degree of diffusion is equal in all the directions, such as in CSF, the diffusion can be represented by a sphere and is referred to as isotropic diffusion. Fractional anisotropy (FA) varies between zero, representing maximal isotropic diffusion, and one, representing maximal anisotropic diffusion. The FA values can also be calculated voxel by voxel, and represented in a map. Areas with high anisotropy (high FA value) are bright (e.g., corpus callosum, internal capsule), and areas with low anisotropy (low FA values) are dark (e.g., CSF or gray matter) [23, 24].

Diffusion tensor also provides information about the principal direction of diffusion. A color code map is used to indicate the direction of the anisotropic diffusion: red indicates left-right, green anterior-posterior, and blue superior-inferior anisotropic diffusion.

Reconstruction of the course of white matter tracts based on the direction and magnitude of anisotropic diffusion is known as fiber tractography.

Tractography is based on the assumption that voxels with a similar orientation of their principal anisotropic diffusion direction are likely to be a part of the same white matter tract [24].

DTI properties of the white matter change with the age. In neonates, white matter anisotropy is relatively low and increases with age. The increase of FA in white matter seems to occur in three stages: fiber organization into fascicles; proliferation and maturation of glial cell bodies and intracellular compartments; and myelination. The most part of fiber organization occurs in utero, and may explain the presence of anisotropy in late intrauterine and premature infants. The following steps, that is maturation of glial cells, development of the cytoskeleton and of various intracellular structures, and finally, the progressive myelination of the white matter are related to a continuous increase in anisotropy. In addition, over time, cells and axonal membranes become more densely packed, resulting in reduced water content and decreased water motion.

Therefore, in evaluating DTI, it is crucial to take into consideration the age of the child: the same image can be normal at a younger age, but abnormal at an older age [23, 24].

The main limitation of diffusion tensor is that it provides a good depiction of the fiber orientation in regions where fibers are aligned along a single axis. DTI fails to represent fiber when they cross, merge, or run adjacent to one another (kissing fibers). To overcome these limitations, high-angular resolution diffusion imaging (HARDI) can better estimate the fiber trajectories, particularly when tracts are intersected. These approaches require longer acquisition times, thus limiting their use in unsedated neonates. However, advances in MRI acquisition techniques, such as neonatal head coils, the use of specific protocols, and multiband MRI together with modern, gradient coil systems now enable acquisition of HARDI in a clinically feasible time.

12.3.4 Compartment Models of Microstructure

Compartment models are aimed to characterize the complexity of grey and white matter tissue by decomposing the signal into compartments describing diffusion within distinct microstructural constituents. The model consists of three compartments: the intracellular, extracellular, and cerebrospinal fluid (CSF) environments [24].

NODDI provides measures of neurite density index (NDI) and orientation dispersion index (ODI).

The intraneurite compartment measures the diffusion inside dendrites and axons. In these compartments, the orientation of diffusion can be highly parallel, such as in corpus callosum or in the internal capsule, or highly dispersed, such as in regions of crossing fibers like the centrum semiovale or in the cortex. The extraneurite compartment represents the space occupied by glial cells, where diffusion is hindered.

The NODDI model has been applied to investigate white and grey matter maturation in the preterm brain. NDI increases in the white matter with increasing maturation. The highest NDI values are observed in primary motor and somatosensory tracts; lower values are observed in association fibers. Cortical maturation is characterized by increasing ODI, related to increased dendritic arborization [24, 25].

At present multicompartmental techniques are confined to research: further development and innovations in MRI techniques will allow reduced time of acquisition and facilitate their use in the study of the neonatal and pediatric brain.

12.3.5 Magnetic Resonance Spectroscopy

Proton MR spectroscopy (MRS) provides measurement of relative metabolite concentrations within a volume of interest. Major metabolite peaks of interest include choline (Cho) at 3.2 ppm from cell membranes; creatine (Cr) at 3.0 ppm, reflecting metabolic activity; and *N*-acetylaspartate (NAA) at 2.0 ppm, reflecting neuronal density.

Other peaks that can be identified in clinical MRS studies include myoinositol (mI) in astroglial cells at 3.5 ppm; glutamate glutamine (Glx) from excitatory neurotransmission at 2.2–2.4 and 3.8 ppm, respectively; lipids (Lip) and macromolecules at 1.3 ppm; and amino acids (AA) at 0.9 ppm. Single-voxel or multi-voxel techniques are usually employed in clinical MRS studies. Single voxel technique is the standard clinical tool for analysis of volumes of about 1 cm^3 within basal ganglia, white matter, and other regions of interest. Multi voxel 2-D or 3-D MRS allow to evaluate metabolite concentrations by comparison across multiple brain regions. With respect to single voxel technique, this approach implies increased imaging time and low signal-to-noise ratio per voxel. Whatever the technique, care should be taken that voxels do not overlap cerebrospinal fluid or scalp tissues, which can introduce artifactual lactate and lipid peaks [26–28].

Different echo times can be selected: short-echo MRS (echo time [TE] = 20–35 ms) is useful to detect minor metabolites at low concentrations.

In neurometabolic disorders, MRS is employed to detect the characteristic lactate (Lac) doublet peak (1.35 ppm), which resonate out of phase and thus invert at intermediate echo times (TE = 144 ms). The same or longer echo MR spectroscopy (TE = 272–288 ms) are useful to assess Cho/CR ratio and the relative concentrations of NAA in tumor imaging or hypoxic–ischemic encephalopathy. Of note, in preterm and near-term infants with immature metabolic pathways, anaerobic glycolysis can cause small lactate peaks and decreased NAA and Cho ratio [26].

12.3.6 Perfusion-Weighted Imaging

Perfusion weighted MRI (PWI) techniques are dynamic susceptibility contrast (DSC), dynamic contrast-enhanced, and arterial spin labeling (ASL).

In DSC, the pass of a bolus of contrast medium gives rise to a modification of signal intensity on T2*-w.i. T2* susceptibility allows to track the signal changes generated by the transit of contrast medium. Different perfusion maps are employed for clinical purposes. Cerebral blood volume (rCBV), is related to neovascular capillary volume in high grade tumors; it is accepted as clinical standard for perfusion weighted MRI studies for differential diagnosis of gliomas, or to distinguish tumors and demyelinating plaques or brain abscess in adult patients. Additional perfusion parameters are relative cerebral blood flow (CBF) and mean transit time (MTT), usually employed in cerebrovascular disorders. Dynamic contrast-enhanced-MRI provides detailed information on the disruption of the blood–brain barrier. This technique uses repeated acquisition of T1-w.i. during the first pass and the recirculation phases in which contrast medium flows into the extravascular compartment. Long imaging times and specialized image post-processing are required, therefore applications are mainly employed in research studies.

However, pediatric applications of DSC are less consistently defined [26, 29, 30].

Arterial spin labeling (ASL) is an MR perfusion imaging technique based on magnetically labeled arterial water molecules in the arteries as endogenous contrast agent. Free-water protons at the base of the brain are tagged by means of an inversion pulse. Then, after a variable post-label delay, a perfusion-sensitive imaging is performed, and is subtracted from a control image. The result is a difference signal proportional to the amount of blood that has entered the brain. By means of a general kinetic model based on the specific tagging approach, this signal can be converted to a map of absolute cerebral blood flow (CBF) and visually displayed in gray scale or various color scales [31].

The absence of exogenous contrast medium is the main advantage in pediatric population in which the use of radioactive tracers or exogenous contrasts agents may be restricted. Furthermore, differently with respect to contrast bolus techniques, ASL can be quantitative and easily repeatable for longitudinal studies. The most common applications of ASL are stroke, vasculopathy, and hypoxic–ischemic encephalopathy. ASL is also employed to characterize areas of hyper-perfusion related to vascular malformations, tumors, epilepsy, infection, and inflammation [26, 32].

12.3.7 Functional Magnetic Resonance Imaging

Task-based functional MRI (fMRI) rely on T2*-weighted blood–oxygen level-dependent (BOLD) imaging.

When a patient is asked to perform a certain task (most commonly a motor or language paradigm), the responsible areas of cortex extract more oxygen from the capillaries. This leads to a transient decrease in oxyhemoglobin-to-deoxyhemoglobin ratio, followed by a compensatory delayed (2–6 s) increase in cerebral blood flow, that results in elevated oxyhemoglobin-to-deoxyhemoglobin ratio and increased tissue signal. By comparing activation and null states, BOLD images can be subtracted, and statistically thresholded to obtain a functional map that highlights the areas of activation for each task. The main application of fMRI is preoperative planning for brain tumor, malformation of cortical development, and vascular or traumatic insults.

fMRI can be also employed in surgical planning in children who have a higher capacity for neuroplasticity and functional reorganization [26].

Compared to adults, the main limitation for pediatric application of BOLD fMRI techniques is the inability to perform task paradigms.

Development and introduction of "resting-state" fMRI techniques (RS fMRI), which do not require task paradigm, are allowed to study and to map functionally specific cortical regions.

RS fMRI rely on BOLD "functional connectivity," namely, phenomenon of temporal synchronization of functionally related brain areas [33].

Two different methods are employed to map functionally connected brain regions: seed-voxel correlation and independent component analysis (ICA) [34].

The motor network represents the temporal synchrony between left and right motor cortical regions; a visual network similarly includes left and right visual cortex. Cortical areas with greatest metabolic activity at rest are referred to as default mode network (DMN). The DMN consists of bilateral posterior cingulate gyrus, precuneus, inferior parietal lobules, ventromedial prefrontal cortex, and variable other regions, including temporal cortex [35, 36].

Pediatric applications of RS fMRI are based on the hypothesis that myelination of white matter tracts correspond to development and strengthening of functional connectivity between intrinsically connected cortical regions. Furthermore, abnormalities of functional connectivity might help to determine the effect of brain injury on brain function, and could be helpful to orientate therapies in neonates and children with brain injury.

Resting state networks, namely, motor, auditory, visual, and DMN, can be detected in premature infants [37], indicating that cortical regions are functionally connected long before the onset of white matter myelination. The DMN could not be detected in premature newborns, but was identified in term-born infants [38]. By 2 years of age, the DMN resembled that of the adult brain.

It is expected that more extensive RS fMRI applications allow to understand progression of cortical and white matter functional activities in developmental age.

12.4 Technical Improvements of Surgical Tools

12.4.1 Operating Microscope

The impact of the operating microscope on neurosurgery has been so important that today it is very difficult to imagine neurosurgery without it. Nevertheless, the process which led to the diffusion of the microscope was long and complex. The operating microscope was firstly used by otolaryngologists for middle ear surgeries in the 1920s [39] (Fig. 12.2).

During the ensuing decades, vascular surgeons demonstrated its utility mainly in experimental models of small vessel anastomosis. The interest toward central nervous system arrived later, in the 1950s, with pioneers such as Theordore Kurze, who performed the excision of a seventh nerve neurinoma and a VII–XII cranial nerve anastomosis with the operating microscope in 1957 [40] (Fig. 12.3).

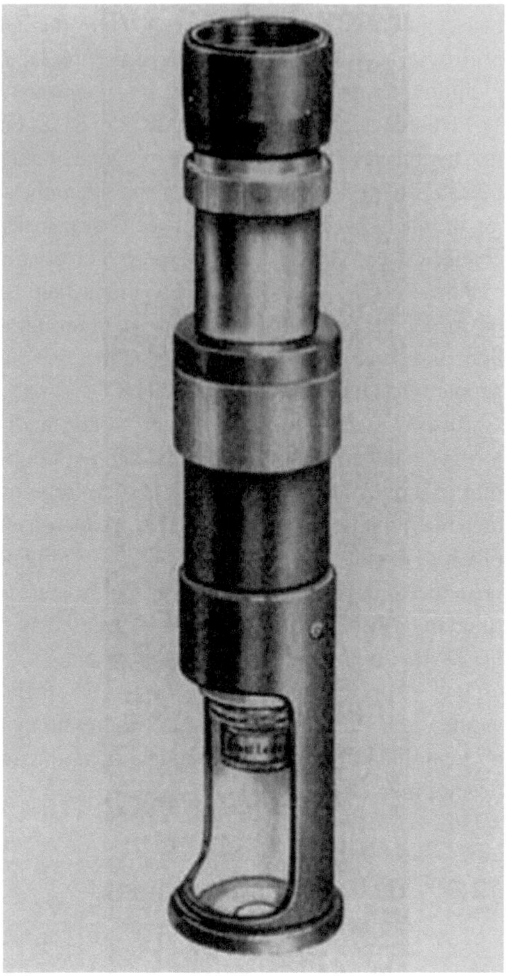

Fig. 12.2 Nylen's Brinell-Leitz monocular microscope (courtesy of Acta Otolaryngol)

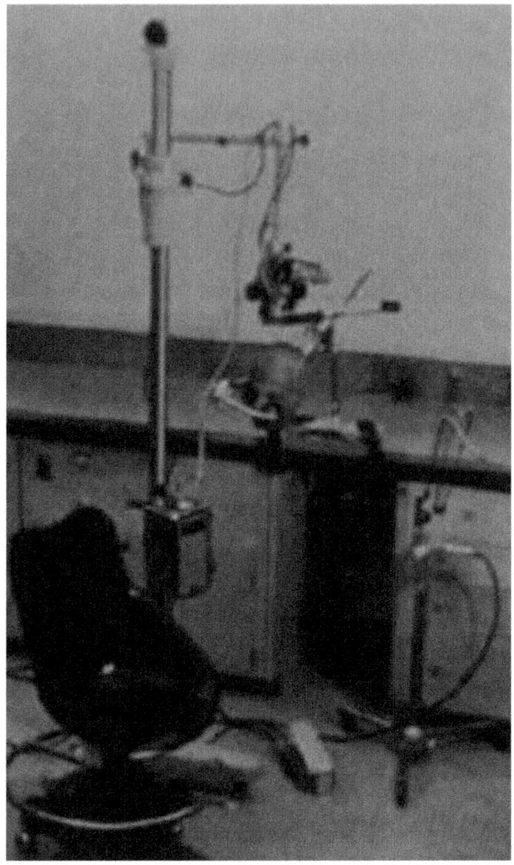

Fig. 12.3 Kurze's microscope in the first cranial base microsurgical laboratory, 1961

The crucial point was the work of Donaghy, who firstly established the world's first microsurgery research and training laboratory in Burlington, Vermont, and then he performed in 1960 the first "microscopic" middle cerebral artery embolectomy. In 1966, M. G. Yasargil spent a year mastering microsurgical techniques in Donaghy's laboratory. In 1967, both Yasargil in Zurich and Donaghy in the USA performed an anastomosis of middle cerebral artery and temporal artery, giving birth to microneurosurgery [41]. In the ensuing years, many neurosurgeons started to admit operating microscope's utility, allowing its diffusion in Europe and in the USA.

Technological innovations allowed progressive improvement and, as a result, the operating microscope has improved tremendously since its invention. Today, the microscope offers good magnification, sufficient illumination and satisfying stability without sacrificing operational flexibility [42] (Fig. 12.4).

The immediate result of microscopy was a reduction of complications, an increase of success probability of surgeries and generally better outcomes. Vascular neurosurgery was the first field to adopt this technique, but in a second moment, it begun to be used for all surgeries that require an invasive operation on the CNS. At the same time, new surgical instrumentation was developed to be used with microscopy. Today, the operating microscope is used for a large

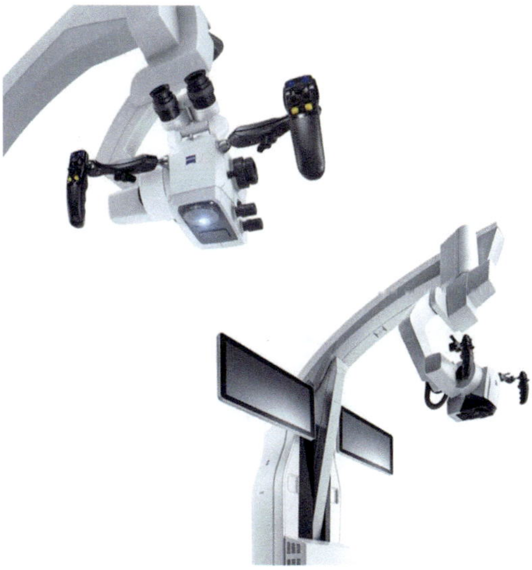

Fig. 12.4 Modern microscope (Zeiss)

spectrum of surgeries, both cranial and spinal. As for vascular neurosurgery, for instance, a rate of 97% efficiency in patients treated with a microscope for vascular disease was observed [43]. Pediatric patients benefit from it for obvious reasons.

High dynamic range imaging (HDR) is a new technology which allows better quality of images with less illumination and allows to capture almost with the same detail brighter and darker parts of the image. Moreover, some microscopes have automatic focusing and some of the new ones can also maintain a good focus also in the deeper layers. In fact, two of the most important problems of the operating microscope are the ability to show the same detail for bright and dark parts of the same image and the fact that zooming induces a narrowing of the focal plane [44]. Modern microscopes allow multiparametric visualization. For example, microscopes can be used during tumoral excision to examine the limits of the resection by using a blue light illumination after the administration of 5-aminolevulinic acid orally [45]. With this technique, the surgeon can differentiate normal tissue from tumor. Another technique is the intraoperative angiography after indocyanine green EV injection.

12.4.2 3-D Exoscope

One of the most recent visualization tools is the 3D exoscope. The exoscope is a system that allows, with polarized eyeglasses, to visualize the smallest details of the surgical field on a wide 4K monitor without any loss of resolution [46]. It is also known as robotized microscope as its central core is made up of a small camera which can be robotically positioned on the surgical field, offering the same magnification as the surgical microscope. Therefore, the surgeon looks directly at the monitor and shares the image with all the surgical staff (surgical assistant, scrub nurses, anesthesiologist, and residents/medical students).

The system is robotized and miniaturized. The robotized arm is controlled through a sterile joypad on the surgical field. Some exoscopes, moreover, can be combined with optical endoscopes both in 3D and 4K.

During the past few years, some centers have already published studies that evaluate its efficacy for the treatment of different neurosurgical conditions [47–52]. Thus, the market already offers various types of exoscopes (e.g., ORBEYE™ Olympus, KINEVO® Carl Zeiss, VITOM® 4K 3D Karl Storz, Modus V™ Synaptive Medical) (Fig. 12.5).

The advantages of the exoscope are mainly user comfort [53], depth perception and reduced light thermal damage [54–57], the possibility to use personal protection devices during neurosurgical procedures on Covid-19 positive patients.

As for disadvantages, prolonged operative time has been described [53, 58]. This has been attributed to the learning curve that surgeons are confronted with, given the need to develop skills of indirect vision tactics and maneuvering hand movements while watching a monitor that is not in line with their hands. In the context of modern neurosurgery, an experienced neurosurgeon who has dedicated training time to neuroendoscopy, won't have any problem with this new technology. For instance, pediatric neurosurgeons, who are keen to perform neuro-endoscopical procedures, might have a less steep learning curve compared to adult neurosurgeons who are more prone to perform microsurgical operations.

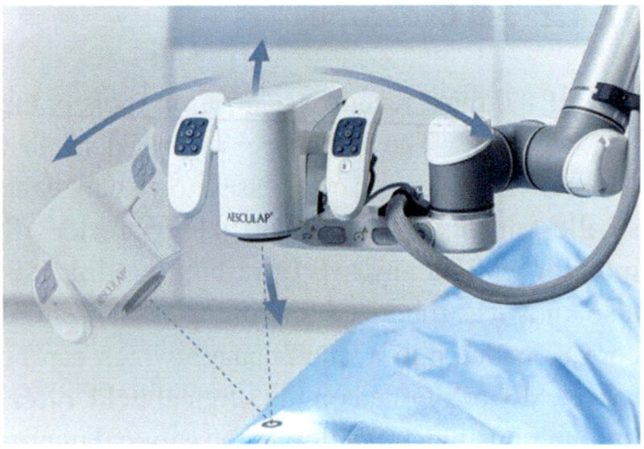

Fig. 12.5 3-D exoscope (Aesculap Aeos®)

In conclusion, 3D-exoscopes might be the future of modern neurosurgery. They will be for sure the tool that actual junior residents will progressively introduce into their daily practice and be the standard for treatment in the next decades.

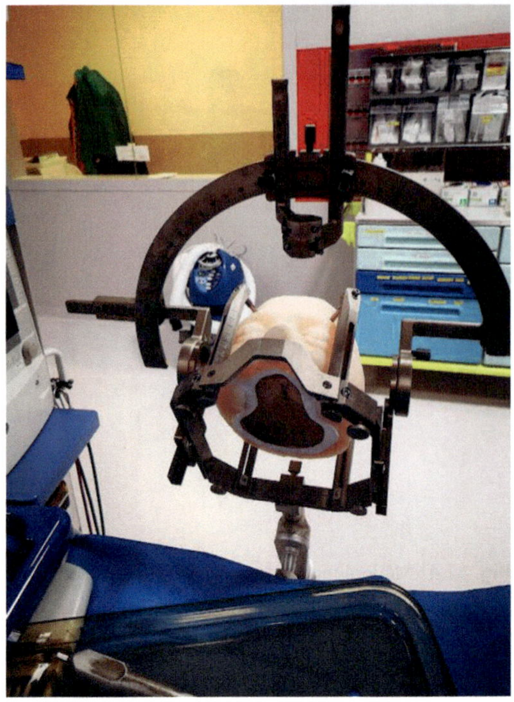

Fig. 12.6 3D model with a stereotactic Leksell frame; pre-operative attempts for ideal targeting of deep-seated lesions

12.4.3 Neuronavigation

Localization techniques represent a revolution in neurosurgery. The first localization technique was frame-based stereotaxis, in which the presence of a frame linked to the patient's head allowed the association between the patient's anatomy and the preoperative images. Frame based techniques are used mostly for biopsy or abscess surgery (Fig. 12.6). The real revolution was allowed by the introduction of frameless stereotaxis, also known as neuronavigation [59, 60]. Neuronavigation is a safe and non-invasive real-time imaging technique, in which it is possible to associate a preoperative imaging to the real anatomy of the patient so that when the surgeon touches the patient's head with a specific probe or pointer, he/she can see on the preoperative image where he/she is touching and the trajectory of that point into the deeper layers. Currently, neuronavigation is indispensable for neurosurgery because it helps to localize a lesion, or a specific region directly on the patient [31, 32] and, at the same time, by this localization, it determines less invasive procedures because the surgeon can use smaller craniotomies and smaller incisions.

Neuronavigation starts with a preoperative imaging. The patient undergoes a dedicated CT or MRI before the surgery, then the image is uploaded onto the neuronavigator. The older navigation systems needed multiple surface references. Those markers were called *fiducials* and they used to be bone screws or adhesive markers [61–64] (Fig. 12.7).

Nowadays, patient's cranial elements are used for the registration process, avoiding the adhesive markers. The use of fiducials is today limited to extremely accurate surgical procedures in which there is need to reach small targets or deep targets, for example, for biopsies, deep brain stimulation, or deep visualase.

Registration is the process through which we create an association between the patient's head and the preoperative imaging. In pediatrics, point pair registration and surface contour registration are the most used. The first one consists in matching at least three non-collinear points such as nasion, lateral canthus, and tragus with a

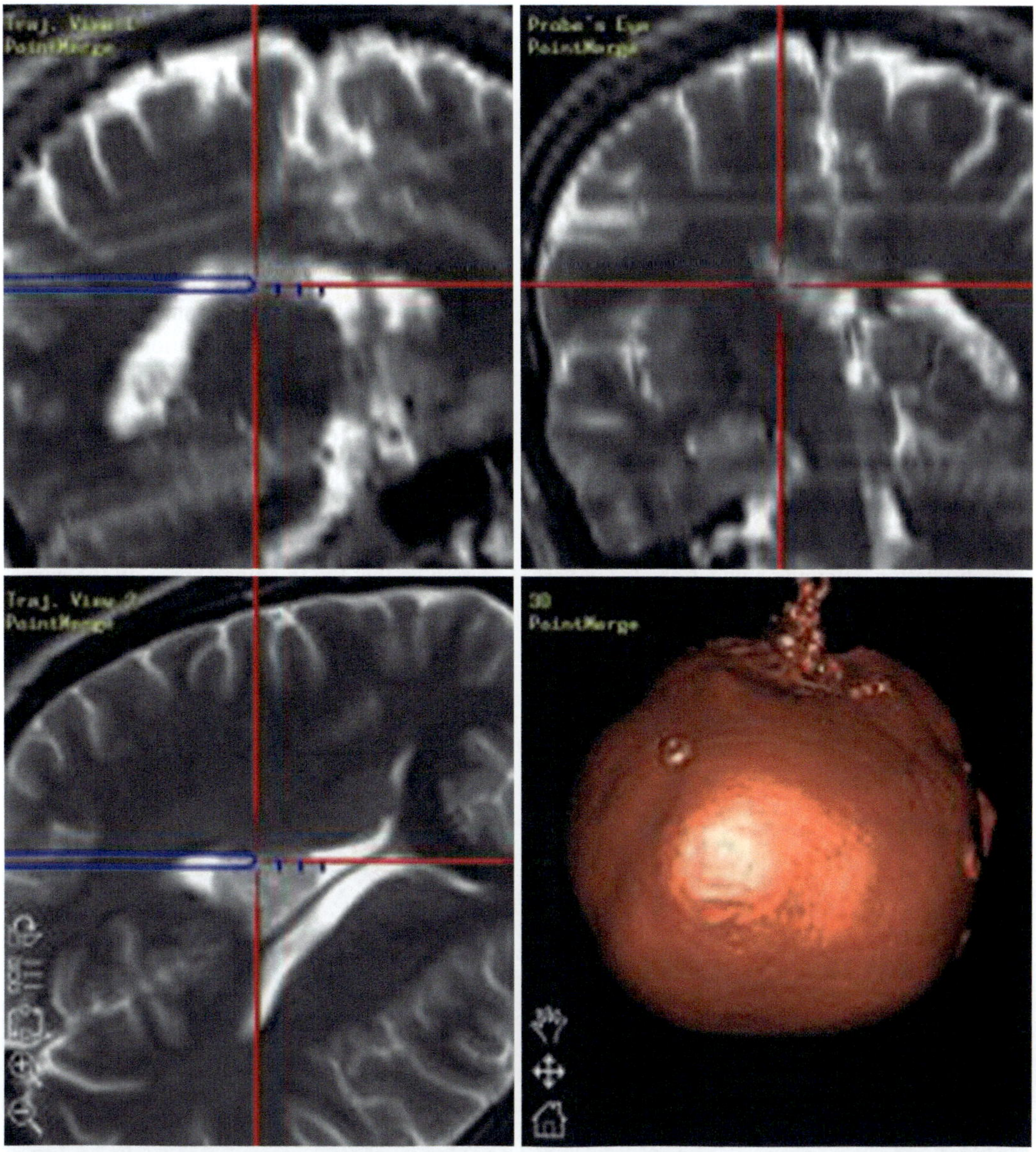

Fig. 12.7 Neuronavigation system. MRI was merged with a CT scan, 3D reconstruction (bottom right) shows adhesive markers (fiducials)

pointer. The latter is done by touching several multiple random points, or by scanning with laser registration [63]. After the registration process, when the pointer touches the patient, the neuronavigator screen shows on the CT/MRI where we are touching and the projection of that point in the deeper layers. This ability of neuronavigation is called *device tracking*. The most used tracking technologies are optical and electromagnetic systems. The first type uses infrared markers on the tracked pointing device so that the tip of the pointer is found by geometric algorithms. The disadvantage of this technique is the need to create a free space between the instrument and the cameras of the neuronavigator. New electromagnetic tracking technology does not need a free space because it uses electromagnetic fields to find the position of the pointer.

Another important concept of neuronavigation is patient head movement. In the first neuronavigator systems, head movement was not allowed because it induced the loss of precise association between real anatomy and the imaging so that patient had to use specific head clamps to immobilize the patient's head [59]. The use of those head-immobilizing devices for children had high taxes of complications due to their skull immaturity (presence of open fontanelle, fragile skull bone, etc.) such as skull bone deformity, fractures, and sometimes epidural hematomas and dural laceration [65]. Today it is possible to use "dynamic reference frames," a reference frame with markers usually attached to the head holder. Another solution is the use of electromagnetic neuronavigation, which does not need absolute immobilization, allowing navigation also in very young patients.

The trajectories described by the neuronavigator allow the surgeon to choose the approach to reach specific regions of the CNS, avoiding important structures of the brain and vessels (Fig. 12.8). Firstly, it allows smaller craniotomies for tumor resection, the assessment of critical brain areas in the surgical trajectory, and the guidance to subcortical lesions. Furthermore, it may allow an improvement in the extent of tumoral removal [61, 66].

It may help neuroendoscopy and all the procedures in proximity of functional areas. Modern frameless methods for localization have a position accuracy within 2–3 mm during surgery. There are some clinical factors that may cause brain shift or lesion shift such as CSF loss, edema, cyst decompression, etc [67]. In the last decade, many authors have implemented the use of intraoperative MRI associated with neuronavigation so that the imaging shown on the neuronavigator is not preoperative but intraoperative, eliminating the problems related to brain shift. Paraskevoloulos et al. showed that iMRI and

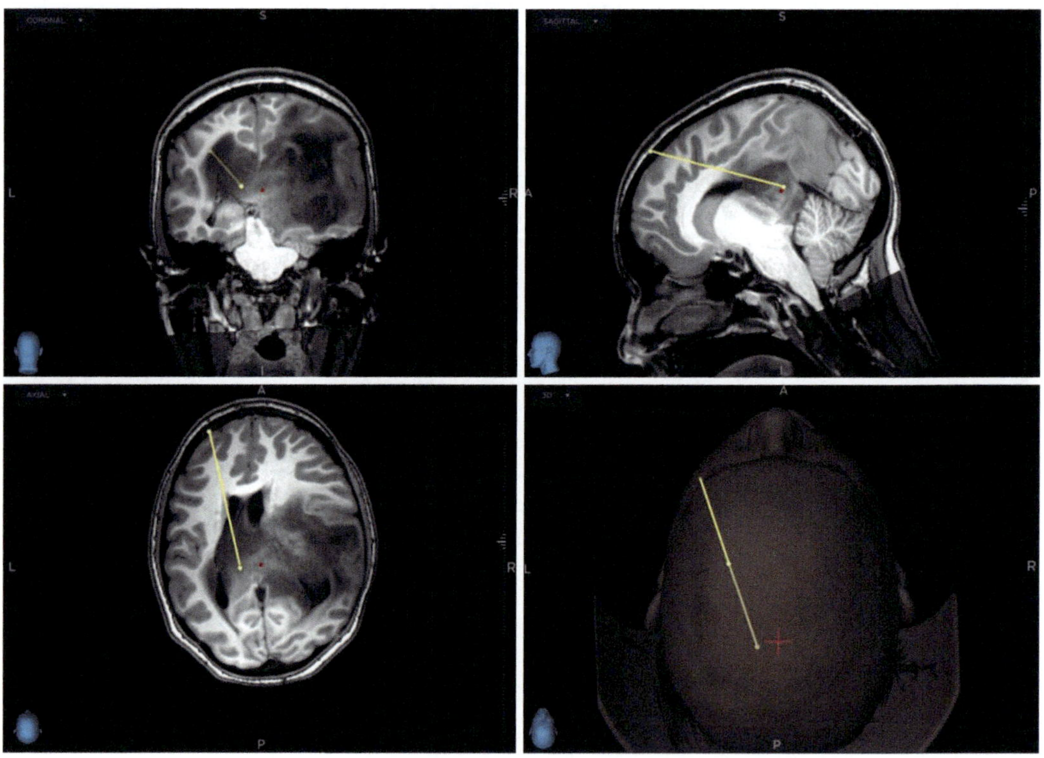

Fig. 12.8 Pre-operative planning for a robot-assisted tumor biopsy (Medtronic)

navigated neuroendoscopy can be used for multicompartmental hydrocephalus and complex cysts in infants [68]. The combination of these two methods have been used also for epilepsy surgery and oncologic neurosurgery.

Robot-assisted surgery can be seen as the evolution of neuronavigation, as the latter is used only for imaging assessment, while the former may perform itself an active part of the surgery. Robot-assisted surgery has spread across several surgical fields and pediatric neurosurgery is one of the most promising (Fig. 12.9). Robotic surgery allows for high accuracy and safety.

De Benedictis et al. showed a series of 128 consecutive pediatric patients operated by ROSA-assisted procedures (neuroendoscopy, implantation of electrodes, shunt placement, deep brain stimulation, biopsy, and stereotactic cyst aspiration) and demonstrated improved safety and feasibility of minimally invasive approaches [69]. Gupta et al. showed no serious complications (only 3 asymptomatic small hematomas and 1 temporary cranial neuropathy) among a series of 23 brainstem and thalamic biopsies done with ROSA-assisted robot with a diagnostic success rate of 91.1% [70]. The ROSA-robot belongs to both supervisory-controlled and shared controlled systems. It can be used for stereotactic and non-stereotactic surgeries. Future perspective are the standardization of robot-assisted surgeries and the use of the robot for further surgeries (such as endoscopic third ventriculostomy, ablation of epileptic foci, implant of intracerebral electrodes for stereo-EEG). Disadvantages of manual arm-based biopsies are larger skin incisions, whilst the advantage of the minimally invasive robotic technique is the precise placement of a small stereotactic stab incision unaffected by the thickness of the skin-muscle layer. Minimally invasive biopsy technique can improve accuracy without increasing operating time and improve cosmetic result, while being equally safe and effective compared to the standard frameless arm-based manual biopsy technique [71].

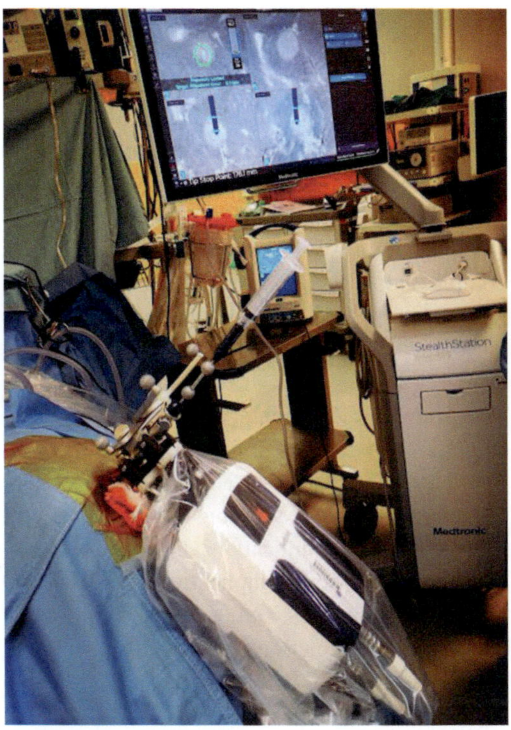

Fig. 12.9 Intraoperative image of a robot-assisted tumor biopsy (Medtronic Autoguide)

12.4.4 Neuroendoscopy

Neuroendoscopy is nowadays a solid neurosurgical reality. The main objectives of this technique are to increase surgical field visualization and to reach deep structures with a less invasive technique. Endoscopes are divided into rod-lens endoscopes and optic fiber endoscopes (also known as fiberscopes). Fiberscopes transmit the image through fiberoptic threads so that they can be rigid or flexible. The quality of the image depends on the number of fibers. Flexible endoscopes have the smallest diameter. Steerable fiberscopes have a working channel to reach the structures that are visualized. Moreover, it is possible to bend the tip in varying degrees. Rigid fiberscopes are available in different lengths and diameters (usually, the increase of the diameter allows better visualization and better quality of

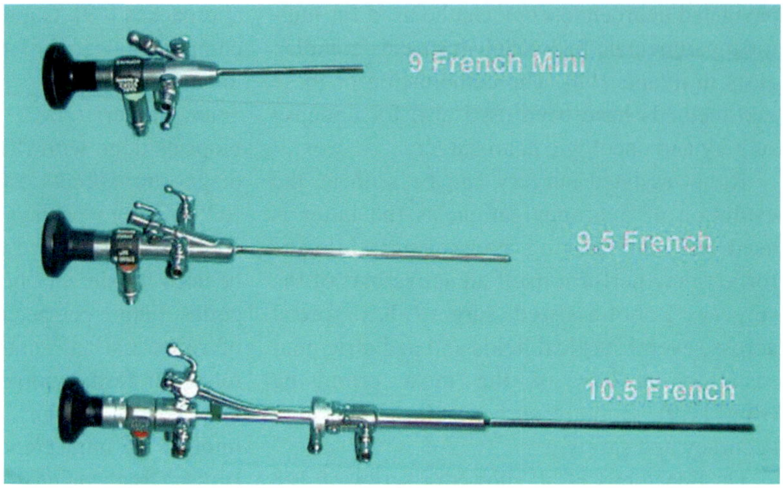

Fig. 12.10 Types of ventricular endoscopes (Genitorishe by Storz)

image) (Fig. 12.10). Rod-lens endoscopes are all rigid with one or two working channels, and they may have different angles (0°-, 30°-, 70°- and 120° angle). They are commonly used in neurosurgery due to their higher quality of image compared to optic fiber endoscopes. Instruments can be used through the working channels or separately, depending on the type of surgery. A light source allows to illuminate the surgical field though the endoscope and the image acquired is sent to a screen in the operating room. Generally, rigid endoscopes are more used than flexible ones, but there are some surgeries in which flexible endoscopes are the main choice, for example, in choroid plexus coagulation with or without ETV for obstructive hydrocephalus treatment [72].

The advantages of neuroendoscopy consist of a less invasive approach compared to microsurgery, an increase of the area of visualization at the surgical site, and the ability to look around corners with angled endoscopes. As mentioned before, rigid endoscopes have different tip angles. The most used are 0°- and 30° angle endoscopes, but specific surgeries might need to inspect surrounding areas with 70°- or 120° endoscopes.

Endoscopes can also be used during craniotomies to enhance the surgeon visualization of the field to understand the next steps. This technique is called endoscope-assisted microneurosurgery [73] (Fig. 12.11).

The disadvantages of neuroendoscopy are the absence of binocular vision, the occupying space in surgical corridor, the limitation of instruments that can be used, and the need of another operator or an endoscope holder to allow bimanual surgery. However, neuroendoscopy has reached optimal results for different pathologies.

Endoscopy has modified obstructive hydrocephalus therapy. Hydrocephalus (HCP) is one of the most common pediatric neurosurgical diseases. Shunting has been the first accepted therapy for hydrocephalus and initially it was used for all types of HCP (Fig. 12.12). Although shunting improves acute patient's conditions, complications have been observed in almost all the patients. Complications are related to mechanical dysfunction, overdrainage, and infections [74], with a rate of 30% in the first years after shunting, a percentage that has not significantly changed over the past 50 years [75, 76]. There are patients that develop multiple episodes of shunt failure [77]. Shunting requires long term follow-up and complications may happen anytime. Shunt-related complications may lead to death even after long time (due to infection, or acute shunt dysfunction); attention to detail and meticulous surgical technique are important if a high rate of shunt infection is to be avoided [78–80].

Therefore, neurosurgeons looked for alternative treatments. Today, endoscopic third ventriculocisternostomy (ETV) is one of the most

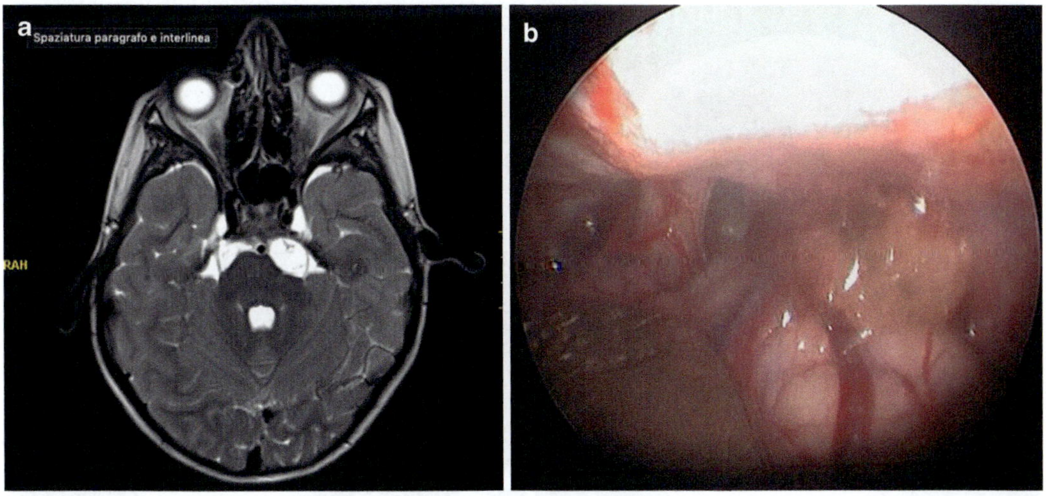

Fig. 12.11 Endoscopic approach to pontocerebellar mass. (**a**) Preoperative T2W RM shows a hyperintense mass of the left pontocerebellar angle in an 8-year-old patient. (**b**) Intraoperative endoscopic image shows the mass on the right. On the left, the trigeminal nerve is visualized

Fig. 12.12 Shunting systems

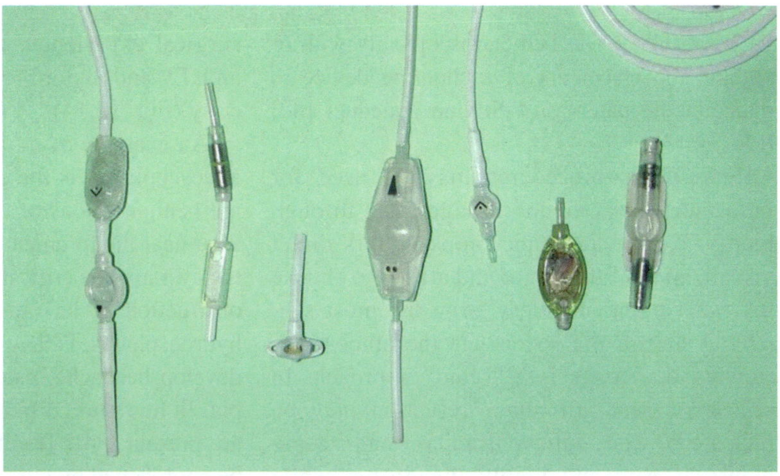

important alternatives for obstructive HCP. ETV failure generally occurs early (about 90% within 3 months), and it is rare to observe failure after 5 years. Most of long-term studies agree with a 70% success rate at 5 years. Age and etiology of HCP are the most important factors in determining success rate. Today, neurosurgeons are trying to understand if ETV can be used for other patients because it is a safe procedure and may allow a shunt-independent life. ETV is the first-line approach to aqueduct stenosis, but it is also effective in tectal plate lesions and midline posterior fossa tumor induced hydrocephalus. The advantages of the ETV over shunt insertion are the lower rate of post-operatory complications and a shunt-free life [81]. ETV is a minimally invasive procedure because it uses small incision and craniotomy. Other advantages are related to the absence of foreign bodies (such as shunt devices) and the establishment of a more physiological CSF circulation rather than the one reached by shunting.

Endoscopy can be used for other forms of HCP such as isolated lateral ventricle (performing a septostomy) and trapped fourth ventricle (performing an aqueductoplasty). Multiloculated

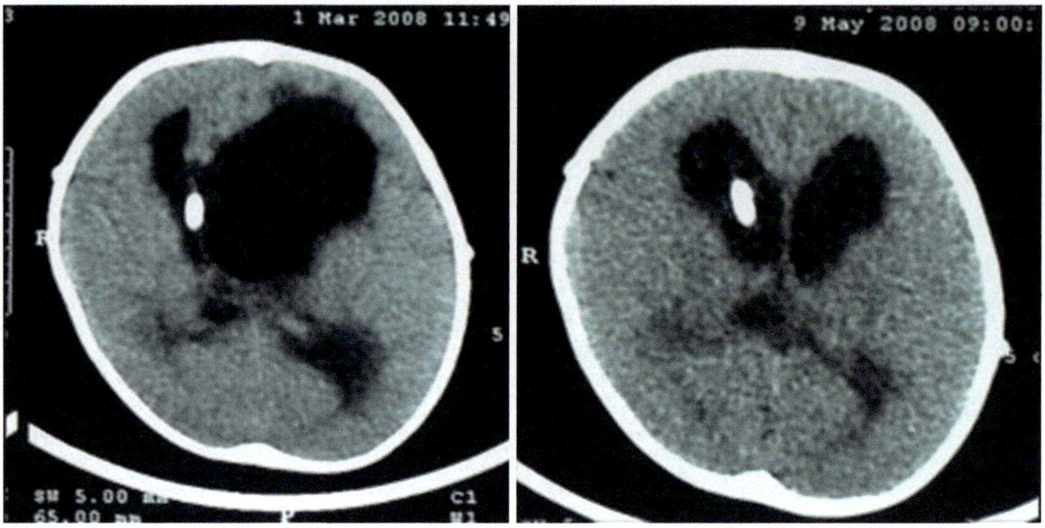

Fig. 12.13 Preoperative and postoperative CT of multiloculated HCP. Lateral ventricle endoscopic fenestration induced an evident reduction of HCP. The post-op CT shows symmetric frontal horns and reduction of occipital horns

HCP can be approached endoscopically with or without the placement of a shunting device to maintain the patency of Silvian aqueduct [82] (Fig. 12.13).

Endoscopic procedures may be used for intraventricular tumor diagnosis through biopsy. Neuroendoscopic biopsy offers direct visualization of the tumor and allows to choose the exact point of biopsy from the most suspicious part of the lesion. On the other hand, stereotactic biopsy is a "blind" approach. In selected cases, full tumor resection may be indicated. The intraventricular endoscopic biopsy is safe and highly diagnostic, while tumor resection is not always possible due to limited instrumentation and poor blood loss control during endoscopy. Tumoral excision depends on tumor characteristics such as density, hardness, and vascularity. In the last years, the introduction of the endoscopic ultrasound aspirator caused an increasing interest toward purely neuroendoscopic total removal of intraventricular and intra-paraventricular tumors and some authors showed the feasibility of these technique for tumors such as subependymal giant astrocytomas, high-grade glioma metastases, and pineal tumors [83]. In selected cases, with opportune anatomy and optimal surgical experience, it is possible to perform an ETV and tumor biopsy with the same endoscopy (Fig. 12.14).

An example of intraventricular lesion treated endoscopically is the colloid cyst. Colloid cysts are benign lesions of the third ventricle situated at or near the foramen of Monro. The position of the cyst may be critical because it may induce an obstruction of lateral ventricles output causing hydrocephalus. Patients may be asymptomatic or develop headache, nausea, vomiting, and diplopia. In literature, different cases of sudden death are present [84]. Traditionally, colloid cysts can be approached by a transcallosal transventricular microsurgery, but there is an increasing interest toward endoscopic treatment [85–87]. The endoscope enters a lateral ventricle and reaches the cyst through the foramen of Monro. Once the cyst is visualized, the first step is the coagulation of the cyst wall. Then, the surgeon opens the cyst, aspirates the content and proceeds with the resection of the walls from the third ventricles' walls and eventually with the removal of the whole cyst. Endoscopy is not always possible. For example, Samadian et al. have shown four cases in which endoscopic approach had to be switched to open microscopic surgery due to incontrollable bleeding during the operation [86, 88].

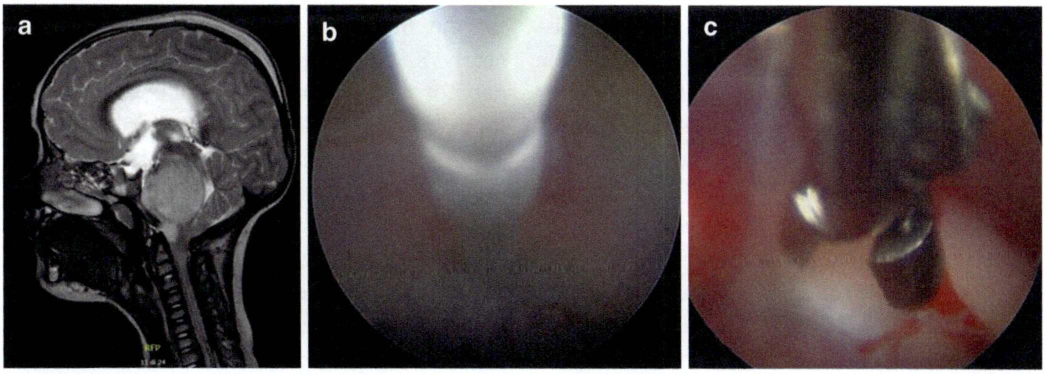

Fig. 12.14 Endoscopic ETV and biopsy of diffuse intrinsic pontine glioma (DIPG). (**a**) Preoperative T2W RM shows a diffuse invasive mass of the brainstem associated with triventricular HCP in a 4-year-old patient. (**b**) Intraoperative endoscopic image shows the creation of ETV by opening the floor of the third ventricle. (**c**) Intraoperative endoscopic biopsy is performed by approaching the tumor from the interpedincular cistern

Arachnoid cysts (AC) may also be treated endoscopically. Arachnoid cysts are congenital malformations which contain CSF and do not communicate with subarachnoid spaces. They can be unloculated or septated. AC can be either asymptomatic or present with headache, intracranial hypertension, focal signs. AC are classified by their position. Middle fossa, suprasellar, quadrigeminal, and posterior fossa cysts can be ideal candidates for endoscopic fenestration [89]. Moreover, the possibility of using lasers to treat arachnoid cysts in selected cases has recently provided good results. Choi et al. [90] performed the largest prospective study assessing the efficacy of laser-assisted endoscopic treatment. A pediatric case report by Van Beijnum et al. [91] also demonstrated successful laser-assisted endoscopic fenestration of a suprasellar arachnoid cyst. However, comparisons of surgical results from laser-assisted endoscopic cyst fenestration with microsurgical cyst excision, stereotactic aspiration, or cystoperitoneal shunting are still lacking in the literature. In experienced hands, the endoscopic technique, as a first line treatment for middle cranial fossa arachnoid cysts, is a reasonable technique to offer in these patients with few neurological sequelae. The families must be warned that with this technique, the cyst may never fully disappear in a significant portion of patients. A second line of repeat endoscopy, craniotomy, or shunt may have to be considered in failures or complications with subdural collections [92–94].

Endoscopic endonasal corridor has been extensively used for skull base surgery in the last two decades [95]. Endoscopic endonasal surgery (EES) is commonly used for the treatment of skull base lesions such as pituitary adenomas, craniopharyngiomas, and Rathke cleft cyst. EES uses the nasal corridor to reach the skull base through a sphenoidotomy [96]. Today pediatric endoscopic skull base surgery is a proven technique, and it is considered safe and useful, but there are no long-term comparison studies between EES and microsurgery techniques [96, 97]. In 2020, a systematic meta-analysis demonstrated the efficacy of EES for craniopharyngiomas in pediatric patients as an optimal alternative to microsurgery [98]. An important issue about EES in pediatrics is the difference between the anatomy of children and adults as the piriform aperture, sphenoid sinus pneumatization, and inter-carotid distance are areas of potential limitation. Piriform aperture width may be a contraindication for EES in the youngest patients (<3 years).

Craniosynostosis consists of a premature fusion of one or more cranial sutures. This condition induces morphologic alterations of skull growth, which may lead to cosmetic alterations but also to diplopia, hydrocephalus, and intracranial hypertension. Craniosynostosis are classified as syndromic and non-syndromic. Another classification of craniosynostosis is based on the localization of the fused suture: different sutures may be involved with different consequent results in term of skull morphology. The treatment is surgical and consists in specific craniectomies which can be done with an open craniectomy or endoscopic strip craniectomy (ESC) [99–104]. The latter is a technique introduced in 1998 by Jimenez and Barone [105]. Its goal is to achieve similar function and cosmetic outcomes minimizing the side effects of open surgery. The targets of this type of surgery are patients younger than 4–5 months with non-syndromic monosynostosis [106] (Fig. 12.15). Over the past two decades, we performed over 2000 procedures for craniosynostosis and we started performing ESC for the treatment of methopic synostosis for nearly 50 cases. Initially, the ESC was indicated only for single suture fusion, but in the last years, it has been used also for more complex stenosis such as bicoronal suture fusion [107], for syndromic craniosynostosis [108], and as single-stage treatment for metopic-sagittal synostosis [109]. The advantages of this technique consist of a reduction of surgical time, blood loss and blood transfusions, reduction of hospitalization, and perioperative complications compared to open surgery [110]. The disadvantages are related to the fact that long-term outcome is still not well understood and, in our experience, according to recent literature, we abandoned this type of approach for sagittal craniosynostosis as we have not encountered any differences in terms of surgical timing,

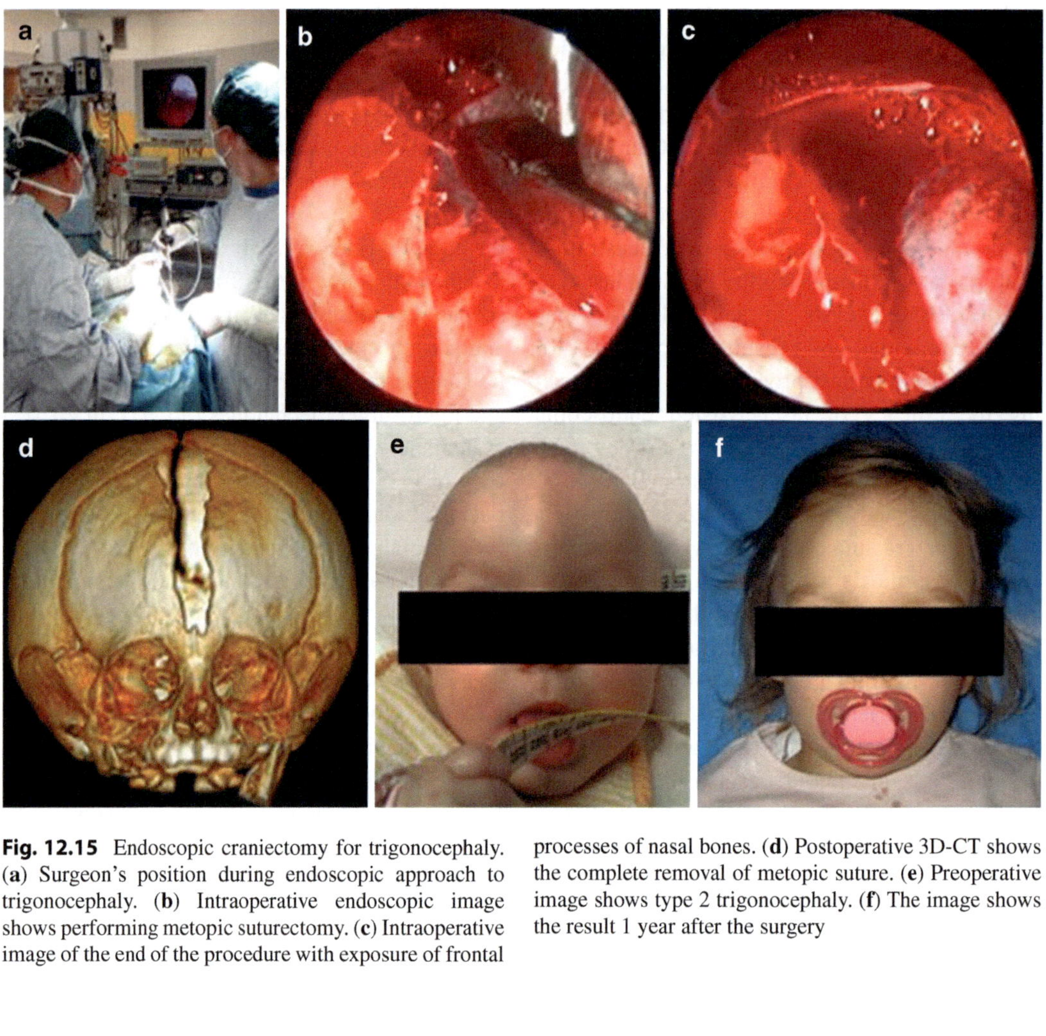

Fig. 12.15 Endoscopic craniectomy for trigonocephaly. (**a**) Surgeon's position during endoscopic approach to trigonocephaly. (**b**) Intraoperative endoscopic image shows performing metopic suturectomy. (**c**) Intraoperative image of the end of the procedure with exposure of frontal processes of nasal bones. (**d**) Postoperative 3D-CT shows the complete removal of metopic suture. (**e**) Preoperative image shows type 2 trigonocephaly. (**f**) The image shows the result 1 year after the surgery

blood loss, and either esthetical or functional outcome [111]. Despite all the advantages, there are no studies on long-term outcome of ESC compared to open technique; therefore, further analysis is required.

12.4.5 Laser Interstitial Thermal Therapy (LITT)

The basic principle of laser interstitial thermal therapy is light amplification by stimulated emission of radiation.

Empirically, atoms' state can be excited under light absorption in special glasses, crystals, or gases. Whenever these atoms go back to their previous state, they dissipate energy as photons or light particles.

These photons, which are produced by all atoms that go back to a previous energy state, act propagating with the same wave length in a physical coherent pattern. Coherence, in physics, means that waves have constant amplitude. Therefore, laser light is compact even when it travels for long distances. As for laser light, all released photons have the same features: the light beam is compact, monodirectional, coherent, monochrome [112].

In medicine, laser can be used to treat tissues with a focalized and regulated dose of energy. As a result, the dose of energy is transferred as heat. The tissue reacts with a protein denaturation process and, thereafter, with cell destruction.

These principles were eventually applied to the treatment of neoplastic lesions affecting the central nervous system [113]. It is possible, in fact, to use laser interstitial thermal therapy with a thin laser fiber in a limited area.

Its functioning is technically easy but, at the same time, technologically and surgically complex.

The surgical technique is based on stereotaxis guided by computerized and automatized systems which can guide the surgeon's hands toward the insertion of a 2 mm diameter fiber laser. The needed burr-hole is about 3.2 mm and the laser energy is concentrated at the tip of the fiber (Fig. 12.16).

The activation of the laser light is made at the same time with the MRI scans, every 3 s.

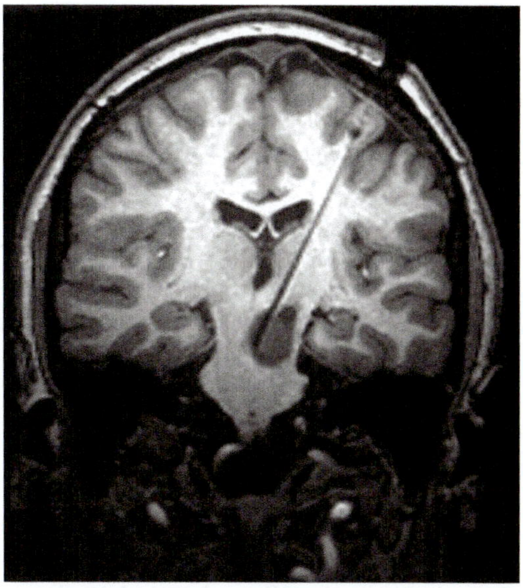

Fig. 12.16 MRI acquired after the insertion of a laser fiber for LITT (laser interstitial thermal therapy)

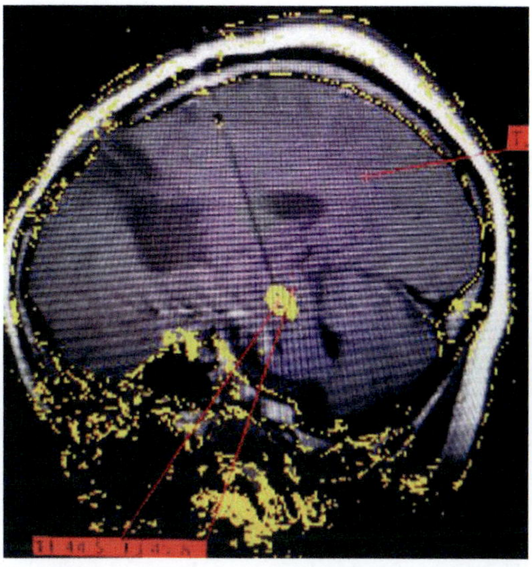

Fig. 12.17 Live thermic map during LITT (temperature around 45 °C at the core of the lesion)

The scans are also translated into a live thermic map (Fig. 12.17).

The neurosurgeon decides when to activate the laser, the power, and timing settings.

The advantages of the procedure are: less hair shaving, patient discharge on second post-operative day, no blood transfusions needed.

The tissue rearrangement starts 1 h after the treatment and can keep on going for months. Follow-up MRIs show, in fact, damage progression even 12 months after the procedure.

The disadvantages of the procedure include risk of bleeding and inaccurate positioning of the fiber.

At our center, five patients underwent a LITT procedure. In one case, we experienced inaccurate fiber positioning. Eventually, after repositioning, the intervention had no further adverse event.

12.4.6 Three-Dimensional (3D) Modeling and Neurosurgical Applications

Three-dimensional (3D) printing has deeply changed the practice of prototyping since its initial usage in the 1980s. This technique has given the possibility to produce physical 3D models from computer-aided designs through additive manufacturing [114]. Applications within clinical medicine are emerging due to 3D printing's ability to produce individualized models, devices, and implants that can potentially improve patient care.

This technology is of particular interest for the production of surgical instruments that can make treatment as much individualized as possible. Moreover, thanks to the most recent advances, biological material can be used to build engineered, inert scaffolds that can be populated with patient cells for the purpose of transplantation.

Studies involving the incorporation of 3D printing in neurosurgery have focused upon the creation of patient-specific anatomical models for surgical planning, training, and education. This type of technology was also used to design neurosurgical devices for assessment and treatment of neurosurgical diseases, and to develop biological tissue-engineered implants [115].

In neurosurgery, physical simulators differ from virtual simulators as they can be directly palpated, easily modified according to the physician's request, incised by real surgical instruments, and manipulated. The combination of virtual and physical simulation enables the identification of a set of surgical approaches that can be objectively compared to find the best intervention strategy. In addition, it gives the chances to clinicians to try the procedure several times and to address its critical steps [116] (Fig. 12.18). Moreover, these models may be extremely useful for surgical residents as they offer a less expensive and more immediate possibility to improve their surgical skills (Fig. 12.19).

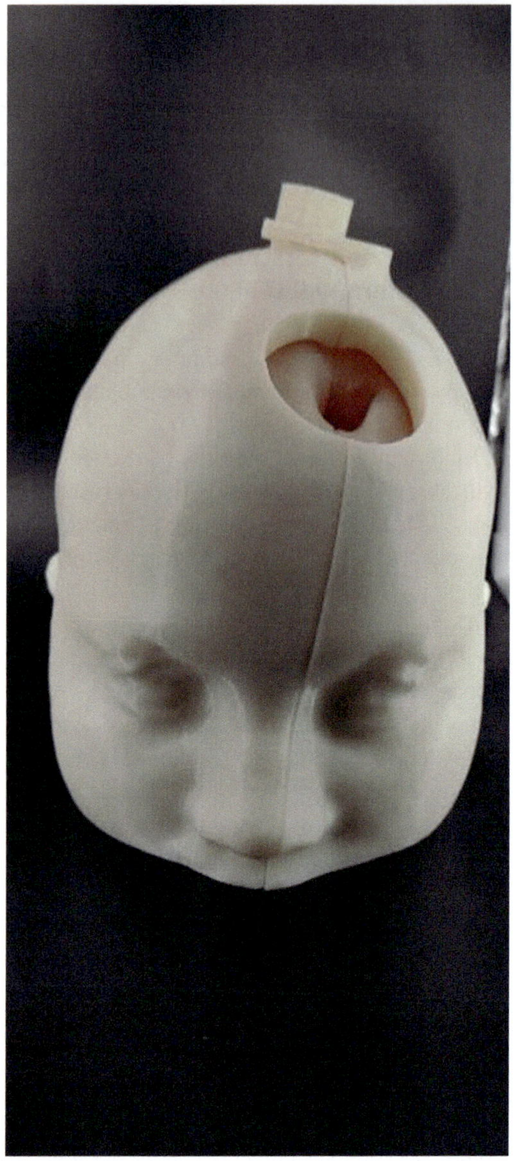

Fig. 12.18 Pre-operative 3D model of a possible neurosurgical approach for a deep-seated lesion

Since 2016, 3D printing entered the daily clinical practice at Meyer Children's Hospital.

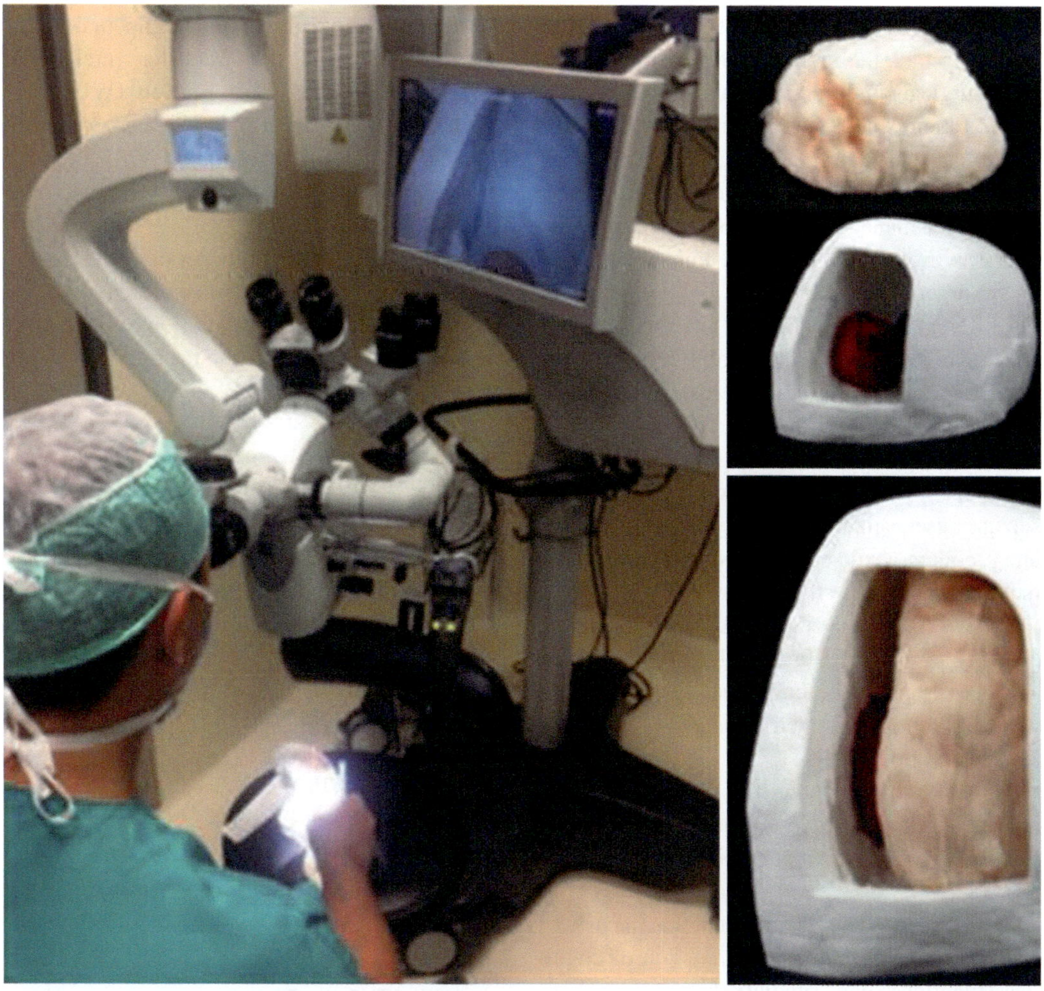

Fig. 12.19 3D printed model. Preoperative attempt of the ideal surgical approach

"T3Ddy" laboratory introduced highly customized medical devices and methods to support the treatment of pediatric diseases. Medical devices for children (implantable or not) often need to follow the child's growth stages. In this context, the use of "tailor-made" production systems for the patient guarantees better functionality and easier installation. By leveraging the unlimited flexibility that modern 3D printing systems make available, the T3Ddy laboratory opened up new opportunities in the advancement of pediatric medicine. By introducing 3D technologies into clinical practice, T3Ddy lays the foundation for the standardization of procedures for the construction of customized medical devices in line with the philosophy of personalized care, where each patient is unique and the solution is built around them. At our center, 3D printing found broad application for customized prostheses, orthoses, cranial vault defects repair, dental replacements, three-dimensional physical models for planning of complex surgical interventions, and small useful objects for nursing practice and simulation [102, 116–118].

12.4.7 Neurocognitive Assessment in Pediatric Neurosurgery

In pediatric neurosurgery, it is mandatory to be aware of the crucial physiological steps of neuropsychological development.

Anomalies of neurocognitive development can be, in fact, the first sign of presentation of a neurosurgical condition not otherwise evident, as well as being the result of surgical therapeutic approaches [119, 120].

For example, neuropsychological assessment has become mandatory for preoperative and postoperative evaluation of patients who undergo epilepsy surgery [121, 122].

Different cognitive domains have been studied and, regardless of that, either stability or improvement has been reported, whereas only in few cases decline has been described [121, 123–129].

Preoperative prognosis factors include age at seizure onset, seizure frequency, duration of epilepsy, epileptogenic etiology. Nevertheless, these factors' influence is still unknown [130].

After surgery, the reported cognitive function changes are variable. In fact, there are considerable variations in the cognitive domain studied with different psychometric tests [131] and follow-up duration [132].

Epilepsy surgery is not the only subspecialty in which neurocognitive evaluation can be considered as part of the diagnostic and therapeutic process.

It has been widely documented that in cases of cerebral tumors, a selective evaluation of cognitive functions can predict the postoperative course and long term evolution [133–135].

There are several possibly contributing factors such as tumor location, developmental stage of the child, chronological age, presence of seizures and age at onset, and histology [136, 137].

The working protocol includes a test battery which differs depending on patient's age.

In pre-scholar age, global developmental quotient is evaluated with the Griffiths Mental Developmental Scale–Revised (GMDS-R) [138], visual attention is evaluated with the selective attention component from the Leiter International Performance Scale–Revised [139], Movement Assessment Battery for Children (M-ABC) test is used to evaluate the preferred hand tasks and the Achenbach Child Behavior Checklist (CBCL 1–5 years) to measure behavioral and affective regulation [140, 141].

In school-age children, the intellectual profile is evaluated using the Wechsler Intelligence Scale for Children–Third Edition (WISC-III), eye-hand coordination is evaluated with the Visual Motor Integration (VMI) [142]. Organization and planning skills with the Tower of London (TOL) test.

Therefore, a detailed preoperative and postoperative behavioral and cognitive evaluation might help firstly to predict the evolution of the pathology and secondly to improve the outcome.

References

1. Morley JE, et al. Frailty consensus: a call to action. J Am Med Dir Assoc. 2013;14(6):392–7. https://doi.org/10.1016/j.jamda.2013.03.022.
2. Pazniokas J, et al. The immense heterogeneity of frailty in neurosurgery: a systematic literature review. Neurosurg Rev. 2021;44(1):189–201. https://doi.org/10.1007/s10143-020-01241-2.
3. Shahrestani S, et al. The role of frailty in geriatric cranial neurosurgery for primary central nervous system neoplasms. Neurosurg Focus. 2020;49(4):E15. https://doi.org/10.3171/2020.7.FOCUS20426.
4. Sastry RA, Pertsch NJ, Tang O, Shao B, Toms SA, Weil RJ. Frailty and outcomes after craniotomy for brain tumor. J Clin Neurosci. 2020;81:95–100. https://doi.org/10.1016/j.jocn.2020.09.002.
5. Gatta G, Caldora M, Galati F, Capocaccia R. Childhood (0–19 years) cancer mortality in Italy, 1970–2008. Epidemiol Prev. 2013;37(1):228–33.
6. Udaka YT, Packer RJ. Pediatric brain tumors. Neurol Clin. 2018;36(3):533–56. https://doi.org/10.1016/j.ncl.2018.04.009.
7. Rosenfeld JV. Minimally invasive neurosurgery. Aust N Z J Surg. 1996;66(8):553–9. https://doi.org/10.1111/j.1445-2197.1996.tb00808.x.
8. Sheinberg MA, Ross DA. Cranial procedures without hair removal. Neurosurgery. 1999;44(6):1263–5. https://doi.org/10.1097/00006123-199906000-00054.
9. Bekar A, Korfall E, Doğan S, Yilmazlar S, Başkan Z, Aksoy K. The effect of hair on infection after cranial surgery. Acta Neurochir. 2001;143(6):533–6. https://doi.org/10.1007/s007010170057.
10. Winston KR. Hair and neurosurgery. Neurosurgery. 1992;31(2):320–9. https://doi.org/10.1227/00006123-199208000-00018.
11. McCann ME, Soriano SG. Progress in anesthesia and management of the newborn surgical patient. Semin Pediatr Surg. 2014;23(5):244–8. https://doi.org/10.1053/j.sempedsurg.2014.09.003.
12. Soriano SG, Eldredge EA, Rockoff MA. Pediatric neuroanesthesia. Neuroimaging Clin N Am.

2007;17(2):259–67. https://doi.org/10.1016/j.nic.2007.03.010.

13. Best C. Paediatric airway anaesthesia. Curr Opin Anaesthesiol. 2012;25(1):38–41. https://doi.org/10.1097/ACO.0b013e32834e63e2.
14. Smith I, et al. Perioperative fasting in adults and children: guidelines from the European Society of Anaesthesiology. Eur J Anaesthesiol. 2011;28(8):556–69. https://doi.org/10.1097/EJA.0b013e3283495ba1.
15. Conroy PH, O'Rourke J. Tumescent anaesthesia. Surgeon. 2013;11(4):210–21. https://doi.org/10.1016/j.surge.2012.12.009.
16. Demaerel P. A. J. Barkovich: Pediatric neuroimaging. Eur Radiol. 2001;11(11):2347. https://doi.org/10.1007/s003300100904.
17. Mathur AM, Neil JJ, McKinstry RC, Inder TE. Transport, monitoring, and successful brain MR imaging in unsedated neonates. Pediatr Radiol. 2008;38(3):260–4. https://doi.org/10.1007/s00247-007-0705-9.
18. Sugahara T, et al. Comparison of HASTE and segmented-HASTE sequences with a T2-weighted fast spin-echo sequence in the screening evaluation of the brain. Am J Roentgenol. 1997;169(5):1401–10. https://doi.org/10.2214/ajr.169.5.9353469.
19. Sargent MA, Poskitt KJ. Fast fluid-attenuated inversion recovery (FLAIR) magnetic resonance imaging of the brain: a comparison of multi-shot echo-planar and fast spin-echo techniques. Pediatr Radiol. 1997;27(6):545–9. https://doi.org/10.1007/s002470050177.
20. Sehgal V, et al. Clinical applications of neuroimaging with susceptibility-weighted imaging. J Magn Reson Imaging. 2005;22(4):439–50. https://doi.org/10.1002/jmri.20404.
21. Agarwal N, Tekes A, Poretti A, Meoded A, Huisman TAGM. Pitfalls in diffusion-weighted and diffusion tensor imaging of the pediatric brain. Neuropediatrics. 2017;48(5):340–9. https://doi.org/10.1055/s-0037-1603979.
22. Le Bihan D, Breton E, Lallemand D, Grenier P, Cabanis E, Laval-Jeantet M. MR imaging of intravoxel incoherent motions: application to diffusion and perfusion in neurologic disorders. Radiology. 1986;161(2):401–7. https://doi.org/10.1148/radiology.161.2.3763909.
23. Feldman HM, Yeatman JD, Lee ES, Barde LHF, Gaman-Bean S. Diffusion tensor imaging: a review for pediatric researchers and clinicians. J Dev Behav Pediatr. 2010;31(4):346. https://doi.org/10.1097/DBP.0b013e3181dcaa8b.
24. Pecheva D, et al. Recent advances in diffusion neuroimaging: applications in the developing preterm brain [version 1; referees: 2 approved]. F1000Research. 2018;7:15073. https://doi.org/10.12688/f1000research.15073.1.
25. Batalle D, et al. Different patterns of cortical maturation before and after 38 weeks gestational age demonstrated by diffusion MRI in vivo. NeuroImage. 2019;185:764–75. https://doi.org/10.1016/j.neuroimage.2018.05.046.
26. Ho ML, Campeau NG, Ngo TD, Udayasankar UK, Welker KM. Pediatric brain MRI, part 2: advanced techniques. Pediatr Radiol. 2017;47(5):544–55. https://doi.org/10.1007/s00247-017-3792-2.
27. Öz G, et al. Clinical proton MR spectroscopy in central nervous system disorders. Radiology. 2014;270(3):658–79. https://doi.org/10.1148/radiol.13130531.
28. Bray MD, Mullins ME. Metabolic white matter diseases and the utility of MR spectroscopy. Radiol Clin N Am. 2014;52(2):403–11. https://doi.org/10.1016/j.rcl.2013.11.012.
29. Cha S. Dynamic susceptibility-weighted contrast-enhanced perfusion MR imaging in pediatric patients. Neuroimaging Clin N Am. 2006;16(1):137–47. https://doi.org/10.1016/j.nic.2005.11.006.
30. Ho CY, Cardinal JS, Kamer AP, Lin C, Kralik SF. Contrast leakage patterns from dynamic susceptibility contrast perfusion MRI in the grading of primary pediatric brain tumors. Am J Neuroradiol. 2016;37(3):544–51. https://doi.org/10.3174/ajnr.A4559.
31. Petcharunpaisan S, et al. Arterial spin labeling in neuroimaging: basic principles, emerging techniques and clinical applications in neuroimaging. World J Radiol. 2010;2(10):384–98.
32. Deibler AR, Pollock JM, Kraft RA, Tan H, Burdette JH, Maldjian JA. Arterial spin-labeling in routine clinical practice, part 1: technique and artifacts. Am J Neuroradiol. 2008;29(7):1228–34. https://doi.org/10.3174/ajnr.A1030.
33. Biswal B, Zerrin Yetkin F, Haughton VM, Hyde JS. Functional connectivity in the motor cortex of resting human brain using echo-planar MRI. Magn Reson Med. 1995;34(4):537–41. https://doi.org/10.1002/mrm.1910340409.
34. McKeown MJ, Sejnowski TJ. Independent component analysis of fMRI data: examining the assumptions. Hum Brain Mapp. 1998;6(5–6):368–72. https://doi.org/10.1002/(SICI)1097-0193(1998)6:5/6<368::AID-HBM7>3.0.CO;2-E.
35. Raichle ME. Cognitive neuroscience. Bold insights. Nature. 2001;412(6843):128–30.
36. Greicius MD, Krasnow B, Reiss AL, Menon V. Functional connectivity in the resting brain: a network analysis of the default mode hypothesis. Proc Natl Acad Sci U S A. 2003;100(1):253–8. https://doi.org/10.1073/pnas.0135058100.
37. Fransson P, et al. Resting-state networks in the infant brain. Proc Natl Acad Sci U S A. 2007;104(39):15531–6. https://doi.org/10.1073/pnas.0704380104.
38. Smyser CD, et al. Longitudinal analysis of neural network development in preterm infants. Cereb Cortex. 2010;20(12):2852–62. https://doi.org/10.1093/cercor/bhq035.
39. Mudry A. The history of the microscope for use in ear surgery. Am J Otol. 2000;21(6):877–86.

40. Kurze T, Apuzzo MLJ, Weiss MH, Heiden JS. Experiences with sterilization of the operating microscope. J Neurosurg. 1977;47(6):861–3. https://doi.org/10.3171/jns.1977.47.6.0861.
41. Kriss TC, Kriss VM. History of the operating microscope: from magnifying glass to microneurosurgery. Neurosurgery. 1998;42(4):899–907. https://doi.org/10.1097/00006123-199804000-00116.
42. Uluç K, Kujoth GC, Başkaya MK. Operating microscopes: past, present, and future. Neurosurg Focus. 2009;27(3):E4. https://doi.org/10.3171/2009.6.FOCUS09120.
43. Sanai N, Spetzler RF. Defining excellence in vascular neurosurgery. Clin Neurosurg. 2010;57:23–7.
44. Richard Winn MH. Youmans and Winn neurological surgery. Amsterdam: Elsevier; 2017.
45. Hadjipanayis CG, Widhalm G, Stummer W. What is the surgical benefit of utilizing 5-aminolevulinic acid for fluorescence-guided surgery of malignant gliomas? Neurosurgery. 2015;77(5):663–73. https://doi.org/10.1227/NEU.0000000000000929.
46. Fiani B, Jarrah R, Griepp DW, Adukuzhiyil J. The role of 3D exoscope systems in neurosurgery: an optical innovation. Cureus. 2021;13:e15878. https://doi.org/10.7759/cureus.15878.
47. Siller S, Zoellner C, Fuetsch M, Trabold R, Tonn JC, Zausinger S. A high-definition 3D exoscope as an alternative to the operating microscope in spinal microsurgery. J Neurosurg Spine. 2020;33(5):705–14. https://doi.org/10.3171/2020.4.SPINE20374.
48. Vetrano IG, Acerbi F, Falco J, D'Ammando A, Devigili G, Nazzi V. High-definition 4K 3D exoscope (ORBEYETM) in peripheral nerve sheath tumor surgery: a preliminary, explorative, pilot study. Oper Neurosurg. 2020;19(4):480–8. https://doi.org/10.1093/ons/opaa090.
49. de Divitiis O, Somma T, Sacco M, d'Avella E, Guizzardi G. VITOM®-3D in lumbar disc herniation: preliminary experience. Interdiscip Neurosurg Adv Tech Case Manag. 2019;18:100547. https://doi.org/10.1016/j.inat.2019.100547.
50. De Divitiis O, D'avella E, Denaro L, Somma T, Sacco M, D'avella D. Vitom® 3D: preliminary experience with intradural extramedullary spinal tumors. J Neurosurg Sci. 2019;66(4):356–61. https://doi.org/10.23736/S0390-5616.19.04666-6.
51. De Divitiis O, et al. The role of Vitom-3D in the management of spinal meningiomas: review of the literature and illustrative case. Mini-Invasive Surg. 2020;4:66. https://doi.org/10.20517/2574-1225.2020.66.
52. Barbagallo GMV, Certo F. Three-dimensional, high-definition exoscopic anterior cervical discectomy and fusion: a valid alternative to microscope-assisted surgery. World Neurosurg. 2019;130:e244–50. https://doi.org/10.1016/j.wneu.2019.06.049.
53. Sack J, et al. Initial experience using a high-definition 3-dimensional exoscope system for microneurosurgery. Oper Neurosurg. 2018;14(4):395–401. https://doi.org/10.1093/ons/opx145.
54. Mamelak AN, Nobuto T, Berci G. Initial clinical experience with a high-definition exoscope system for microneurosurgery. Neurosurgery. 2010;67(2):476–83. https://doi.org/10.1227/01.NEU.0000372204.85227.BF.
55. Muhammad S, Lehecka M, Niemelä M. Preliminary experience with a digital robotic exoscope in cranial and spinal surgery: a review of the Synaptive Modus V system. Acta Neurochir. 2019;161(10):2175–80. https://doi.org/10.1007/s00701-019-03953-x.
56. Panchal S, et al. A practice survey to compare and identify the usefulness of neuroendoscope and exoscope in the current neurosurgery practice. Asian J Neurosurg. 2020;15(3):601. https://doi.org/10.4103/ajns.ajns_339_19.
57. Wanibuchi M, Komatsu K, Akiyama Y, Mikami T, Mikuni N. Effectiveness of the 3D monitor system for medical education during neurosurgical operation. World Neurosurg. 2018;109:e105–9. https://doi.org/10.1016/j.wneu.2017.09.113.
58. Rossini Z, Cardia A, Milani D, Lasio GB, Fornari M, D'Angelo V. VITOM 3D: preliminary experience in cranial surgery. World Neurosurg. 2017;107:663–8. https://doi.org/10.1016/j.wneu.2017.08.083.
59. Haase J. Neuronavigation. Childs Nerv Syst. 1999;15(11–12):755–7. https://doi.org/10.1007/s003810050466.
60. Enchev Y. Neuronavigation: geneology, reality, and prospects. Neurosurg Focus. 2009;27(3):E11. https://doi.org/10.3171/2009.6.FOCUS09109.
61. Willems PWA, Van Der Sprenkel JWB, Tulleken CAF, Viergever MA, Taphoorn MJB. Neuronavigation and surgery of intracerebral tumours. J Neurol. 2006;253(9):1123–36. https://doi.org/10.1007/s00415-006-0158-3.
62. Barnett GH, Kormos DW, Steiner CP, Weisenberger JRT. Use of a frameless, armless stereotactic wand for brain tumor localization with two-dimensional and three-dimensional neuroimaging. Neurosurgery. 1993;33(4):674–8. https://doi.org/10.1227/00006123-199310000-00017.
63. Pfisterer WK, Papadopoulos S, Drumm DA, Smith K, Preul MC. Fiducial versus nonfiducial neuronavigation registration assessment and considerations of accuracy. Neurosurgery. 2008;62(3 Suppl. 1):ONS201–8. https://doi.org/10.1227/01.neu.0000317394.14303.99.
64. Mongen MA, Willems PWA. Current accuracy of surface matching compared to adhesive markers in patient-to-image registration. Acta Neurochir. 2019;161(5):865–70. https://doi.org/10.1007/s00701-019-03867-8.
65. Mert A, Gan LS, Knosp E, Sutherland GR, Wolfsberger S. Advanced cranial navigation. Neurosurgery. 2013;72(Suppl. 1):A43–53. https://doi.org/10.1227/NEU.0b013e3182750c03.
66. LoPresti MA, Nguyen J, Lam SK. Pinning in pediatric neurosurgery: the modified rubber stopper technique. J Neurosurg Pediatr. 2020;26(1):98–103. https://doi.org/10.3171/2020.1.PEDS19541.

67. Orringer DA, Golby A, Jolesz F. Neuronavigation in the surgical management of brain tumors: current and future trends. Expert Rev Med Devices. 2012;9(5):491–500. https://doi.org/10.1586/erd.12.42.
68. Paraskevopoulos D, Biyani N, Constantini S, Beni-Adani L. Combined intraoperative magnetic resonance imaging and navigated neuroendoscopy in children with multicompartmental hydrocephalus and complex cysts: a feasibility study—clinical article. J Neurosurg Pediatr. 2011;8(3):279–88. https://doi.org/10.3171/2011.6.PEDS10501.
69. De Benedictis A, et al. Robot-assisted procedures in pediatric neurosurgery. Neurosurg Focus. 2017;42(5):E7. https://doi.org/10.3171/2017.2.FOCUS16579.
70. Gupta M, et al. Robot-assisted stereotactic biopsy of pediatric brainstem and thalamic lesions. J Neurosurg Pediatr. 2021;27(3):317–24. https://doi.org/10.3171/2020.7.PEDS20373.
71. Minchev G, et al. A novel robot-guided minimally invasive technique for brain tumor biopsies. J Neurosurg. 2020;132(1):150–8. https://doi.org/10.3171/2018.8.JNS182096.
72. Okano A, Ogiwara H. Long-term follow-up for patients with infantile hydrocephalus treated by choroid plexus coagulation. J Neurosurg Pediatr. 2018;22(6):638–45. https://doi.org/10.3171/2018.6.PEDS1840.
73. Gallieni M, Del Maestro M, Luzzi S, Trovarelli D, Ricci A, Galzio R. Endoscope-assisted microneurosurgery for intracranial aneurysms: operative technique, reliability, and feasibility based on 14 years of personal experience. Acta Neurochir Suppl. 2018;129:19–24.
74. Drake JM. The surgical management of pediatric hydrocephalus. Neurosurgery. 2008;62(Suppl. 2):SHC633–42. https://doi.org/10.1227/01.neu.0000316268.05338.5b.
75. Hanak BW, Bonow RH, Harris CA, Browd SR. Cerebrospinal fluid shunting complications in children. Pediatr Neurosurg. 2017;52(6):381–400. https://doi.org/10.1159/000452840.
76. Stein SC, Guo W. Have we made progress in preventing shunt failure? A critical analysis. J Neurosurg Pediatr. 2008;1(1):40–7. https://doi.org/10.3171/PED-08/01/040.
77. Rocque BG, et al. Shunt failure clusters: an analysis of multiple, frequent shunt failures. J Neurosurg Pediatr. 2021;27(3):287–93. https://doi.org/10.3171/2020.7.PEDS20199.
78. Gmeiner M, et al. Long-term mortality rates in pediatric hydrocephalus—a retrospective single-center study. Childs Nerv Syst. 2017;33(1):101–9. https://doi.org/10.1007/s00381-016-3268-y.
79. Vinchon M, Rekate H, Kulkarni AV. Pediatric hydrocephalus outcomes: a review. Fluids Barriers CNS. 2012;9(1):18. https://doi.org/10.1186/2045-8118-9-18.
80. Choux M, Genitori L, Lang D, Lena G. Shunt implantation: reducing the incidence of shunt infection. J Neurosurg. 1992;77(6):875–80. https://doi.org/10.3171/jns.1992.77.6.0875.
81. Gholampour S, Bahmani M, Shariati A. Comparing the efficiency of two treatment methods of hydrocephalus: shunt implantation and endoscopic third ventriculostomy. Basic Clin Neurosci. 2019;10(3):185. https://doi.org/10.32598/bcn.9.10.285.
82. Shim KW, Park EK, Kim DS, Choi JU. Neuroendoscopy: current and future perspectives. J Korean Neurosurg Soc. 2017;60(3):322–6. https://doi.org/10.3340/jkns.2017.0202.006.
83. Cinalli G, et al. Initial experience with endoscopic ultrasonic aspirator in purely neuroendoscopic removal of intraventricular tumors. J Neurosurg Pediatr. 2017;19(3):325–32. https://doi.org/10.3171/2016.10.PEDS16352.
84. Turillazzi E, Bello S, Neri M, Riezzo I, Fineschi V. Colloid cyst of the third ventricle, hypothalamus, and heart: a dangerous link for sudden death. Diagn Pathol. 2012;7(1):1–5. https://doi.org/10.1186/1746-1596-7-144.
85. Greenlee JDW, Teo C, Ghahreman A, Kwok B. Purely endoscopic resection of colloid cysts. Neurosurgery. 2008;62(3 Suppl. 1):ONS51–6. https://doi.org/10.1227/01.neu.0000317373.00018.6f.
86. Samadian M, et al. Colloid cyst of the third ventricle: long-term results of endoscopic management in a series of 112 cases. World Neurosurg. 2018;111:e440–8. https://doi.org/10.1016/j.wneu.2017.12.093.
87. Kumar V, Behari S, Kumar Singh R, Jain M, Jaiswal AK, Jain VK. Pediatric colloid cysts of the third ventricle: management considerations. Acta Neurochir. 2010;152(3):451–61. https://doi.org/10.1007/s00701-009-0531-y.
88. Longatti P, et al. Cooperative study by the Italian neuroendoscopy group on the treatment of 61 colloid cysts. Childs Nerv Syst. 2006;22(10):1263–7. https://doi.org/10.1007/s00381-006-0105-8.
89. Gangemi M, Seneca V, Colella G, Cioffi V, Imperato A, Maiuri F. Endoscopy versus microsurgical cyst excision and shunting for treating intracranial arachnoid cysts: clinical article. J Neurosurg Pediatr. 2011;8(2):158–64. https://doi.org/10.3171/2011.5.PEDS1152.
90. Choi JU, Kim DS, Huh R. Endoscopic approach to arachnoid cyst. Childs Nerv Syst. 1999;15(6–7):285–91. https://doi.org/10.1007/s003810050396.
91. Van Beijnum J, Hanlo PW, Sen Han K, Van Der Pol WL, Verdaasdonk RM, Van Nieuwenhuizen O. Navigated laser-assisted endoscopic fenestration of a suprasellar arachnoid cyst in a 2-year-old child with bobble-head doll syndrome: case report. J Neurosurg Pediatr. 2006;104(Suppl. 5):348–51. https://doi.org/10.3171/ped.2006.104.5.348.
92. Spacca B, Kandasamy J, Mallucci CL, Genitori L. Endoscopic treatment of middle fossa arachnoid cysts: a series of 40 patients treated endoscopically in two centres. Childs Nerv Syst. 2010;26(2):163–72. https://doi.org/10.1007/s00381-009-0952-1.

93. Xu S, Wang Y, Luo Q, Jiang J, Zhong C. Endoscopic fenestration of 26 patients with middle fossa arachnoid cyst. J Craniofac Surg. 2016;27(4):973–5. https://doi.org/10.1097/SCS.0000000000002624.
94. Peretta P, et al. Complications and pitfalls of neuroendoscopic surgery in children. J Neurosurg Pediatr. 2006;105(Suppl. 3):187–93. https://doi.org/10.3171/ped.2006.105.3.187.
95. Cappabianca P, et al. Endoscopic endonasal transsphenoidal approach. In: Midline skull base surgery. Cham: Springer International Publishing; 2016.
96. Munson PD, Moore EJ. Pediatric endoscopic skull base surgery. Curr Opin Otolaryngol Head Neck Surg. 2010;18(6):571–6. https://doi.org/10.1097/MOO.0b013e3283401fdc.
97. Giovannetti F, et al. Endoscopic endonasal skull base surgery in pediatric patients. A single center experience. J Cranio-Maxillofac Surg. 2018;46(12):2017–21. https://doi.org/10.1016/j.jcms.2018.09.013.
98. Soldozy S, et al. Endoscopic endonasal surgery outcomes for pediatric craniopharyngioma: a systematic review. Neurosurg Focus. 2020;48(1):E6. https://doi.org/10.3171/2019.10.FOCUS19728.
99. Denis D, Genitori L, Conrath J, Lena G, Choux M. Ocular findings in children operated on for plagiocephaly and trigonocephaly. Childs Nerv Syst. 1996;12(11):683–9. https://doi.org/10.1007/BF00366151.
100. Giordano F, Serio P, Savasta S, Oliveri G, Genitori L. Craniofacial surgery in fibrous dysplasia. J Pediatr Endocrinol Metab. 2006;19(Suppl. 2):595–604. https://doi.org/10.1515/jpem.2006.19.s2.595.
101. Spinelli G, et al. Complex craniofacial advancement in paediatric patients: piezoelectric and traditional technique evaluation. J. Cranio Maxillofac Surg. 2015;43(8):1422–7. https://doi.org/10.1016/j.jcms.2015.07.012.
102. Volpe Y, et al. Surgery of complex craniofacial defects: a single-step AM-based methodology. Comput Methods Prog Biomed. 2018;165:225–33.
103. Mannelli G, Arcuri F, Spacca B, Genitori L, Spinelli G. Respiratory and volumetric changes of the upper airways in craniofacial synostosis patients. J Cranio-Maxillofac Surg. 2019;47(4):548–55. https://doi.org/10.1016/j.jcms.2019.01.042.
104. Genitori L, Cavalheiro S, Lena G, Dollo C, Choux M. Skull base in trigonocephaly. Pediatr Neurosurg. 1991;17(4):175–81. https://doi.org/10.1159/000120591.
105. Jimenez DF, Barone CM. Endoscopic craniectomy for early surgical correction of sagittal craniosynostosis. J Neurosurg. 1998;88(1):77–81. https://doi.org/10.3171/jns.1998.88.1.0077.
106. Nelson JH, Menser CC, Reddy SK. Endoscopic craniosynostosis repair. Int Anesthesiol Clin. 2019;57(4):61–71. https://doi.org/10.1097/AIA.0000000000000246.
107. Williams CT, et al. Evaluation of endoscopic strip craniectomy and orthotic therapy for bilateral coronal craniosynostosis. J Craniofac Surg. 2019;30(2):453. https://doi.org/10.1097/SCS.0000000000005118.
108. Hersh DS, Hoover-Fong JE, Beck N, Dorafshar AH, Ahn ES. Endoscopic surgery for patients with syndromic craniosynostosis and the requirement for additional open surgery. J Neurosurg Pediatr. 2017;20(1):91–8. https://doi.org/10.3171/2017.2.PEDS16710.
109. Zubovic E, Skolnick GB, Naidoo SD, Bellanger M, Smyth MD, Patel KB. Endoscopic treatment of combined metopic-sagittal craniosynostosis. J Neurosurg Pediatr. 2020;26(2):113–21. https://doi.org/10.3171/2020.2.PEDS2029.
110. Goyal A, Lu VM, Yolcu YU, Elminawy M, Daniels DJ. Endoscopic versus open approach in craniosynostosis repair: a systematic review and meta-analysis of perioperative outcomes. Childs Nerv Syst. 2018;34(9):1627–37. https://doi.org/10.1007/s00381-018-3852-4.
111. Kung TA, Vercler CJ, Muraszko KM, Buchman SR. Endoscopic strip craniectomy for craniosynostosis: do we really understand the indications, outcomes, and risks? J Craniofac Surg. 2016;27(2):293–8. https://doi.org/10.1097/SCS.0000000000002364.
112. Patel NV, et al. Laser interstitial thermal therapy technology, physics of magnetic resonance imaging thermometry, and technical considerations for proper catheter placement during magnetic resonance imaging-guided laser interstitial thermal therapy. Clin Neurosurg. 2016;79:S8–16. https://doi.org/10.1227/NEU.0000000000001440.
113. Melnick K, et al. Role of laser interstitial thermal therapy in the management of primary and metastatic brain tumors. Curr Treat Options Oncol. 2021;22(12):1–17. https://doi.org/10.1007/s11864-021-00912-6.
114. Liew Y, Beveridge E, Demetriades AK, Hughes MA. 3D printing of patient-specific anatomy: a tool to improve patient consent and enhance imaging interpretation by trainees. Br J Neurosurg. 2015;29(5):712–4. https://doi.org/10.3109/02688697.2015.1026799.
115. Randazzo M, Pisapia J, Singh N, Thawani J. 3D printing in neurosurgery: a systematic review. Surg Neurol Int. 2016;7(34):S801–9. https://doi.org/10.4103/2152-7806.194059.
116. Mussi E, et al. Current practice in preoperative virtual and physical simulation in neurosurgery. Bioengineering. 2020;7(1):7. https://doi.org/10.3390/bioengineering7010007.
117. Marzola A, Governi L, Genitori L, Mussa F, Volpe Y, Furferi R. A semi-automatic hybrid approach for defective skulls reconstruction. Comput Aided Des Appl. 2020;17(1):190–204. https://doi.org/10.14733/cadaps.2020.190-204.
118. Buonamici F, et al. Reverse engineering techniques for virtual reconstruction of defective skulls: an overview of existing approaches. Comput Aided

Des Appl. 2018;16(1):112. https://doi.org/10.14733/cadaps.2019.103-112.

119. Rønning C, Sundet K, Due-Tønnessen B, Lundar T, Helseth E. Persistent cognitive dysfunction secondary to cerebellar injury in patients treated for posterior fossa tumors in childhood. Pediatr Neurosurg. 2005;41(1):15–21. https://doi.org/10.1159/000084860.
120. Maddrey AM, et al. Neuropsychological performance and quality of life of 10 year survivors of childhood medulloblastoma. J Neuro-Oncol. 2005;72(3):245–53. https://doi.org/10.1007/s11060-004-3009-z.
121. Laguitton V, et al. Intellectual outcome from 1 to 5 years after epilepsy surgery in 81 children and adolescents: a longitudinal study. Seizure. 2021;91:384–92. https://doi.org/10.1016/j.seizure.2021.07.010.
122. Baxendale S, et al. Indications and expectations for neuropsychological assessment in epilepsy surgery in children and adults: report of the ILAE Neuropsychology Task Force Diagnostic Methods Commission: 2017–2021 neuropsychological assessment in epilepsy surgery. Epileptic Disord. 2019;21(3):221–34. https://doi.org/10.1684/epd.2019.1065.
123. Westerveld M, et al. Temporal lobectomy in children: cognitive outcome. J Neurosurg. 2000;92(1):24–30. https://doi.org/10.3171/jns.2000.92.1.0024.
124. Viggedal G, Olsson I, Carlsson G, Rydenhag B, Uvebrant P. Intelligence 2 years after epilepsy surgery in children. Epilepsy Behav. 2013;29(3):565–70. https://doi.org/10.1016/j.yebeh.2013.10.012.
125. Skirrow C, Cross JH, Cormack F, Harkness W, Vargha-Khadem F, Baldeweg T. Long-term intellectual outcome after temporal lobe surgery in childhood. Neurology. 2011;76(15):1330–7. https://doi.org/10.1212/WNL.0b013e31821527f0.
126. Klajdi P, Smith ML. Predictors of long-term quality of life after pediatric epilepsy surgery. Epilepsia. 2015;56(6):873–81.
127. Korkman M, et al. Two-year follow-up of intelligence after pediatric epilepsy surgery. Pediatr Neurol. 2005;33(3):173–8. https://doi.org/10.1016/j.pediatrneurol.2005.04.006.
128. Helmstaedter C, Beeres K, Elger CE, Kuczaty S, Schramm J, Hoppe C. Cognitive outcome of pediatric epilepsy surgery across ages and different types of surgeries: a monocentric 1-year follow-up study in 306 patients of school age. Seizure. 2020;77:86–92. https://doi.org/10.1016/j.seizure.2019.07.021.
129. Gleissner U, Clusmann H, Sassen R, Elger CE, Helmstaedter C. Postsurgical outcome in pediatric patients with epilepsy: a comparison of patients with intellectual disabilities, subaverage intelligence, and average-range intelligence. Epilepsia. 2006;47(2):406–14. https://doi.org/10.1111/j.1528-1167.2006.00436.x.
130. Moosa ANV, Wyllie E. Cognitive outcome after epilepsy surgery in children. Semin Pediatr Neurol. 2017;24(4):331–9. https://doi.org/10.1016/j.spen.2017.10.010.
131. Sim LP. Cognitive dysfunction in children with temporal lobe epilepsy. Paediatr Child Adolescent Health. 2006;46(3):180–2.
132. Lou Smith M. Neuropsychology in epilepsy: children are not small adults. Epilepsia. 2010;51(Suppl. 1):68–9. https://doi.org/10.1111/j.1528-1167.2009.02451.x.
133. Chieffo D, Tamburrini G, Caldarelli M, Di Rocco C. Preoperative neuropsychological and behavioral evaluation of children with thalamic tumors: clinical article. J Neurosurg Pediatr. 2014;13(5):507–13. https://doi.org/10.3171/2014.2.PEDS13352.
134. Di Rocco C, Chieffo D, Frassanito P, Caldarelli M, Massimi L, Tamburrini G. Heralding cerebellar mutism: evidence for pre-surgical language impairment as primary risk factor in posterior fossa surgery. Cerebellum. 2011;10(3):551–62. https://doi.org/10.1007/s12311-011-0273-2.
135. Di Rocco C, Chieffo D, Pettorini BL, Massimi L, Caldarelli M, Tamburrini G. Preoperative and postoperative neurological, neuropsychological and behavioral impairment in children with posterior cranial fossa astrocytomas and medulloblastomas: the role of the tumor and the impact of the surgical treatment. Childs Nerv Syst. 2010;26(9):1173–88. https://doi.org/10.1007/s00381-010-1166-2.
136. Dennis M. Language disorders in children with central nervous system injury. J Clin Exp Neuropsychol. 2010;32(4):417–32. https://doi.org/10.1080/13803390903164355.
137. Chieffo D, Tamburrini G, Frassanito P, Arcangeli V, Caldarelli M, Di Rocco C. Preoperative neurocognitive evaluation as a predictor of brain tumor grading in pediatric patients with supratentorial hemispheric tumors. Childs Nerv Syst. 2016;32(10):1931–7. https://doi.org/10.1007/s00381-016-3170-7.
138. Cirelli I, Bickle Graz M, Tolsa JF. Comparison of Griffiths-II and Bayley-II tests for the developmental assessment of high-risk infants. Infant Behav Dev. 2015;41:17–25. https://doi.org/10.1016/j.infbeh.2015.06.004.
139. Farmer C. Leiter International Performance Scale-Revised (Leiter-R). In: Encyclopedia of autism spectrum disorders. Cham: Springer Nature; 2021.
140. Achenbach T. Manual for the ASEBA school-age forms and profiles an integrated system of multi-informant assessment. Res Cent Child. 2007;1617(82):238.
141. Achenbach TM. Manual for the child: behavior checklist and revised child behavior profile. Encycl Psychol. 2004;2(8):230.
142. Valverde AA, Araújo CRS, de Castro Magalhães L, Cardoso AA. Relationship between visual-motor integration and manual dexterity in children with developmental coordination disorder. Braz J Occup Ther. 2020;28(3):AO1999. https://doi.org/10.4322/2526-8910.CTOAO1999.

13 Fragility of Children with Severe Early Onset Scoliosis

Description and Analysis of Innovative Techniques with "Growing Systems"

Tiziana Greggi and Maria Renata Bacchin

13.1 Introduction

Background Early-onset scoliosis (EOS) is defined as a spinal deformity which occurs clinically before the age of 5 years. It can be classified as idiopathic, neuromuscular/syndromic, and congenital, according to etiology. Many patients may have congenital spinal malformations; others may have severe scoliosis, rapidly evolving, which occurs early as a phenotypic feature of rare diseases with major comorbidities or serious health problems. Treatment of non-idiopathic spine deformities in young children is very demanding. Rare syndromes are various clinical conditions, heterogeneous in terms of clinics, but associated with spinal deformities in a large percentage of cases. Scoliosis is the most common early-onset deformity, sometimes present at birth and often rapidly evolving.

Methods The literature on the treatment of EOS was reviewed and the authors' experience summarized.

Results Conventional management tools, such as bracing and fusion, are not always effective. The natural syndromic scoliosis is highly dependent on the natural history of the underlying disorder. Scoliosis often affects children's life early, creating situations of discomfort and isolation, making it difficult to treat the problem and sometimes opening the way to difficult and ineffective paths.

Conclusion While lack of treatment has been shown to lead to increased mortality, extensive early definitive fusion may lead to thoracic insufficiency. There are a number of surgical techniques to treat severe and developmental spine deformities (EOS) and control growth without fusion with the aim to delay definitive surgery with fusion. Delaying definitive surgery and using growing instrumentation may provide benefit in maintaining pulmonary health. The genetic and molecular study of syndromic diseases associated with rapidly evolving scoliosis may lead to early diagnosis. Even the study of idiopathic scoliosis (certainly of a polygenic nature) will help to deal with the pre-symptomatic situation and better control the severity of the evolution. Children that need spinal surgery for early-onset scoliosis (EOS) may have a wide

T. Greggi (✉)
Orthopedics and Traumatology, Physical Medicine and Rehabilitation, University of Bologna, Bologna, Italy

M. R. Bacchin
Department of Anesthesia, Intensive Care and Reanimation, Rizzoli Orthopedic Institute, Bologna, Italy
e-mail: mariarenata.bacchin@ior.it

M. Lima, M. C. Mondardini (eds.), *Frailty in Children*,
https://doi.org/10.1007/978-3-031-24307-3_13

range of underlying conditions, including congenital defects, tumors, arteriovenous malformations (AVMs) and consequences from other primary diseases. The most common diseases that require surgery on the spinal cord are neural tube defects and their associations, namely, tethered cord syndrome, diastematomyelia, and syringomyelia. Tumors in children presenting for spinal surgery are a less common occurrence, while vascular disease of the spine (e.g., AVMs) is rare.

Young patients with neuromuscular scoliosis often have critical issues at heart level and sometimes may show the need for implantation of intrathecal baclofen pumps to control muscle spasm (cerebral palsy [CP]). Sometimes, neuromuscular patients have major allergies (latex). Anesthesia during spinal surgery in children must address surgical requirements for positioning and monitoring in addition to taking into consideration the associated medical problems, age-related pathophysiology, and the potential for blood loss and vascular injury of the spinal cord. The pediatric anesthesiologist is presented with a wide spectrum of underlying pathology of variable range of age and size. New surgical techniques with "growing rod" systems help are often non-aggressive as opposed to instrumented fusion. However, the fragility of a child requires not only an experienced vertebral surgeon, but also multidisciplinary study and strict collaboration (vertebral surgeon, anesthesiologist, pediatrician, neurosurgeon, neurologist).

Clinical Relevance Multidisciplinary collaboration with translational research has brought more specialized fields closer to new knowledge on severe early onset scoliosis: innovative surgical techniques are employed that allow a rapid correction of a developing scoliosis in a child, thus giving to the vertebral surgeon everything to ensure adequate growth of the trunk and respiratory capacity, avoiding, or at least limiting, the neurological consequences of spinal deformity, providing these children the best opportunity for a safe operation and recovery.

13.2 Multidisciplinary Evaluation

Multidisciplinary preoperative evaluation is essential. The main actors are the anesthesiologist and the vertebral surgeon, in addition to the little patient and their family. Quite often, when dealing with syndromic situations, other specialists should be consulted, such as the pediatrician, pediatric surgeon, cardiologist, neurosurgeon, child neuropsychiatrist: very close communication and specific dedication are mandatory. The clinical and instrumental investigations carried out in this phase are listed in Table 13.1.

Meeting for preoperative assessment is also fundamental for the informational interview with the little patient and their family. For an experienced vertebral surgeon, the technical aspect of the surgical treatment of EOS is less important and is lost in the complexity of the multidisciplinary evaluation. In the context of severe early-onset scoliosis, the most frequently associated

Table 13.1 Preoperative multidisciplinary evaluation

Fundamental investigations	What should be evaluated
• Blood chemistry tests • Echocardiogram • Spirometry • Spine MRI with encephalo-spinal passage • Full blood count • Urea and electrolytes • Clotting profile test • Liver function tests • Chest X-rays • Baseline arterial blood gas analysis • Spirometry, when possible • Imaging of the cervical spine • ECG and echocardiogram	• All organ systems to detect other congenital defects • The nervous system and documentation of neurological deficit • Anatomical abnormalities leading to 'airway challenge' • Specific age-related anesthetic considerations (e.g., neonates) • Awareness of associated pathology (e.g., Arnold-Chiari malformation, CP) • Respiratory and cardiovascular status • Previous anesthetic records • Awareness of potential for latex allergy • Psychological potential for latex allergy status • Premedication • Preoperative investigations

severe malformations are the myelo-radicular ones: the vertebral surgeon and the anesthesiologist should have a clear knowledge of them before undertaking surgery [1, 2].

13.3 Comorbidities of Early-Onset Scoliosis

A percentage of children who require spinal surgery will have other underlying medical conditions, such as neural tube defects (myelodysplasia). The systemic MRI study conducted by Bradford on 42 congenital scoliosis revealed 38% of spinal anomalies and, of these, 56% were negative on standard clinical and radiographic examination [3]. **Myelodysplasia** is an abnormality in fusion of the embryologic neural groove during the first month of gestation. The incidence is 1 per 1000 live births. Failure of neural tube closure results in a sac-like herniation of the meninges (meningocele) or a herniation of neural elements. Scoliosis associated with myelomeningocele and spina bifida is often severe and developmental with an indication to be treated in the pediatric age. **Myelomeningocele** can happen anywhere along the spinal cord, though it is most common in the lumbosacral area. High thoracic defects will result in severe neurological deficit.

Spina bifida refers to a failure of the fusion of the vertebral arches and is often associated with myelomeningocele [4, 5].

In 5–10% of the patients, it occurs as spina bifida occulta, in which the defect is covered by the skin and soft tissues, usually at L5. A surface abnormality, which may be either a skin dimple or a hairy patch, is usually observed. The defect in the vertebral arches communicates with the meningocele or myelomeningocele in spina bifida aperta. **Tethered cord** results when a thick rope-like filum terminale persists and anchors the conus at or below the L2 level. Neurological signs may develop because of abnormal tension on the spinal cord, especially during flexion and extension [6, 7]. Surgical transection of the thick filum terminale tends to halt the progression of neurological signs. Orthopedic and urological symptoms may develop. **Diastematomyelia** refers to the division of the spinal cord into two halves by a projection of a fibrocartilaginous or bony septum originating from the posterior vertebral body and extending posteriorly. It represents a disorder of neural tube fusion with persistence of mesodermal tissue from the primitive neurenteric canal. The majority of cases involve the lumbar vertebrae and tend to be associated with abnormalities of the vertebral bodies, including fusion defects, hemivertebra, hypoplasia, kyphoscoliosis, spina bifida, and myelomeningocele [8]. Neurological signs result from flexion and extension movements of the cord. Diastematomyelia may coexist with a tethered cord. The condition is likely to be picked up in the preschool age. The treatment of symptomatic patients is the excision of the bony spur or septum and lysis of the adherent structures.

Syringomyelia is defined as a cystic cavity within the spinal cord, which may communicate with the cerebrospinal fluid pathways or remain localized and non-communicating. The central canal of the spinal cord is normally obliterated after birth by the cellular proliferation of the spinal cord, and the ventricular system terminates at the obex on the caudal floor of the fourth ventricle. The disturbed embryology of the caudal cerebellum in the spina bifida–Arnold-Chiari malformation complex frequently alters the spinal cord and causes the central canal to remain enlarged and patent, causing symptomatic hydrosyringomyelia [9]. Knowledge of the status of the central nervous system (CNS) aids understanding of the above conditions and related investigations are summarized in Table 13.1. **Chiari malformations** are a group of anatomic abnormalities that include displacement of the cerebellar vermis through the foramen magnum, elongation of the brainstem and fourth ventricle, and non-communicating hydrocephalus. Most children with myelomeningocele have an associated Arnold-Chiari malformation (Chiari II) and ultimately develop hydrocephalus, usually within the first month of life. This will necessitate a drainage procedure to be performed—either a ventriculoperitoneal shunt or a ventriculostomy [10, 11].

Tumors Primary spinal cord tumors can develop in association with severe and rapidly progressive scoliosis in children. These constitute a fifth of all CNS tumors in children. They are either intramedullary or extramedullary, which, in turn, can be either intradural or epidural [12, 13]. The most common intramedullary tumors are low grade astrocytomas and ependymomas [14, 15]. Extramedullary intradural tumors are usually benign and arise from neural crest tissue. They include neurofibromas, ganglioneuromas, and meningiomas. Extramedullary epidural tumors are usually metastatic lesions arising from primary neuroblastomas, sarcomas, and lymphomas. This condition must be addressed along with correction of spinal deformity. With modern surgical techniques, many tumors can be safely and totally resected. Surgical removal of benign extramedullary tumors is associated with a good prognosis [16, 17].

13.4 Complex Syndromes with Multi-Organ Compromise

Scoliosis is a fixed, structural, lateral curvature of the spine with associated rotation of the vertebrae. It often occurs in **Down syndrome**, where a malformation with instability at the occipitocervical junction resulting from a vertebral formation defect is commonly found [2, 18]. Congenital scoliosis is often part of a generalized condition, such as in, for example, **Spina Bifida** and **Goldenhar syndrome,** and may be associated with abnormalities in the renal, cardiac, respiratory, or neurological systems [4]. Indication for surgery is documented progression at any age. Most acquired scoliosis is idiopathic. Infantile onset idiopathic scoliosis (before the age of 8 years) carries the most serious prognosis and, if left unchecked, is likely to result in cardiopulmonary failure in middle age [12]. **Vascular disease of the spine** [19, 20]. This is rare, but may cause spinal compression, vascular steal, and spinal cord ischemic damage. The maintenance of spinal cord perfusion pressure (SCPP) and avoidance of cord compression are crucial considerations.

The VACTERL Syndrome Vertebral, anorectal, cardiovascular, tracheoesophageal, genitourinary, and limb malformations are seen in 13% of children with tracheoesophageal fistula. Meningoceles and myeloceles are usually repaired within the first day of life to minimize bacterial contamination of the exposed spinal cord and subsequent sepsis, which is the most common cause of death in this population during the newborn period. Many genitourinary and orthopedic procedures may be needed in the future and the threat of developing latex allergy is real. The main latex exposure is in the surgeons' gloves and ideally all gloves and equipment used in these children should be latex-free from the first exposure [17, 21].

13.5 Anesthetic Technique

13.5.1 Introduction

Children may present for spinal surgery at any age from infancy to adolescence. The anesthesiologist should consider age-related pathophysiology while choosing the appropriate anesthetic technique. Anesthetic management requires a meticulous approach to safety, positioning, and spinal cord perfusion, with maintenance of normothermia and normovolemia [22]. Neurological deficit can be minimized by careful attention to preoperative assessment, good surgical technique, good hemodynamic management through cardiovascular monitoring, and continuous monitoring of spinal cord function.

13.5.2 Preoperative Considerations

When assessing a child for spinal surgery, it is important to adopt a holistic approach. Vertebral defects ad scoliosis in pediatric age may be associated with other congenital anomalies. Many children present with congenital problems and may be candidates for multiple procedures. Associated medical conditions, details of previous medical and surgical procedures, previous anesthetic records, and details of ongoing treatments should be sought and evaluated. Special attention should be paid to the respiratory and cardiovascular systems, as well as the CNS, since any function impairment can be associated with or result from the condition requiring spinal surgery. Preoperative assessment of patients with neuromuscular disease or who are immobile is more difficult. They are neither able to do exercise tolerance testing nor to perform spirometry adequately. Muscular dystrophies may be complicated by a subclinical cardiomyopathy. More than 50% of patients with Duchenne muscular dystrophy have some degree of dilated cardiomyopathy and an ejection fraction of less than 45%. Any reduction in ejection fraction may mean difficulties coping with the rapid fluid shifts during surgery. Echocardiography is required to assess the left ventricular function in these patients; however, a normal function does not exclude significant pathology. An accurate cardiac assessment becomes indispensable and a specialized pediatric heart center is recommended for intra- and postoperative consultation [4].

Table 13.2 Preoperative anesthetic planning and monitoring

- Induction of anesthesia
- Consider fiber-optic intubation to manage difficult airways or unstable spinal injuries
- Consider intubation in lateral position to protect the neuroplaque
- Secure safe venous access
- Routine monitoring: include invasive BP monitoring where appropriate
- Airway management: secure the tube well
- Prone positioning: ensure safety
- Use appropriate agents to maintain anesthesia
- Facilitation of spinal cord monitoring
- Maintenance of SCPP
- Prevention of hypothermia
- Maintenance of volume status
- Awareness of potential for blood loss—blood/products organized
- Blood conservation techniques where appropriate
- Antibiotic prophylaxis after discussion with surgical team
- Oximetry, capnography, and gas monitoring
- ECG, BP (usually invasive), and core temperature
- Monitoring of neuromuscular block. Postoperative considerations
- High dependency unit/intensive care nursing where appropriate
- Postoperative analgesia

13.5.3 Anesthetic Aspects, Intra- and Perioperative Monitoring

Pediatric spine surgery, especially the correction of scoliosis, has now become a routine component of pediatric anesthesia practice. Pediatric patients undergoing scoliosis surgery present unique physiological and pharmacological challenges for the anesthesiologist. Pediatric anesthesia is rapidly advancing, along with new anesthetic techniques, pharmacological options, blood-replacement modalities, and neurophysiological monitoring. At the same time, new surgical spinal techniques and new instrumentation have become available [1, 2]. Therefore, it is fundamental to have a team of expert anesthesiologists who can assess the young patient preoperatively with all the instruments for adequate intra- and postoperative treatment (Table 13.2).

Spinal surgery is performed in children of all age groups; some of them will have other severe conditions. Most operations will be performed with the patient in the prone position. Blood loss may be high for some types of surgery and patients will benefit from blood-sparing techniques. Many of them will require spinal cord monitoring to assess cord function and prevent neurological deficit [23].

13.5.4 Induction and Maintenance of Anesthesia

General anesthesia with intubation and mechanical ventilation is common in spinal surgery and may be induced with IV or inhalation (Table 13.3). Patients are placed in the prone position and the tracheal tube and lines should be well secured before and after turning the patient. The use of an armored tracheal tube minimizes the risk of kinking. Protection of the eyes and pressure points must be ensured. Syndromic patients may experience difficulties in intubation and/or ventilation due to the presence of craniofacial malformations, cervical spine motility abnormalities, mouth opening, and bone fragil-

Table 13.3 Child's spine surgery and anesthetic aspects and monitoring

- Hypercarbia stimulates respiration to a lesser extent in infants than in adults
- Hypoxia leads to severe respiratory depression
- Tendency to periodic breathing and increased risk of postoperative apnea up to 60 weeks after conceptual age
- Newborns at increased risk of atelectasis
- Diaphragm is susceptible to fatigue
- Increased risk of airway obstruction and thoracoabdominal asynchrony under anesthesia. Characteristics of the neonatal circulation and myocardial function
- Limited functional reserve
- Myocardium less able to generate force
- Myocardium more dependent on extracellular calcium
- Balance in favor of the parasympathetic system. Immature hepatic function
- Require adjustment and maintenance of drug dosing intervals
- Immature renal function tolerates fluid restriction and fasting poorly and may lead to higher incidence of intraoperative complications
- Dislodgement of the tracheal tube
- Obstruction of tracheal tube
- Bronchial intubation
- Pneumothorax
- Failure of anesthetic equipment
- Hypothermia

ity. In particular, airway management problems are often encountered in patients suffering from mucopolysaccharidosis (Morquio), Apert syndrome, Klippel Feil syndrome, Prader–Willi syndrome, Trisomy 21, and osteogenesis imperfecta. Some patients have reduced esophageal tone (e.g., Prader–Willi, Rett, Trisomy 21) and are at increased risk of inhalation. Proper management of these patients requires the presence of an experienced anesthesiologist, advanced equipment for difficult pediatric airway management (fibrobronchoscope, video laryngoscope, intubating LMA), and all necessary time. It would be advisable to schedule the intervention as the first of the operating session. Patients with severe scoliosis have restrictive syndrome of varying severity and are often subject to recurrent lower respiratory tract infections. Furthermore, some syndromes (trisomy 21, Prader–Willi, etc.) are associated with OSAS. Postoperatively, respiratory function may worsen due to pain and also use of opioid drugs with subsequent need for ventilatory support. In these patients, early specialist assessment is appropriate to allow optimization of respiratory function through physiotherapy and, when required, the use of non-invasive ventilation devices that will also be useful in the postoperative period. To repair meningocele and myelomeningocele, tracheal intubation may need to be performed with the child in the supine or lateral decubitus position using a padded ring in order to protect the neuroplaque [24]. Muscle relaxation is normally achieved with a nondepolarizing neuromuscular blocking agent. In neonates, the onset of action of atracurium is slightly longer than that of suxamethonium. If a nerve stimulator is to be used to identify functioning nerve tissue, then suxamethonium is the relaxant of choice. Venous access needs to be secured in all children. In those cases where major blood loss may be expected, more than one large cannula will be needed. Blood loss may be excessive in children undergoing extensive and aggressive spine surgery, especially when treating scoliosis secondary to neoplastic lesions. Blood loss depends on the complexity and duration of the procedure. Any standard technique can be used for maintenance of anesthesia; however, when performing intraoperative monitoring with somatosensory- and motor-evoked potentials, intravenous anesthesia becomes mandatory. The focus of intraoperative management is minimizing spinal cord ischemia and compression on the spinal cord. These are accomplished maintaining SCPP through control of blood pressure (BP) and minimizing venous congestion by careful positioning of the patient to prevent compression of the abdomen. We need to ensure spinal cord perfusion while producing a bloodless surgical field.

The most commonly used drug is remifentanil that is becoming increasingly popular for this purpose. Remifentanil is an ultra-short-acting opioid, which produces profound analgesia, has a rapid onset, excellent titrability, and a rapid offset. It can be used as part of either an inhalation or an IV maintenance regimen. Propofol and remifentanil can be used together for total IV anesthesia in children older than 2 years [25]. Monitoring during spinal surgery should routinely include ECG, pulse oximetry, capnography, anesthetic agent monitoring, temperature (core and peripheral), neuromuscular block and BP (usually invasive). Central venous pressure monitoring should be undertaken in patients with associated cardiac disease and where major blood loss is anticipated. In addition to routine monitoring and vascular access, placement of an arterial line should be considered in long surgical cases. It is wise to place a urinary catheter in such cases. Frequent evaluation of acid–base status, hemoglobin, hematocrit, and coagulation profiles may be needed in some patients. Monitoring for air embolus will also need to be undertaken in scoliosis surgery in pediatric age [26]. The state-of-the-art management for pediatric spinal cord injuries in the operating theater mandates control of the airway while the patient is under spontaneous ventilation and, optimally, with continuous somatosensory evoked potential (SSEP) monitoring. Accurate monitoring during extension and positioning is of prime importance, because this phase may lead to catastrophic spinal movement and irreversible injuries. Spinal electrical monitoring should be part of the perioperative care of these patients and should be used throughout the procedure until the patient is turned supine, the trachea is extubated, and the integrity of the spinal cord confirmed.

Decisions about where the child should be cared for after operation depends on the pre-existing cardiac and respiratory function, duration of the procedure, intraoperative events, extent of blood loss, hypothermia, and analgesic requirements. Some children need postoperative ventilation and intensive-care nursing [27, 28]. General considerations on anesthesia for spinal surgery in children are summarized in Table 13.2.

The Prone Position The majority of spinal surgery in children is performed in the prone position. The prone position refers to a patient placed face down with supports beneath the upper chest, shoulders, and iliac crests, allowing freedom of abdominal movement to facilitate ventilation and reduce intra-abdominal pressure so as to reduce bleeding from the epidural plexus. The head is usually placed in a headrest in neutral position or turned to one side while resting on the pillow. A padded foam or jelly pad may be used to protect the ear and eyes. In younger patients, bolsters or jelly rolls may be used to provide support to the torso while lifting the abdomen free from the surface of the operating table and stabilizing the patient. These usually consist of four adjustable posts designed to hold the patient while prone: two posts support the upper chest and the other two support the iliac crests (Fig. 13.1a, b). You should be aware of the

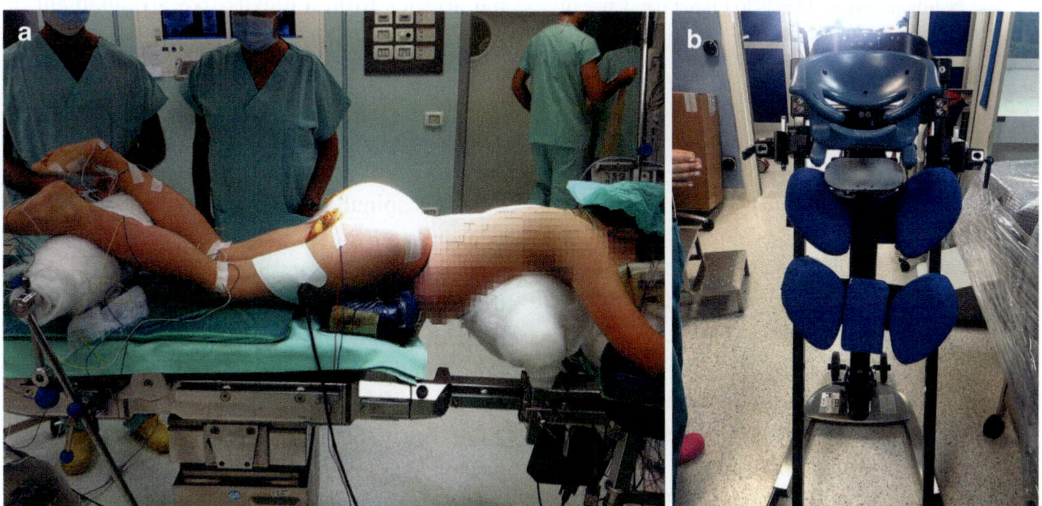

Fig. 13.1 (**a**) (male, 12 years) Neuromuscular scoliosis, preoperative prone position on a previous generation surgical table, with customized padding. Electrodes placed for SEEP and MEP neurophysiological monitoring can be seen. (**b**) A surgical table for spine surgery, equipped with support devices adaptable to very small somatic measurements, particularly suitable for pediatric scoliosis surgery

Table 13.4 Complications of prone position

- Unintentional extubation
- Eye complications: corneal abrasions, conjunctival and periorbital edema, retinal ischemia, postoperative loss of vision due to ischemic optic neuropathy (ION)
- Cable entanglement: accidental dislodgement of access and monitoring lines
- Abdominal compression leading to impaired ventilation, increased bleeding from epidural plexus, and decreased cardiac output
- Improper head and neck positioning leading to venous and lymphatic obstruction
- Macroglossia

Monitoring

- Hypercarbia stimulates respiration to a lesser extent in infants than in adults
- Hypoxia leads to severe respiratory depression
- Tendency to periodic breathing and increased risk of postoperative apnea up to 60 weeks after conceptual age
- Newborns at increased risk of atelectasis
- Diaphragm is susceptible to fatigue
- Increased risk of airway obstruction and thoracoabdominal asynchrony under anesthesia. Characteristics of the neonatal circulation and myocardial function
- Limited functional reserve
- Myocardium less able to generate force
- Myocardium more dependent on extracellular calcium
- Balance in favor of the parasympathetic system. Immature hepatic function
- Require adjustment and maintenance of drug dosing intervals
- Immature renal function tolerates fluid restriction and fasting poorly and leads to higher incidence of intraoperative complications
- Dislodgement of the tracheal tube
- Obstruction of tracheal tube
- Bronchial intubation
- Pneumothorax
- Failure of anesthetic equipment
- Hypothermia

complications that can occur in the prone position (Table 13.4). Meticulous attention to detail can prevent their occurrence.

Temperature Maintenance Infants are more susceptible to hypothermia, because they have little subcutaneous (s.c.) fat and a greater surface area-to-body mass ratio. Hypothermic children are more prone to apnea, bradycardia, hypotension, and acidosis [12]. Infants maintain normothermia by a combination of vasoconstriction and brown fat thermogenesis, but cannot increase their metabolic rate in response to mild intraoperative hypothermia. Hypothermia also prolongs recovery from neuromuscular block, impairs platelet function, and leads to a higher incidence of wound infections. Devices available to minimize intraoperative hypothermia include warming mattresses and hot air warming blankets, such as the Bair hugger device and warmed fluids [29]. Conservation of body heat is important for infants with myelomeningocele, especially because autonomic control below the level of the defect is abnormal. Operating theater temperature should be 27 °C and radiant heat lamps should be used during positioning and skin preparation.

13.6 Spinal Cord Blood Flow—Vascular Anatomy—Blood Flow Regulation

The spinal cord vascular anatomy comprises separate anterior and posterior circulations that arise from the vertebral arteries and are supplemented by intercostal and lumbar vessels from the descending aorta. A single anterior spinal artery supplies the ventral two-thirds of the spinal cord, which includes the corticospinal tracts and motor neurons. Paired posterior spinal arteries form a plexus-like arrangement on the surface of the cord and supply the dorsal one-third of spinal cord parenchyma, which transmits proprioception and light touch. There is essentially no collateral flow between the anterior and posterior circulations [30]. The anterior spinal artery, which supplies motor neurons and tracts, is of uneven caliber and is not functionally continuous. The blood flow to the anterior spinal cord is supplemented by collateral flow through radicular arteries arising from the aorta. Only 6–8 of the 62 radicular vessels present during development persist into adult life. The large distance between these radicular arteries leaves watershed areas at the upper thoracic and lumbar levels, thus making the spinal cord particularly vulnerable to ischemia. The great radicular artery of Adamkiewicz arises from the aorta between the T8 and L3 nerve roots, and supplements the blood flow to the anterior portion of the distal thoracic spinal cord and lumbar enlargement [31]. It provides up to 50% of the entire spinal cord blood flow [32, 33]. The venous outflow of the spinal cord is divided into two systems called the vertebral and venous plexuses. These internal and external plexuses communicate with each other and with the segmental systemic veins. Literature review suggests that spinal cord blood flow is controlled by the same factors and general physiological principles as cerebral blood flow (CBF) [34, 35]. Spinal cord blood flow is lower than CBF, because absolute spinal cord metabolism is lower than that of the brain. Blood flow to the spinal grey matter is about half that to the cerebral cortex and the flow to the white matter is about one-third of that to spinal grey matter. SCPP equals mean arterial pressure minus extrinsic pressure on the spinal cord. Pressures exerted by local extrinsic mechanical compression, such as tumor, hematoma, spinal venous congestion, and increased intraspinal fluid pressure can be important determinants of the SCPP. Spinal blood flow is maintained constant by vasodilation or vasoconstriction of the vasculature of the cord to accommodate for changes in mean arterial BP. Limits of autoregulation of spinal cord blood flow are 45–180 mmHg. Conditions that affect this autoregulatory mechanism include severe hypoxia, hypercapnia, and trauma [15, 36]. The spinal cord vasculature and cerebral vasculature react to changes in oxygen and carbon dioxide concentrations in a similar fashion. Epidural anesthesia may affect the spinal fluid pressure.

13.6.1 Spinal Cord Monitoring

Intraoperative monitoring of spinal cord function is considered a standard of care in spinal surgery [37]. Spinal cord monitoring usually forms a part of the surgical procedure for spinal injuries and for scoliosis correction. Techniques to monitor the integrity of spinal cord function intraoperatively include the wake-up test [2], SSEP [3], motor-evoked potentials (MEPs), and [4] dermatomal responses.

The Wake-Up Test It was first described 20 years ago [38]. Before the introduction of electrical monitoring, it was used to evaluate spinal cord function during corrective procedures of the spine [39]. The major advantage is that it assesses anterior spinal cord function (i.e., motor function). The hazards of this test include accidental extubation, air embolism during deep inspiration, and dislodgement of fixators. Its major limitation is that it assesses spinal cord function only at one specific time (i.e., during the wake-up test) and not continuously during the procedure. False negatives are reported. Both inhalation and IV anesthetic techniques are suitable for the 'wake-up' test. A standard wake-up test cannot be performed in infants and small children.

Somato-Sensory-Evoked Potentials SSEPs are a more widespread method of electrical monitoring of the spinal cord. SSEPs measure the electrical potentials evoked by stimulation of the sensory system [23]. The response of constant current stimulation of the median, tibial, and, rarely, the sural nerve is recorded at the cortex using surface electrodes or a bipolar electrode placed epidurally by the surgeon. Baseline SSEPs are recorded in order to exclude neurological dysfunction and also to determine the feasibility of operative monitoring. Neurophysiology technicians monitor the latency and amplitude of the recordings continuously during anesthesia and surgery. A 50% decrease in SSEP amplitude is deemed significant. Numerous anesthetic agents interfere with the latency and amplitude of the SSEPs. Surgical stimulation level and hypothermia also interfere with SSEPs. Volatile agents, cold, hypoxia, hypercarbia, and spinal ischemia suppress both SSEPs and motor-evoked potentials (MEPs) [40, 41]. Responses recorded from the cerebral cortex are more sensitive to the effects of anesthetic agents than epidurally recorded responses. Neuromuscular block reduces muscle artifact on the recorded SSEPs. SSEP monitoring is a pathway-specific method; an injury not involving the sensory pathway will not be detected. Global cord monitoring may be possible with combined SSEPs and MEPs [41]. Motor-evoked potentials (MEPs) may be either evoked EMGs or compound muscle action potentials (CMAPs) [42]. They assess function of the motor cortex and the descending motor pathways. They may be obtained by stimulation of the motor areas of the brain or spinal cord through the intact skin, direct stimulation of the exposed neuronal tissue, or direct root stimulation (e.g., during the release of a tethered cord) through recording of a stimulus-related response either as a CMAP or as an efferent compound nerve action potential (CNAP). CNAPs allow the patient to have neuromuscular blocking agents. Multiple pulse transcranial stimulation involves cortical stimulation with progressive energy aimed at detecting the threshold needed to achieve peripheral muscular signal. A modification of this threshold is a sensitive marker of spinal compromise.

Dermatomal Responses Pudendal nerve responses are a special case of dermatomal responses that are particularly useful, especially in patients with neuromuscular diseases [43]. The pudendal nerve carries sensory fibers from the penis, urethra, anus, and pelvic floor muscles and supplies motor innervation to the bulbocavernosus and pelvic floor muscles, external urethral sphincter, and external anal sphincter. Cortical responses to the electrical stimulation of the dorsal nerve of the penis, urethra, and urinary bladder have all been described. Pudendal nerve responses are of similar morphology to the tibial nerve SEP and are best recorded from the same area of the scalp. Intraoperative neurophysiological monitoring is mandatory in a patient with neuromuscular scoliosis, who does not walk but has sphincter control, to avoid any neurological aggravation during scoliosis treatment.

13.6.1.1 Intra-op Neuromonitoring for Neuromuscular Scoliosis

Cerebral palsy (CP), for instance, includes a group of non-progressive, but often changing, motor impairment syndromes secondary to lesions or anomalies of the brain arising in the early stage of its development. It is often associated with progressive scoliosis. The motor defect may be spasticity, ataxia, or dyskinesia. CP children may be treated with different types of medications. Baclofen is an agonist at the GABA-b receptor, acting in the spinal cord to inhibit the release of excitatory neurotransmitters and thereby reducing the muscle tone. It is the only medication currently used intrathecally with a demonstrable reduction in spasticity. Baclofen may be administered intrathecally via a programmable pump, which is implanted surgically [44]. Children with rapidly developing neuromuscular scoliosis often go directly to the vertebral surgeon for spinal surgery. Their most common medical issues may include difficult venous access, limb contractures making positioning difficult, epilepsy, gastro-esophageal reflux, chronic upper airway obstruction, and difficulty in pain assessment which is crucial if pain management is to be effective [45]. Evaluation of perioperative risk is very difficult, especially in children with severe disability.

13.6.2 How to Control Pain and Anemia in the Postop

Blood Conservation Spinal surgical procedures have the potential for massive hemorrhage. Preoperative planning for spinal surgery should always include cross-matching of two or more units of blood. Preoperative supplementation with oral iron and possibly s.c. erythropoietin is mandatory. In addition, the following should be carefully evaluated: predonation of blood, acute normovolemic hemodilution, good surgical technique and hemostasis, correct positioning of the patient when prone, hypotensive anesthesia (only with adequate cord monitoring), use of cell saver, aprotinin [42, 45], tranexamic acid [44], intrathecal opiates, and monitored use of coagulation products [42, 44–48]. Acceptance of a lower postoperative hemoglobin level should reduce the need for postoperative transfusions. Homologous blood transfusion is also associated with the risks of transmission of bacterial and viral infections, alloimmunization, immunomodulation, graft vs. host disease (GvHD), metabolic imbalance, and transfusion mismatch [47, 49].

There is a growing medical and parental concern about these potential hazards.

Management of Postoperative Pain Pain management after spine surgery usually requires opioid-based protocols: in younger children, either a morphine infusion or a nurse-controlled analgesia. Children aged 7 years or more may be able to use patient-controlled analgesia. Infiltration of the wound at the end of surgery with local anesthetic will help relieve pain in the immediate postoperative period. Opioids should be supplemented with regular paracetamol and non-steroidal anti-inflammatory drugs, if there are no contraindications to their use. In case of scoliosis surgery, an additional solution involves the placement of an epidural catheter by the surgeon at the end of the procedure [50].

13.7 Surgical Treatment

13.7.1 Introduction

Early onset scoliosis (EOS) is defined as a spinal deformity diagnosed before the age of 5 (Fig. 13.2a, b). The etiology of EOS can be idiopathic, neuromuscular/syndromic, and congenital. These patients may have congenital spinal abnormalities associated with rare diseases with thoracic malformations, such as fused or missing ribs, and neuromuscular syndromes with severe breathing difficulties. However, they may also have normal vertebral formation as it happens with idiopathic scoliosis in children. It is a rare condition: the incidence of idiopathic scoliosis is 1.5% and idiopathic scoliosis in children accounts for 4% of this population. However, early-onset scoliosis is an important health issue. These children develop spinal deformities at a young age and, if left untreated, are at risk of rapid progression with impaired physiological growth and cosmetic appearance and, most of all, lung failure. In patients with untreated scoliosis, mortality rate is reported to increase: this occurs more frequently in scoliosis with childhood-onset (first 5 years of life), followed by juvenile scoliosis (6–10 years), and is mainly due to respiratory failure. EOS often leads to severe deformities developing at an early age. Clinically, most of them are spinal deformities with double main curves and some have significant thoracolumbar hyperkyphosis [51, 52].

13.7.2 Treatment

There are no guidelines for treatment: when they see children with mild deformities presenting non-congenital progressive curves, most clinicians will just observe them and prescribe physical activity or treatment with brace. Unfortunately, the use of orthopedic braces and plaster casts in the treatment of congenital and neuromuscular scoliosis is known not to be effective. This is especially true for those patients with a rib-vertebral angle (Metha angle) >20°, indicative of a highly progressive curve. The orthopedic corset is commonly used for minor angular curves with a Cobb angle of 20°–30°. Treatment with orthopedic corsets requires prolonged use, especially in patients with early scoliosis, and effectiveness often depends on the collaboration of patients and families. In many cases, the orthopedic corset is not accepted or is poorly tolerated, especially when small patients with proximal thoracic curves have to wear a tall Milwaukee brace [52, 53].

13.7.3 Vertebral Fusion

In the past, definitive early fusion (or vertebral arthrodesis) has been advocated for children with severe progressive scoliotic curves, in particular congenital deformities. However, there is a growing consensus that early spinal fusion produces (excluding very selected congenital deformities) adverse pulmonary consequences [54]. Most spine surgeons who are experienced in scoliosis now use fusion as a last resort in pediatric patients. A literature review of the long-term results after fusion in patients with early scoliosis showed that in 37.2–39.3% of cases, it was necessary to re-intervene for the progression of the deformity. This has also occurred in some patients treated with anterior and posterior fusion during

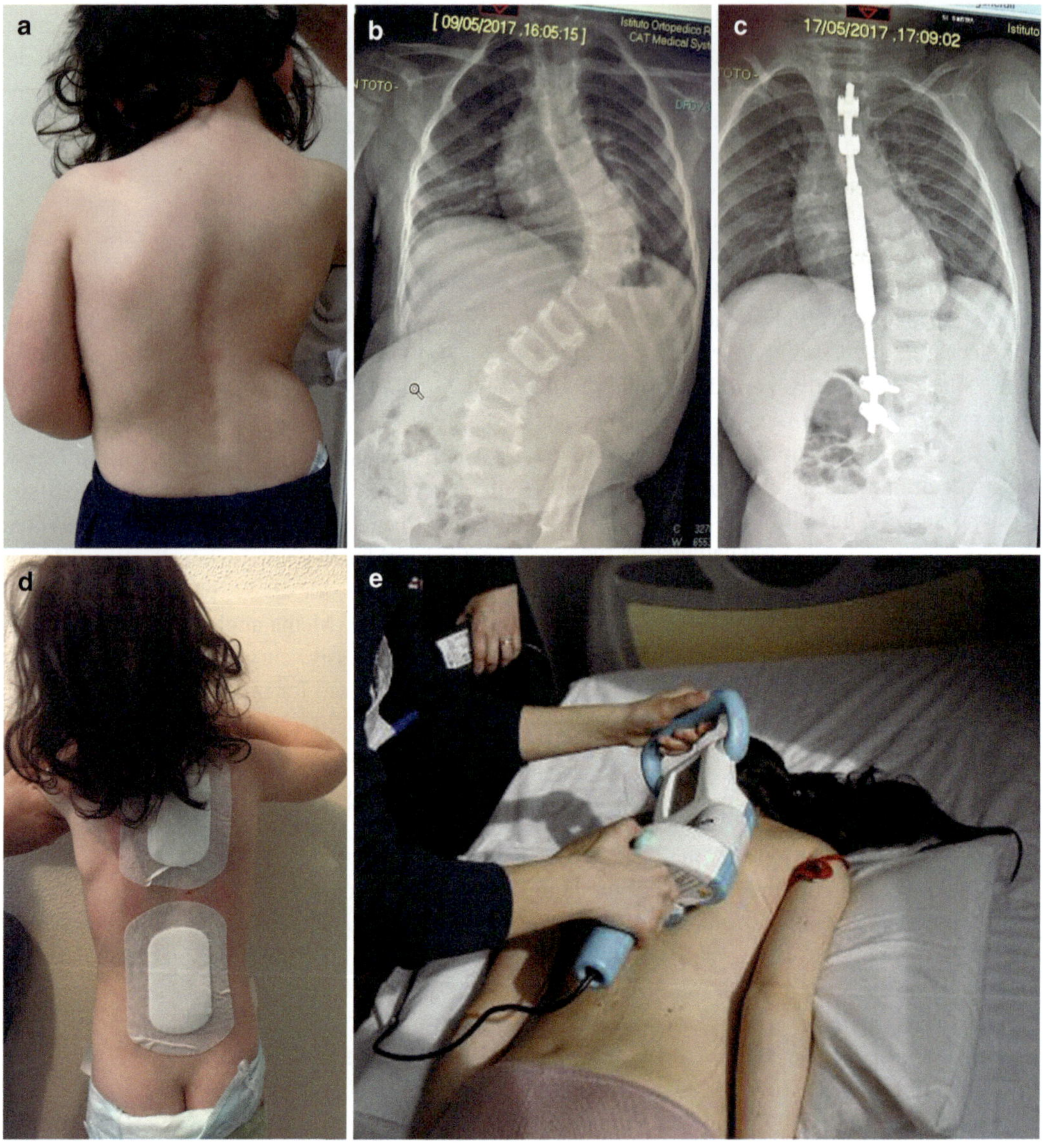

Fig. 13.2 (**a**) (female, 26 months) Severe idiopathic infantile scoliosis, clinical picture. (**b**) (female, 26 months) Severe idiopathic infantile scoliosis, pre-op radiographic picture. (**c**) Severe idiopathic infantile scoliosis, post-op radiographic picture. Implantation of a magnetic extendable bar. (**d**) Severe idiopathic infantile scoliosis, clinical picture on post-op day 3 after minimal access surgery. (**e**) System lengthening every 2 months and as day surgery. Bars are distracted using an external remote controller

growth, theoretically to achieve circumferential stability [55, 56]. In addition to its failure to control spinal deformity, fusion can have negative consequences on the overall growth of the child. Prof. A. Di Meglio has conducted numerous studies on spinal growth and observed that the fastest period of spinal growth occurs in the first 5 years of life, when the spine increases by 50% of its length. It was also found that between the ages of 5 and 10, the spine continues to grow, albeit at a slower rate. The height of the thoracic spine is on average 11 cm in the newborn, 18 cm from the age of 5 and 22 cm at the age of 10 [57]. All of this makes it clear why treating early scoliosis with spinal fusion in a 5-year-old child can result in a loss of spinal growth of more than

12.5 cm. Additionally, the presence of congenital rib fusions associated with congenital scoliosis in growing children can lead to arrested lung development. This leads to chest failure syndrome or the inability of the chest to sustain normal breathing [58, 59]. Pulmonary function has been studied in patients who underwent early spinal fusion for scoliosis, and inhibition of normal thoracic growth was observed. The normal development of the lungs in children is determined, in fact, by an increase in the number of alveoli in the first years of life and an increase in lung volumes up to adolescence [60, 61]. For this reason, surgery with definitive arthrodesis of the spine at this age can be a great limitation on lung development [62, 63].

13.7.4 Growing Rods

To address limitations after spinal fusion for early scoliosis, growth-friendly implants have been developed since a long time. The instrumentation techniques initially included those of the last century, such as the Harrington system (widely studied and used as an extendable bar by the Italian Masters Marchetti and Faldini), Cotrel-Dubousset, or Luque devices. More recently, the friend and colleague Prof. B. Akbarnia (San Diego Center of Spinal Disorders, University of California, former president of SRS) disseminated the technique of the dual growing rod, first mechanically then magnetically controlled. The mechanical dual growing rod system, we have been using for over 10 years, consists of two extendable bars that we apply via a minimally invasive subfascial route to a spinal segment with deformity without fusion. The anchors for the bars, either hooks or pedicle screws, are placed only at the proximal and distal end of the segment. Distraction of the bars for lengthening over time occurs with minimally invasive surgical access, usually every 6–8 months. Once maximum spinal growth or skeletal maturity is reached, then final fusion surgery is performed. With this approach, the stretchable bars control the progression of the spinal deformity and gradually correct it.

13.7.5 The Vertical Expandable Prosthetic Titanium Rib (VEPTR) Device

When the main deformity is not the spinal one, but it is associated with an important thoracic deformity with onset in the pediatric age, a specific spine-rib device called VEPTR and developed by R. Campbell in 2004 can be used. The length of the device can be expanded as the patient grows, just as with the growing rods (Fig. 13.3a–e). Clearly, a treatment path with extendable systems is very demanding for the patient and their family, especially for the scheduled repeated surgeries to be added to the unscheduled procedures following mechanical failures (mobilization and breakage of the bars) [64, 65]. The need for repeated surgery under general anesthesia required by growing-rods and VEPTR is a major drawback. A high number of operations involves a greater number of anesthetic and surgical complications. In addition, various socioeconomic concerns are associated, including longer periods of hospitalization and more time away from school and work for the child and parents, respectively. Repeated operations, hospitalization, and the appearance of a cosmetically unacceptable surgical scar can also affect the child's psychological well-being [66].

13.7.6 Magnetically Controlled Growing Rods (MGRs)

Due to the aforementioned drawbacks associated with the use of mechanical extendable bars, technological development over the last decade has led to the construction of systems that allow lengthening without surgery. MCGRs reproduce the effectiveness of the mechanical growing rod and can be controlled by an external magnet. This new device eliminates the need for frequent hospitalizations and repeated interventions under general anesthesia, thus reducing wound-related complications, as well as psychological and socioeconomic problems (Fig. 13.2a–e). Stretching is performed in clinics with the patient awake in a few minutes, on average every

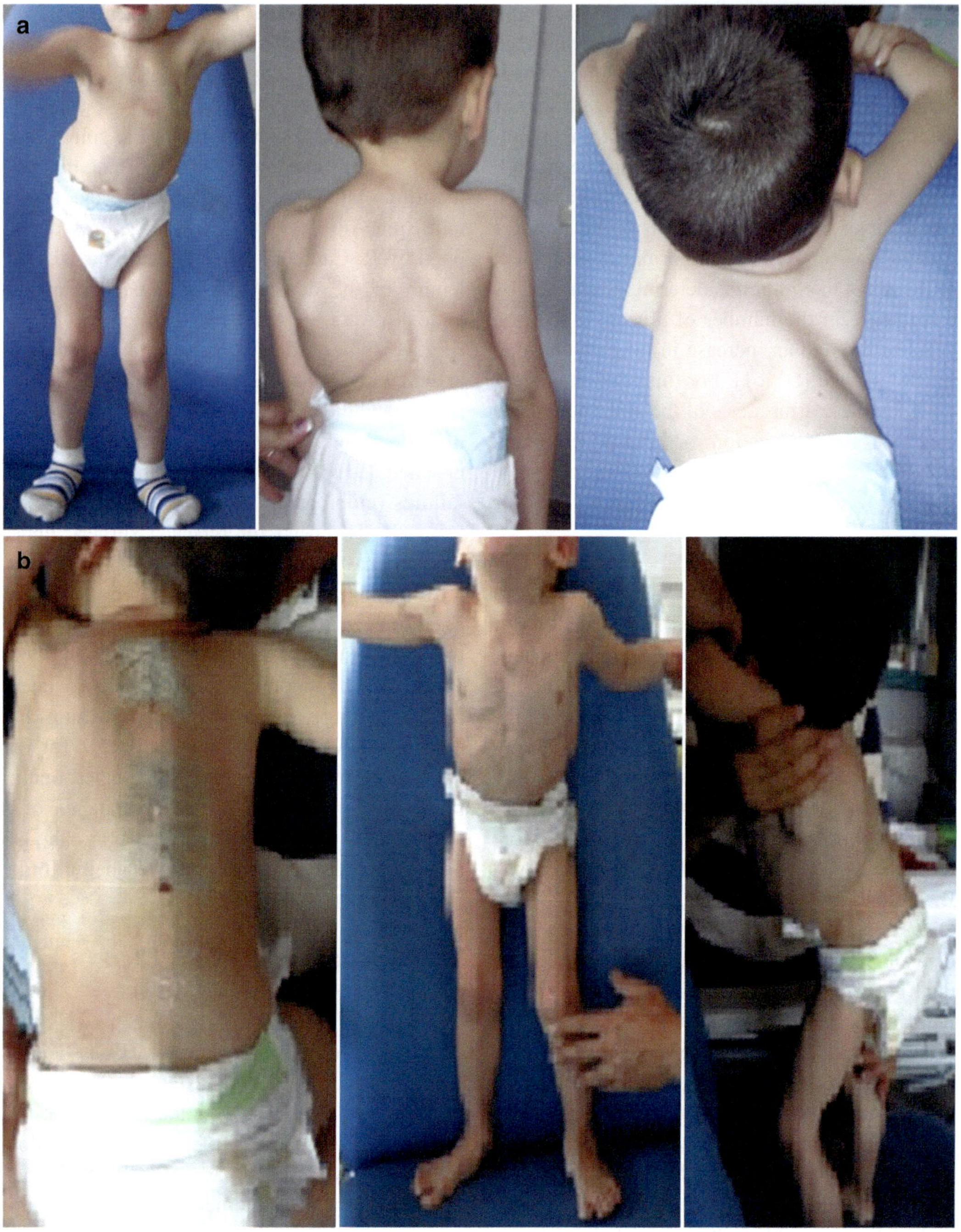

Fig. 13.3 (**a**) (male, 2.5 years) Preoperative clinical picture of severe congenital kyphoscoliosis with respiratory insufficiency equal to PO_2 71 mmHg (spirometry cannot be performed). (**b**) (male, 2.5 years) Severe congenital kyphoscoliosis. Post-op clinical picture after surgery with VEPTR rib-spine instrumentation via minimal access surgery. After surgery, the respiratory function has improved to PO_2 90 mmHg. (**c**) On the left, post-op radiographic picture, LL and AP views, after surgery with VEPTR instrumentation. On the right, radiographic picture, AP view, showing the VEPTR rib-spine bar after three lengthening procedures 2 years after first surgery. (**d**) On the left, a scheme illustrating the VEPTR lengthening procedure. On the right, intra-op picture of the surgical lengthening of an extendable bar. (**e**) (male, 6 years) Congenital kyphoscoliosis with severe respiratory insufficiency. At the age of 2.5 years, he was implanted with the VEPTR device. Clinical picture at 6 years, after five lengthening procedures, plus one replacement of the bar. Spirometry result was FV1 81%

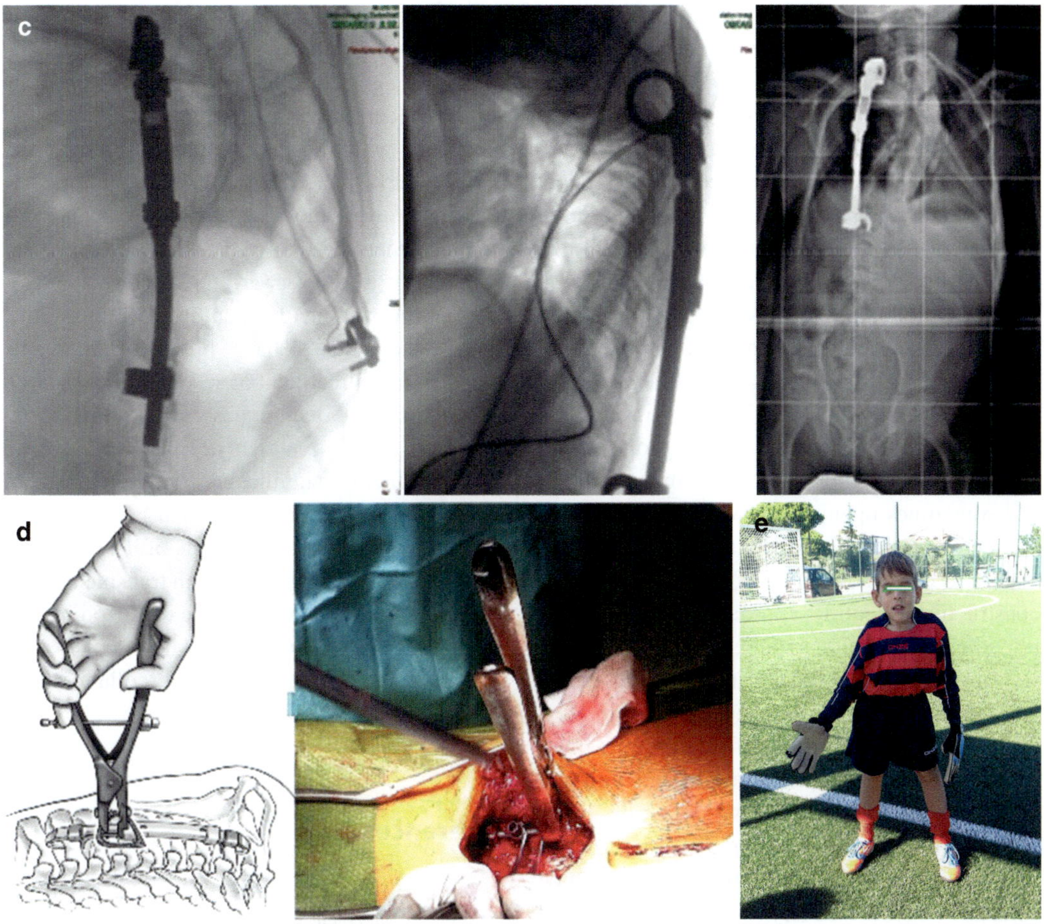

Fig. 13.3 (continued)

2 months [67, 68]. In addition to the cost of the implant, another negative aspect of the magnetic system is the contraindication to its use in patients who need high intensity MRI controls (e.g., myeloradicular malformations associated with scoliosis). However, there are studies that have demonstrated that MRI has no harmful effects on MCGRs and that there is no distortion for imaging of the head and neck [20].

13.8 Conclusion

Early-onset scoliosis is a difficult challenge. These patients are young, with significant growth potential. As a result of scoliosis, they can develop progressive deformities with extremely negative consequences on cosmetic appearance and cardiopulmonary function. Surgical treatment of non-idiopathic spine deformities in young children is very demanding. Rare syndromes are various clinical conditions, heterogeneous in terms of clinics but associated with spinal deformities in a large percentage of cases.

Scoliosis is the most common early-onset deformity, sometimes present at birth and often rapidly evolving. Conventional management tools, such as bracing and fusion, are not always effective. Additionally, fusion can also cause significant inhibition of normal spinal and thoracic growth [69, 70]. Extendable bars are currently the treatment of choice for early scoliosis since they are distracted at intervals to allow for growth. However, the need for repeated interventions is associated with an exponential increase in complications.

With the development of the magnetic extendable system, non-invasive stretches can be performed, thus reducing the need for frequent interventions and, consequently, the incidence of the aforementioned negative aspects for children and parents. However, as it always happens with any new technology, more studies are needed to further reduce complications and improve outcomes in children undergoing treatment for early-onset scoliosis [71, 72]. Scoliosis often affects children's life early, creating discomfort and isolation, making surgical treatment painful, and sometimes opening the way to difficult and ineffective paths. The dialogue with other specialists to discuss the state of the art is always a constructive scientific approach. I believe that providing information to patients and families, as well involving other specialists, can be an added value to our research. Growing systems are good devices which have proved effective in the treatment of early onset scoliosis associated with rare syndromes: they should be used when the peculiar features of the syndromes make deformities very aggressive and consequently, difficult to be controlled conservatively. Both clinical and instrumental evaluation tailored to fit the patient's needs are of the utmost importance: an overall assessment of the peculiar features of each syndrome along with the common characteristics of scoliosis should be made.

PFR evaluates young patients' life quality indirectly; cardio-US and abdominal US are useful in the study of visceral malformations; brain and spine MRI can detect spinal cord malformation, that is to say contraindications to surgery and therefore, they are all mandatory for thorough preoperative planning. The indication for traditional growing rod, magnetic rod, or VEPTR, should be given according to patient's age and considering the presence of thoracic hyperkyphosis or chest deformities.

Multidisciplinary collaboration with translational research will bring more specialized fields closer to new knowledge on scoliosis and in particular on severe early onset spinal deformities. The genetic and molecular study of syndromic diseases and rapidly evolving scoliosis may lead to early diagnosis. Even the study of idiopathic scoliosis (certainly of a polygenic nature) will help deal with the pre-symptomatic stage and better control the severity of the evolution. The use of the most modern "imaging" technology, such as dynamic MRI for the study of the thorax, will take us a step forward to the correct assessment of thoracic involvement in EOS. Innovative surgical techniques have brought remarkable changes in the treatment of severe scoliosis. Even the "non-fusion" techniques are currently a viable option for the treatment of EOS. Although we are still facing significant complications, we should not be discouraged. This situation, as Prof. Akbarnia says, reminds us of the first steps taken on the path towards "organ transplantation" [1]: a lot of efforts are still to be made to improve results and aggregate strengths and experiences with national and international collaborations [18, 73].

References

1. Akbarnia BA, Yazici M, Thompson GH. The growing spine management of spinal disorders in young children. Berlin: Springer; 2016.
2. Greggi T. Surgical treatment of severe early onset scoliosis (idiopathic and associated with rare diseases). Surg Case Stud Open Access J. 2020;5(5):22. https://doi.org/10.32474/SCSOAJ.2020.05.00022.
3. Bradford DS, Heithoff KB, Cohen M. Intraspinal abnormalities and congenital spine deformities: a radiographic and MRI study. J Pediatr Orthop. 1991;11(1):36–41. https://doi.org/10.1097/01241398-199101000-00009.
4. Kaufman BA. Neural tube defects. Pediatr Clin N Am. 2004;51:389–419.
5. Glenn OA, Barkovich J. Magnetic resonance imaging of the fetal brain and spine: an increasingly important tool in prenatal diagnosis: part 2. Am J Neuroradiol. 2006;27:1807–14.
6. Michelson DJ, Ashwal S. Tethered cord syndrome in childhood: diagnostic features and relationship to congenital anomalies. Neurol Res. 2004;26:745–53.
7. Warder DE. Tethered cord syndrome and occult spinal dysraphism. Neurosurg Focus. 2001;15:E1.
8. Greggi T, Barbanti Brodano G, Tabarroni M, Parisini P. Diastematomyelia in congenital scoliosis. A review of the literature and description of one clinical case. Chir Organi Mov. 1997;82(1):83–9.

9. Platt JH Jr. Syringomyelia complicating myelomeningocele: review of the evidence. J Neurosurg. 2004;100:101–9.
10. Stevenson KL. Chiari type II malformation: past, present and future. Neurosurg Focus. 2004;15:E5.
11. Vandertop WP, Asai A, Hoffman HJ, et al. Surgical decompression for symptomatic Chiari II malformation in neonates with myelo-meningocele. J Neurosurg. 1992;77:521–4.
12. Wazeka AN, DiMaio MF, Boachie-Adjei O. Outcome of pediatric patients with severe restrictive lung disease following reconstructive spine surgery. Spine. 2004;29:528–34.
13. Rosemberg S, Fujiwara D. Epidemiology of pediatric tumors of the nervous system according to the WHO 2000 classification: a report of 1195 cases from a single institution. Childs Nerv Syst. 2005;21:940–4.
14. Auguste KI, Gupta N. Pediatric intramedullary spinal cord tumors. Neurosurg Clin N Am. 2006;17:51–61.
15. Jallo GI, Freed D, Epstein F. Intramedullary spinal cord tumours in children. Childs Nerv Syst. 2003;19:641–9.
16. Acaroglu RE, Demirikiran HG, Ghermandi R, Boriani S. Management of spine tumors in young children. In: Akbarnia BA, Yazici M, Thompson GH, editors. The growing spine management of spinal disorders in young children. Berlin: Springer; 2016.
17. T. Greggi, L. Boriani, et al. Unusual presentation of a medulloblastoma mimicking an AARS (Atlanto axial rotatory subluxation). A case report. Medicine Published 2020. Corpus ID: 229492465, https://doi.org/10.21203/rs.3.rs-110593/v1.
18. Ali FE, Al-Bustan MA, Al-Busairi WA, Al-Mulla FA, Esbaita EY. Cervical spine abnormalities associated with down syndrome. Int Orthop. 2006;30(4):284–9. https://doi.org/10.1007/s00264-005-0070-y.
19. Deutsch H, Shrivistava R, Epstein F, Jallo GI. Pediatric intramedullary spinal cavernous malformations. Spine. 2001;26:E427–31.
20. Nagib MG, O'Fallon MT. Intramedullary cavernous angiomas of the spinal cord in the pediatric age group: a pediatric series. Pediatr Neurosurg. 2002;36:57–63.
21. Milstein JM, Lau M, Bickers RG. Tracheal agenesis in infants with VATER association. Am J Dis Child. 1985;139:77–80.
22. Bacchin R, Feoli A, Morigi A, Ghisi D, Greggi T. Liver and skeletal muscle injury in a 12-year-old female patient after scoliosis correction in prone position: a case report. Spine Deform. 2020;8(2):345–8.
23. Pastorelli F, Di Silvestre M, Plasmati R. The prevention of neural complications in the surgical treatment of scoliosis: the role of the neurophysiological intraoperative monitoring. Eur Spine J. 2011;20:105–14.
24. Soundararajan N, Cunliffe M. Anaesthesia for spinal surgery in children. Br J Anaesth. 2007;99(1):86–94. https://doi.org/10.1093/bja/aem120.
25. Eyres R. Update on TIVA. Paediatr Anaesth. 2004;14:374–9.
26. Fassett DR, McCall T, Brockmeyer DL. Odontoid synchondrosis fractures in children. Neurosurg Focus. 2006;20:E7.
27. Frankel AS, Holzman RS. Air embolism during posterior spinal fusion. Can J Anaesth. 1988;35:511–4.
28. Almenrader N, Patel D. Spinal fusion surgery in children with non-idiopathic scoliosis: is there a need for routine postoperative ventilation? Br J Anaesth. 2006;97:851–7.
29. Mural I, Berniere J, Constant I. Evaluation of the efficacy of a forced-air warmer (Bair Hugger) during spinal surgery in children. J Clin Anesth. 1994;6:425–9,
30. Standring S. Gray's anatomy: the anatomical basis of medicine and surgery. 39th ed. Edinburgh: Churchill-Livingstone; 2004.
31. Alleyne CH Jr, Cawley CM, Shengelaia GG, Barrow DL. Microsurgical anatomy of the artery of Adamkiewicz and its segmental artery. Neurosurgery. 1998;89:791–5.
32. Servais LJ, Rivelli SK, Dachy BA, Christophe CD, Dan B. Anterior spinal artery syndrome after aortic surgery in a child. Pediatr Neurol. 2001;24:310–2.
33. Stocki B, Wimmer C, Innerhofer P, Kofler M, Behensky H. Delayed anterior spinal artery syndrome following posterior scoliosis correction. Eur Spine J. 2005;14:906–9.
34. Holtz A, Nystrom B, Gerdin B. Regulation of spinal cord blood flow in the rat as measured by quantitative autoradiography. Acta Physiol Scand. 1988;133:485–93.
35. Rubinstein A, Arbit E. Spinal cord blood flow in the rat under normal physiological conditions. Neurosurgery. 1990;27:882–6.
36. Gibson PR. Anaesthesia for correction of scoliosis in children. Anaesth Intensive Care. 2004;32(4):548–59. https://doi.org/10.1177/0310057X0403200413.
37. Sale F, Krzan MJ, Deletis V. Intraoperative neurophysiological monitoring in pediatric neurosurgery: why, when, how? Childs Nerv Syst. 2002;18:264–87.
38. Accadbled F, Henry P, de Gauzy JS, Cahuzac JP. Spinal cord monitoring in scoliosis surgery using an epidural electrode. Results of a prospective, consecutive series of 191 cases. Spine. 2006;31:2614–23.
39. Dorgan JC, Abbott TR, Bentley G. Intra-operative awakening to monitor spinal cord function during scoliosis surgery. Description of the technique and report of four cases. Bone Jt Surg Br. 1984;66:716–9.
40. Boisseau N, Madany M, Staccini P, Armando G, Martin F, Grimaud D, et al. Comparison of the effects of sevoflurane and propofol on cortical somatosensory evoked potentials. Br J Anaesth. 2002;88:785–9.
41. Costa P, Bruno A, Bonzanino M, et al. Somatosensory and motor evoked potential monitoring during spine and spinal cord surgery. Spinal Cord. 2007;45:86–91.
42. Macdonald DB. Intraoperative motor evoked potential monitoring: overview and update. J Clin Monit Comput. 2006;20:347–77.
43. Cohen BA, Major MR, Huizenga BA. Pudendal nerve evoked potential monitoring in procedures involving low sacral fixation. Spine. 1991;16:S375–8.
44. Albright AL, Ferson SS. Intrathecal baclofen in children. Neurosurg Focus. 2006;21:3.

45. Wongprasartsuk P, Stevens J. Cerebral palsy and anaesthesia. Paediatr Anaesth. 2002;12:296–303.
46. Samama CM. Aprotinin and major orthopedic surgery. Eur Spine J. 2004;13:S56–61.
47. Sethna NF, Zurakowski D, Brustowicz RM, Bacsik J, Sullivan LJ, Shapiro F. Tranexamic acid reduced intra-operative blood loss in pediatric patients undergoing scoliosis surgery. Anesthesiology. 2005;102:727–32.
48. Shiga T, Wajima Z, Inoue T, Sakamoto A. Aprotinin after major orthopaedic surgery: a systematic review of randomized controlled trials. Anesth Analg. 2005;101:1602–7.
49. Stainsby D, Jones H, Asher D, et al. SHOT Steering Group. Serious hazards of transfusion: a decade of hemovigilance in the UK. Transfus Med Rev. 2006;20:273–82.
50. O'Hara JF Jr, Cywinski JB, Tetzlaff JE, Xu M, Gurd AR, Andrish JT. The effect of epidural vs intravenous analgesia for posterior spinal fusion surgery. Paediatr Anaesth. 2004;14:1009–15.
51. Campbell RM. Spine deformities in rare congenital syndromes: clinical issues. Spine. 2009;34:1815–27.
52. Giacomini S, Greggi T, Maredi E, Di Silvestre M, Vommaro F, et al. Treatment of early onset scoliosis associated with rare diseases. In: 2nd World congress on rare diseases and orphan drugs. 2017.
53. Fletcher ND, McClung A, Rathjen KE. Serial casting as a delay tactic in the treatment of moderate-to-severe early-onset scoliosis. J Pediatr Orthop. 2012;32:664–71.
54. Dubousset J, Herring JA, Shufflebarger H. The crankshaft phenomenon. J Pediatr Orthop. 1989;9:541–50.
55. Goldberg CJ, Moore DP, Fogarty EE. Long-term results from in situ fusion for congenital vertebral deformity. Spine. 2002;27:619–28.
56. Chang DG, Kim JH, Ha KY. Posterior hemivertebra resection and short segment fusion with pedicle screw fixation for congenital scoliosis in children younger than 10 years: greater than 7-year follow-up. Spine. 2015;15:E484–91.
57. Dimeglio A, Bonnel F. Le rachis en croissance. Paris: Springer; 1990.
58. Yaszay B, O'Brien M, Shufflebarger HL. Efficacy of hemivertebra resection for congenital scoliosis. Spine. 2006;36(24):2052–60.
59. Bollini G, Docquier PL, Viehweger E. Lumbar hemivertebra resection. J Bone Jt Surg Am. 2006;88:1043–52.
60. Campbell RM, Smith MD, Mayes TC. The characteristics of thoracic insufficiency syndrome associated with fused ribs and congenital scoliosis. J Bone Jt Surg Am. 2003;85:399–408.
61. Burri PH, McDonald JA. Structural aspects of prenatal and postnatal development and growth of the lung. Lung growth and development. New York: Dekker; 1997. p. 1–35.
62. Thurlbeck WM. Postnatal human lung growth. Thorax. 1982;37:564–71.
63. Johnston CE, Tran DP, McClung A. Functional and radiographic outcomes following growth-sparing management of early-onset scoliosis. J Bone Jt Surg Am. 2017;99:1036–42.
64. Campbell RM, Hell-Vocke AK. Growth of the thoracic spine in congenital scoliosis after expansion thoracoplasty. J Bone Jt Surg Am. 2003;85:409–20.
65. Campbell RM, Smith MD, Hell-Vocke AK. Expansion thoracoplasty: the surgical technique of opening-wedge thoracostomy. Surgical technique. J Bone Jt Surg Am. 2004;86(A):51–64.
66. Greggi T, Lolli F, Di Silvestre M. Complications incidence in the treatment of early onset scoliosis with growing spinal implants. Stud Health Technol Inform. 2012;176:334–7.
67. Bess S, Akbarnia BA, Thompson GH. Complications of growing-rod treatment for early-onset scoliosis: analysis of one hundred and forty patients. J Bone Jt Surg Am. 2010;92(15):2533–43.
68. Upasani VV, Parvaresh KC, Pawalek JB. Age at initiation and deformity magnitude influence complication rates of surgical treatment with traditional growing rods in early-onset scoliosis. Spine Deform. 2016;4:344–50.
69. Pehrsson K, Larsson S, Oden A. Long-term follow-up of patients with untreated scoliosis: a study of mortality, causes of death, and symptoms. Spine. 1992;17:1091–6.
70. Thompson GH, Lenke LG, Akbarnia BA. Early onset scoliosis: future directions. J Bone Jt Surg Am. 2007;89(1):163–6.
71. Vitale MG, Gomez JA, Matsumoto H. Variability of expert opinion in treatment of early-onset scoliosis. Clin Orthop Relat Res. 2011;469:1317–22.
72. Tis JE, Karlin LI, Akbarnia BA. Early onset scoliosis: modern treatment and results. J Pediatr Orthop. 2012;32:647–57.
73. Alvarez AG, Dearn KD, Lawless BM, Lavecchia CE, Vommaro F, et al. Design and mechanical evaluation of a novel dynamic growing rod to improve the surgical treatment of early onset scoliosis. Mater Des. 2018;155:334–45.

Medical and Rehabilitation Interventions in Children with Frailty

14

Rossana Toglia, Eleonora Lovardi, and Enrico Castelli

14.1 Introduction

Frailty is a multidimensional syndrome characterized by a reduced ability to deal with acute, physical, psychological and socioeconomic stressors, and/or to perform daily living activities.

It is essential that the type of approach to the fragile child is multidisciplinary given the high clinical complexity of the underlying pathologies.

In these children, the most observable problems are neurological, sensory, cognitive and secondarily musculoskeletal, gastrointestinal problems, psychological difficulties and problems in the inter-family and social areas [1].

Growth abnormalities are frequently observed, these children very often present a delay in the growth curve with disharmony in somatic development. For example, the presence of chronic diseases (lung, kidney, liver diseases, etc.) changes the correct absorption and supply of nutrients essential for growth, with a significant negative impact on the child's somatic development; another example is the child with neurological affections (cerebral palsy, spastic-dystonic quadriplegia with high caloric consumption due to the great pathological neuromuscular commitment), often presenting signs of malnutrition; patients with spastic hemiparesis may have a reduced rate of growth of the paretic limb compared to the contralateral.

Sensory deficits include primary and/or secondary visual difficulties (central visual blindness, visual-perceptual disturbances), auditory deficits (cortical deafness, sensorineural and transmissive deafness), proprioceptive disorders deriving from the difficulty of analysing and integrating external stimulations; all these sensory deficits can also occur as a complication of the underlying pathology and often represent an obstacle to the success of the rehabilitation process.

Frailty patients often have a cognitive disability, deriving from primary neurological damage or, for example, in the case of a non-neurological patient, from prolonged hospitalization. Hospitalization in long-term care facilities leads to environmental deprivation, the child is exposed to the poverty of stimulations that delay cognitive development, this has also an impact on behavioural, social and family points of view. The delay in the acquisition of the stages of psychomotor development concerning all areas of competence of the child (cognitive, language, social, motor), early rehabilitation intervention aimed at supporting the stages of psychomotor development has as its main objective the functional recovery of emerging abilities.

The family environment in which the patient is placed cannot be neglected, parents often need

R. Toglia (✉) · E. Lovardi · E. Castelli
Dipartimento di Neuroriabilitazione Intensiva e Robotica, Ospedale Pediatrico Bambino Gesù, Rome, Italy
e-mail: rossana.toglia@opbg.net; eleonora.lovardi@opbg.net; enrico.castelli@opbg.net

M. Lima, M. C. Mondardini (eds.), *Frailty in Children*,
https://doi.org/10.1007/978-3-031-24307-3_14

support and assistance to reshape their parenting style to the child's fragility; support for the extended family (grandparents, relatives, siblings) is also useful so that all the figures around the child and the parental couple are supportive and must move in the same direction, to foster the growth of the fragile child in an environment that is as serene and favourable as possible.

The diagnosis of the child's frailty must be made early to allow the immediate start of the rehabilitation treatment and the achievement of the best outcome.

14.2 Rehabilitation Framework and Individual Rehabilitation Project

Rehabilitation is a complex process aimed at promoting the best possible participation and quality of life for the frailty child and the family. Through direct and indirect actions, it focuses on the individual in all his dimensions, physical, mental, emotional, communicative and relational (holistic approach), and it involves the whole family, social and environmental contexts (ecological approach).

It is achieved through the formulation of the rehabilitation plan and of the various treatment programmes for three areas: re-education, care and education. Re-education is the responsibility of health workers, and its aim is to promote the development and improvement of adaptive functions. It is a discontinuous process that is limited in time and must necessarily end when it is ascertained, concerning the most up-to-date knowledge of biological processes of recovery, that the patient has not, over a reasonable period, shown any significant changes in either the development or the use of adaptive functions; education is a responsibility that lies with the family, with health workers and with teachers and educators; care has as its objective the well-being of the child and his family, and is the responsibility of health personnel and social workers.

The aim is twofold: to prepare the child to play his role in society (i.e. to educate the disabled person) and to teach the community, beginning with schools, to welcome and integrate him (i.e. to educate about disabled people), to increase his resources and the effectiveness of the re-education treatment. Social integration is, throughout the rehabilitation process and at all ages, a priority objective that must not be subject to the prior achievement of certain therapeutic goals. It must be provided to the child and his family uninterruptedly from the moment they are informed that they have been diagnosed as disabled. The resources for the family must be calibrated according to the needs expressed and not the modifiability of the child's paralysis.

The rehabilitation plan and the various treatment programmes formulated must naturally include integrated interventions to be made, necessarily, in the three areas mentioned: re-education, education and care. We wish to emphasize, however, that it is not re-education (physiotherapy, speech therapy, etc.) that represents the element of continuity in the entire rehabilitation process, but rather care; this is particularly true in "severe" cases, in which, very often, re-education rapidly proves ineffective and there emerges a growing need for a care-based approach implemented through sometimes-complex interventions. This distinction is crucial as it justifies the difficulty in evaluating the work of health and social service technicians (effectiveness, efficiency and appropriateness).

A precise functional profile of the patient must be formulated at the beginning of the rehabilitation treatment. To this end, a classification of the consequences of diseases and traumas called "International Classification of Impairment, Disabilities and handicap" (ICIDH) is used, which joins the etiological reference model called International Classification of Disease, as established by the WHO in 1980.

The ICIDH defines three dimensions of the consequences of disease and trauma

1. Impairment: temporary or permanent anomaly, defect or loss of a limb, organ or body structure or a defect of a system of bodily function, for example, nerve functions; represents the externalization of a pathological

condition; the interventions aimed at it are medical and rehabilitative.
2. Disability: limitation or loss resulting from impairment of the ability to carry out an activity in the way considered normal for a human being, it can be temporary or permanent, reversible or irreversible, progressive or regressive. It represents the objectification of impairment and can be minimized through adaptive aids or therapeutic rehabilitation practices.
3. Handicap: situation of social disadvantage resulting from impairment or disability, which prevents the development of a role considered normal for an individual, depending on his age, sex, cultural and social factors; represents the socialization of an impairment or disability, reflecting the consequences they have for the individual.

In 2001, the second revision of the ICIDH was issued with an innovative title: International Classification of Functioning, Disability and Health (ICF) [2].

The innovation of this version is the positive description of residual abilities, which replaces the term disability with ability, handicap with participation. The process leading to handicap represents a malfunction for the individual and can occur at three levels:

1. Loss or abnormality of anatomical structures (impairments).
2. Limitation of activities.
3. Restriction of participation.

Seven dimensions in the health condition are defined in this new classification

1. Body functions: physiological or psychological functions of body systems
2. Body structures: anatomical parts of the body (organs, limbs)
3. Impairments: Problems in body functions and/or structures, defined as deviations or losses
4. Activity or ability to perform a task by an individual
5. Limitation of activity: difficulties that an individual may encounter in carrying out activities
6. Participation: involvement of individuals in life situations: it is related to health conditions, functions, body structures, activities and contextual factors
7. Restriction of participation: problems that an individual may have in life situations

In 2007, the WHO published the "International Classification of the Functioning of Disability and Health for Children and Adolescents" (ICF-CY), developed to supply the need for a version of the ICF that could be universally used for children and adolescents in sectors of health, education and social services. This new version identifies innovative factors such as modification and expansion of descriptions, modification of the inclusion and exclusion criteria and expansion of qualifiers to allow for the inclusion of aspects related to the development of the child. Therefore, new terms belonging to the world of the child are taken into account such as cognition, language, play, attitude and behaviour [3].

On the operational level, medical rehabilitation interventions (rehabilitation medicine) and social interventions (social rehabilitation) are distinguished. Medical rehabilitation operates in the fields of impairment and disability, while social rehabilitation in the field of handicap and participation; it is therefore essential to draw up a complete rehabilitation project that includes an integrated social and health path that develops all the residual potential of the individual in functional skills.

Rehabilitation represents a development process aimed to realize the physical, psychological, relational, social, professional, occupational, educational potential of the frailty patients, compatibly with the anatomical psychological impairments and environmental limitations.

The rehabilitation project is defined as individual as it sets realistic goals for the individual that must guide the various curative and assistance interventions.

For the most serious disabilities and therefore also in the case of highly frailty patients, the rehabilitation project must also involve the family and the living environment, for example, the school, to operate to achieve optimal function independent of the residual disability.

The complexity of the global rehabilitation approach means that many professionals turn around the patient, who work in a coordinated and integrated way. The rehabilitation team is made up of the patient, his family members and the professional team, a group of healthcare professionals with different professional skills who work to achieve common goals. In this way, the patient receives global management.

The decision-making process of the rehabilitating physician, the patient's clinical manager, in determining the Individual Rehabilitation Project (IRP) must take into account the functional prognosis and the modifiability margin of the disability framework, the degree of clinical stability of the patient and his possible participation in the programme. The doctor guarantees, with the involvement of the team's professionals, a constant flow of information to the patient, family, caregivers and family doctor.

Members of the rehabilitation team are

- Physiatrist—physician specialized in rehabilitation activities, responsible for the rehabilitation project and whose task is the evaluation, diagnosis, prognosis and treatment of the consequences of diseases and traumas.
- Child neuropsychiatrist—doctor who deals with the diagnosis and medical management of developmental delays.
- Paediatrician—doctor who manages any acute and systemic diseases and baby feeding problems.
- Physiotherapist—who assists the patient in the functional recovery process and takes care of impairments and motor disabilities, according to the indications of the physiatrist.
- Nurse—deals with medical treatments during hospitalization in health or social-health structures and the patient's care needs.
- Speech therapist—supports the patient with linguistic and communication problems, memory, thinking and swallowing.
- Psychologist—who provides support and education to help the patient and the family.
- Psychomotor therapist—specific for the developmental age.
- Occupational therapist—supports the individual to recover autonomy in the activities of daily life;
- Orthopaedic technician—responsible for the evaluation, design and manufacture of prostheses and orthoses.
- Social worker.
- Professional educator.

The professional responsible for the individual area of intervention has the task of drawing up the individual rehabilitation programme, in which the short-, medium- and long-term objectives are defined based on the specific disabilities and residual abilities of the patient; the times for achieving the objectives, the types of rehabilitation intervention and the measures to be used to verify compliance are defined.

There must be periodic checks and reassessments of the programme, and updates of the individual rehabilitation project, based on the changes of the patient and their specific needs during the medical follow-up.

14.3 Medical and Surgical Interventions

As mentioned in the introductory part, many medical problems can fall within the description of a fragile child, the area of interest of physiatry, a branch of specialist medicine in neurorehabilitation. These children have high clinical frailty due to neurological disorders and/or all conditions that alter their physiological development, with particular regard to motor functions.

Therapeutic interventions after brain damage aim, in the acute phase, to reduce the injury and increase the survival of the damaged brain tissue. Subsequent interventions are aimed at recovering motor functions by taking advantage of neuronal plasticity. The earlier, more intensive and more targeted the therapeutic/rehabilitative intervention, the greater the chances of recovery.

One of the main consequences of brain and spinal cord injuries in the paediatric patient is the alteration of muscle function, in particular spasticity, dystonia and hypotonia.

- **Spasticity** is a clinical phenomenon in which muscles overreact to rapid stretch. Spasticity determines, together with the dyskinetic component, involuntary movements and postures that affect motor control, cause pain and, over time, lead to the onset of antalgic postures and osteoarticular retractions. To treat correctly the spasticity, a correct medical examination is primarily necessary.

The signs useful for diagnosis observable during the visit are

- Increase of reflexes that the doctor evokes by hitting the knee with the hammer, for example.
- Clonus (fast and repeated muscle contractions).
- Babinski's sign. Normally, when rubbing the lateral edge of the sole of the foot, the toes bend (Babinski negative). If there is a neurological problem, by rubbing the sole the big toe extends upwards and the other toes fan out (Babinski positive). However, it should be remembered that the Babinski sign is of little significance in children under the age of 1 or 2 years, due to the immaturity of the corticospinal pathways that control the stretch reflex.

Muscle spasticity is controlled with the use of muscle relaxant drugs, taken by mouth or locally infiltrated, according to the severity of the spasticity and depending on the muscle groups most involved.

General pharmacological treatments, to be administered several times a day, are indicated in situations where it is necessary to obtain a relaxation of all the muscles of the body but, at higher doses, side effects may occur. The most used are baclofen, diazepam, trihexyphenidyl hydrochloride and tizanidine.

Local or focal drug treatments are useful when spasticity particularly affects certain muscle groups. Among the drugs used, botulinum toxin has assumed an important role in the treatment of spasticity because it gives the children the opportunity to modify their motor control, expanding the "therapeutic window" of the rehabilitation process.

The treatment of spasticity can also be performed by surgery, with the implantation of a pump for the intrathecal infusion of baclofen or with the intervention of Selective Dorsal Rhizotomy (SDR).

Intrathecal baclofen infusion consists of the surgical implantation, in the abdomen, of a pump that infuses continuously, through a catheter, baclofen directly into the cerebrospinal fluid, the fluid that surrounds and protects the brain and spinal cord. Baclofen is a drug that relaxes muscles by counteracting the release of excitatory stimuli from the central nervous system.

The SDR surgery consists of cutting a portion of the dorsal (posterior) roots of the nerves of the spinal cord. The excitatory stimuli passing through the spinal cord are thus reduced. This surgery reduces hypertonicity and spasticity of the lower limb muscles more than any other therapy or intervention. Patients eligible for SDR are generally selected in a clinic dedicated to the assessment of spasticity through standardized international functional assessment scales and quality-of-life rating scales. The post-surgical course is characterized by 3 days of bed rest in the supine position; on the third day, the patient is assisted in assuming the semi-sitting position. For neuropathic pain, gabapentin and paracetamol are given for 3 weeks; urinary retention may occur in the first weeks and spontaneously regresses. To facilitate the stretching of the muscles of the lower limbs, knee pads are used in extension and leg–foot braces at 90°. On the fifth day, the loading exercises begin based on the patient's tolerance, the first week of rehabilitation is totally focused on the passive and active lengthening of the muscles of the lower limbs, followed by muscle strengthening exercises and selective recruitment until the progressive recovery of the load.

14.3.1 Movement Disorders

The child with high clinical neurological frailty, especially in the posture-motor forms of spastic-dystonic quadriplegia, presents a clinical picture considerably complicated by the presence of *dystonia*. The causes can be numerous. We distinguish forms due to mutation of specific genes, forms in which the cause is not known and forms, more frequent, due to "external" factors such as perinatal asphyxia, drugs, infections and tumours.

Dystonia is defined as a movement disorder characterized by sustained or intermittent muscle contractions or co-contractions (that is, simultaneous activation of muscle groups across one or more joints) causing abnormal and repetitive movements and/or postures.

Dystonia can be classified according to the aetiology, the distribution of symptoms and the age of onset.

They are distinguished by

- The primary forms (on a genetic or idiopathic basis).
- The secondary forms ranging from perinatal suffering to progressive encephalopathies, up to dystonia induced by neuroleptic drugs.

In dystonia we can identify

- Focal forms (the scribe's cramp is an example).
- Segmental forms, where the disorder is limited to a single body segment.
- Generalized forms, frequent in early childhood cases, characterized by involvement of the cervical area, trunk, limbs and the area of the mouth and jaw.

The treatment of dystonia involves an early therapeutic approach that allows avoiding the establishment of musculoskeletal alterations, to promote psychic and behavioural development and adequate school and social integration. Medical therapy includes several drugs, often administered in combination, including anticholinergics, dopamine agonists, but also dopamine antagonists and benzodiazepines. Satisfactory results have been achieved, especially for focal forms or those with prevalent involvement of a body segment, by administering botulinum toxin. The efficacy of medical therapy is generally partial and, in relation to the high doses of the drug required, the appearance of unwanted side effects is frequent.

In drug-resistant cases, it is now possible to consider a series of surgical options that include peripheral denervation (useful in focal forms), intrathecal baclofen infusion and surgical procedures on the basal nuclei. In particular, a neurosurgical procedure defined as pallidotomy, which consists of the ablation of both internal pale globes (GPi), is performed with benefit. More recently, the technique of deep brain stimulation (DBS) has become widespread in the field of movement disorders, a reversible procedure that allows adjusting the stimulation parameters to the patient's clinical needs.

Dystonia and spasticity have distinct pathophysiological features that require different management strategies as they can lead to skeletal deformities, contractures or spasms, changes in passive components of muscle or muscle activity elicited by sensory triggers.

The use of orthoses is fundamental, a device applied directly to the patient's body and used in order to modify the structural or functional characteristics of the neuro-musculoskeletal system. The orthoses, like the aids we will discuss later, are developed by the professional figure of the orthopaedic technician who must collaborate closely with the physician (physiatrist, neurologist or orthopaedist, as appropriate) who is responsible for the medical prescription.

If tendon retraction or skeletal deformity does not respond to the various treatments listed above or causes significant pain, functional orthopaedic surgery is chosen, which acts on the tendon and myoarticular structures with the aim of improving their conformation and functionality. This approach emphasizes the importance of a multidisciplinary team that revolves around the fragile child.

Among the orthopaedic interventions most performed among children suffering from spasticity is the tenotomy, in which one or more tendons of the retracted spastic muscles are sectioned and/or stretched. These interventions, in the most severe forms of disability, allow better management of the patient from a postural point of view and for assistance. More frequently, we intervene on adductors muscles, hamstring muscles (flex the knee), ileo-psoas muscles (hip flexor) and Achilles tendon (muscle that allows you to extend the ankle).

The intervention on skeletal deformities of the spine is also fundamental, as they affect respiratory mechanics and/or gastroenterological functionality, as well as structure dysfunctional analgesic positions for the child, especially in the case of serious secondary alterations on respiratory mechanics. In neurological patients, not adequately postured over the years or with severe spasticity, another possible complication is the mono or bilateral subluxation of the hip; also in this case, there is the onset of pain (with subsequent worsening of the spastic symptoms and/or dystonic due to the constant presence of the trigger) or important functional deficits affecting walking; the subluxations must therefore be treated with corrective interventions on the skeletal system.

After surgery, there are three recovery phases:

1. The phase of bone and/or soft tissue healing. It lasts about 6 weeks and is characterized by the implementation of particular precautions and/or by the application of means of immobilization, which can be cast or orthotic appliances; depending on the tissues undergoing surgery, the type of orthosis needed will change; it will also be necessary to establish together with the surgeon the degree of intensity of the mobilization and the maximum possible joint excursion.
2. The stage of muscular recovery. It lasts about 12 weeks. It concerns the muscle area directly affected by the surgery, and the surrounding areas. In this phase, the rehabilitator's activity begins: the programme will vary according to the patient's pre-existing conditions and the intervention immediately; the rehabilitator will have to collaborate with the surgeon to decide the times and methods of recovery and the new objectives will be defined from time to time; essential in the case of operations on the lower limbs, define the times and methods of recovery of the load.
3. The phase of functional recovery correlated with the patient's skills. Functional improvements can occur up to 12 months after surgery.

14.4 Role of AIDS and Orthoses

Orthoses are defined as devices applied directly to the patient's body and used in order to modify the structural or functional characteristics of the neuro-musculoskeletal system. Orthoses are essential to keep a bone segment in a precise position or, in case of walking disturbance, to compensate for muscle activation deficits, both from cause primary cortical and secondary from prolonged immobilization, or contrast conditions of muscle hyperactivity. Finally, they are useful in case of prolonged bed rest to prevent tendon retractions.

Orthoses are classified into

- Static orthoses, which maintain correct joint alignment avoiding retractions of muscles or tendons and skeletal deformities or support the load of the body in an upright position; they can also be useful in the case of surgical interventions in which it is necessary in the first postoperative period to maintain certain positions or in the case of interventions on the tendon system to favour the recovery of a correct length.
- Dynamic orthoses, which compensate for impaired function or provide forces that replace muscle contraction.

The most used orthoses in neurological rehabilitation are

- Upper limb orthosis, for example, to the forearm–hand district. These are static orthoses, day or night, which aim to reduce the development of deformities, maintaining correct alignment of the joints and favouring the elongation of the muscle-tendon structures; they can also be functional, stabilizing the carpus and thus allowing the action of the flexor muscles of the fingers.
- Trunk orthosis: there are corsets of different typologies made with various materials; they are used to contain spinal deformities, to promote trunk control and correct scoliosis.
- Lower limb orthoses, which are mainly used
  - To prevent muscular-tendon retractions and skeletal deformities.

  - To promote the stability of the limb when it is under load.
  - To allow walking; in this case, the orthosis will be tailored to the functional alteration to be corrected.

The main lower limb orthoses are the following:

- Insoles or Foot Orthosis that exert a corrective or compensatory action in case of altered support of the foot.
- Ankle Foot Orthosis (AFO): these are orthoses applied to the leg–foot segment. They are used in cases of hyperactivity of the triceps surae muscle to contrast the equinus foot (the tip of the foot falls down while the heel remains raised), or when the lower limb is unable to support the load of the body.
- Knee Ankle Foot Orthosis (KAFO): an orthosis that runs from the root of the thigh to the heel. The static variant is used, for example, after surgical elongation of tendons when it is necessary to maintain the knee in extension for most of the day. The dynamic variant, jointed at the knee, is used when there is a weakness of the quadriceps muscle, or when it is necessary to maintain the correct alignment of the knee joint during walking.
- Hip Knee Ankle Foot Orthosis, HKAFO: it consists of two KAFOs joined to each other and fixed to the pelvis; in some cases, it can reach a large part of the trunk. They are used in cases of spinal or neuromuscular diseases to allow standing and walking.

Another fundamental aid for supporting frailty children is the use of appropriate facilities; it is defined in this way of any product, tool, equipment or technological system that can be used by a disabled person to prevent, compensate, alleviate or eliminate an impairment or disability.

Often the frailty child has a delay in the acquisition of head and trunk control: therefore commercial high chairs cannot be used, but postural seats are necessary: these are chairs equipped with a seat that allows correct containment of the pelvis and alignment of the lower limbs, with straps to give greater stability; rigid back that can be equipped with lateral supports for a correct alignment of the trunk; headrests in case of lack of control of the head; in the same way, commercial strollers cannot be used, but postural strollers are more appropriate; these are strollers equipped with the same support systems of the postural seat.

Frailty child may also present a delay in the acquisition of an upright position and, in some cases, this can never be achieved; to allow the child to experience the standing position with its known benefits on breathing, intestinal transit and bone growth, stabilizing aids are produced, where the child is passively positioned in an upright position and is supported at the level of the lower limbs, pelvis, trunk and possibly head.

The child can acquire walking, but support may be required. We have walkers, systems equipped with wheels, more or less simple, depending on the characteristics of the patient: from the type open on the front without any support to walkers with pelvic and thoracic support in case of poor trunk and pelvis control; other walking aids are tripods and quadripods, sticks with three or four feet, which allow greater stability by increasing the support base, compared to the one-footed cane.

Often a child with frailty, even if they have reached walking, may present difficulties in moving for long distances, both for structural deficits and easy fatigue: therefore, adequate aids are necessary, such as wheelchairs, which also in this case can present different characteristics depending on the patient clinic features; they can allow to push yourself or be pushed by the caregiver, they can be more or less light, they can be foldable to facilitate transport; they can be equipped with a postural system in case of significant axial hypotonia with containment systems similar to those of postural high chairs; finally, they can be electric, to allow greater autonomy to a patient with difficulty in using the upper limbs. There are also removable devices on the market, which can transform a manual wheelchair into an electric one.

14.5 Management of Dysphagia and Sialorrhea

Fragile children with central nervous system diseases may have a delay or impairment in the development of motor control, which, in some cases, also causes dysphagia. In particular, this is frequent in children with quadriplegia, genetic syndromes or oral–facial malformations. Often they have partial or incomplete swallowing capacity, not only of the food material but also of the salivary secretion.

Dysphagia is a very common disorder among children with clinical frailty; it is a pervasive disorder because, in most cases, it affects all phases of the deglutition process: chewing, lingual movements, the deglutition reflex, which can be delayed or weak, the closing of the glottis (partial or none), the persistence of residues in the oro-pharyngeal canal. It is also present in subjects with cognitive disabilities as there is an alteration of behavioural acts (foraging for food, food selectivity, inappetence, refusal of food), of preliminary sensory and motor information for swallowing (visual and olfactory recognition of food), of organization, chewing and propulsion of the bolus [4].

Frequently there is a massive presence of salivary secretions, poorly managed by the patient due to swallowing difficulties, defined as sialorrhea. One of the most important complications of drooling is the inhalation of saliva into the respiratory, bronchial and pulmonary tracts, which causes recurrent chemical pneumonia. Chemical pneumonia occurs when inhaled material, in this case saliva, has a direct toxic effect on the lungs. In the neurological patient, in whom the general and respiratory clinical conditions are already considerably compromised, sialorrhea causes continuous episodes of inhalation pneumonia which can significantly aggravate the already precarious clinical conditions.

Sialorrhea is also an important social and management problem for those who care for the patient and, in the child, for the parents. It can be a source of embarrassment, as well as create significant relationship and language problems. It is therefore a form of severe discomfort that considerably limits the social life of the patient and the family [5].

The specific treatment for chronic sialorrhea is divided into two different therapeutic options: medical and surgical. Medical treatment is conservative and is based on the use of medical aids, such as the use of transdermal scopolamine, glycopyrrolate, trihexyphenidyl hydrochloride and/or inoculation of botulinum toxin type A in the salivary glands [6, 7].

Surgery is a secondary therapeutic option that is used when sialorrhea, in addition to representing a social and interpersonal disorder, involves serious respiratory risks for the patient due to continuous salivary inhalations and when pharmacological treatment does not provide adequate and time-maintained clinical results. The surgery consists of the isolation and subsequent ligation of the salivary ducts [8].

The management of dysphagia is extremely important as the major complication of oral incoordination is bronchial aspiration which involves respiratory complications and puts the patient's life at risk (pneumonia ab ingestis, airway obstruction, need for oro-tracheal intubation and subsequent tracheostomy) [9–11].

The anatomical-functional differentiation of dysphagia is essential to define the diagnostic-therapeutic approach in order to intervene effectively with speech therapy rehabilitation techniques, improve the patient's quality of life, and minimize the complications (suffocation, aspiration pneumonia and malnutrition).

The radiological methods used for the diagnosis of a swallowing disorder or a silent aspiration are the Video Fluoroscopic Swallow Study (VFS) or the Fibreoptic Endoscopic Evaluation of Swallowing (FEES). VFS is a method that involves the use of X-rays and shows the physiology of all the structures involved in swallowing; allows to highlight the inability or delay in starting pharyngeal swallowing, aspiration of ingests, nasopharyngeal or gastroesophageal reflux, residual bolus in the pharyngeal cavity after swallowing. The FESS investigates laryngeal penetration, aspiration and the presence of residues inside the pharyngeal cavity after swallowing. It also allows you to observe the movements of the bolus in the hypopharynx and calibrate the success of the protection manoeuvres [12].

Based on the results of the instrumental tests, a multidisciplinary intervention plan is developed, which involves various professional figures, as well as the active education of the patient, family members and/or caregivers:

- Dietary approach: it is essential to intervene in the characteristics of food such as consistency, cohesion, homogeneity, viscosity and temperature. Nutrition must not only respond to strictly rehabilitative needs but must also satisfy the correct caloric and water intake, therefore collaboration with the dietician/nutritionist is essential.
- Assumption of a correct posture: the correct alignment of the head and trunk while taking meals is essential; it has been shown that this causes a temporary change in the size of the pharynx and the flow of the bolus, resulting in an improvement in the oropharyngeal transit time, a reduction in the risk of aspiration and a decrease in post-swallowing residues. It is therefore essential that the physiatrist prescribe a postural system suitable for the patient.
- Artificial feeding techniques: they must be used if it is impossible to feed orally the child due to severe dysphagia, or oral feeding alone does not satisfy a correct caloric intake; among the artificial feeding techniques, we start using the gastric-nose tube for patients who are unable to feed themselves orally or in whom there is a high risk of aspiration and worsening of dysphagia; this device is generally poorly tolerated by the patient as it causes hypersalivation, frequent dislocations, ulceration of the airways and pain; in case of persistent dysphagia beyond 4 weeks and/or severe calorie-protein malnutrition, the most used and best method to guarantee a correct nutritional intake is Percutaneous Endoscopic Gastrostomy (PEG). PEG also reduces the risk of aspiration. It is useful to consider a Percutaneous Endoscopic Jejunostomy (PEJ) in case of severe gastroesophageal reflux and high gastric stagnation to further reduce the risk of inhalation. Through the PEG, it is possible to administer food more easily without necessarily having to resort to hospital preparations; moreover, the administration of drugs is made easier and more absorbable [13, 14].
- Specific speech therapy for dysphagia makes use of the following methods [15, 16]:
  - Use of foods treated with thickeners
  - Mechanical and sensorial oral stimulations
  - Reduction of drooling with drugs such as scopolamine, glycopyrrolate, trihexyphenidyl hydrochloride and, in severe cases, surgery such as ligation of the salivary ducts or injection of botulinum toxin in salivary ducts
  - Oral electrostimulation to improve chewing kinetics in combination with oral sensorial stimulations
  - Functional chewing therapy (FuCT): a technique that improves chewing ability and reduces lingual thrust and, indirectly, also drooling

14.6 Motor Rehabilitation, Speech and Neuropsychological Aspects

It is fundamental that the rehabilitation intervention focused on the fragile child is as early as possible and oriented towards functional motor recovery based on active motor learning strategies. Active motor intervention, unlike the conventional one based on passive movement techniques, improves the type and harmony of movement starting from a cognitive approach, stimulating what we can define as motor intentionality [17].

The traditional techniques of passive movement do not produce an improvement in motor skills like an active motor learning, which takes advantage of the mechanisms of cerebral plasticity. The latter allow the reorganization of damaged neural networks which, from a clinical point of view, translate into a targeted motor activity. Through active motor learning, the child acquires new motor patterns and this, if carried out consistently and through an intensive rehabilitation intervention, allows brain reorganization towards non-pathological movement and behaviour patterns.

At present, the most effective rehabilitation interventions are those that have the following characteristics:

- Carrying out tasks and activities typical of daily life that allow an easier internalization; the child focuses on a purpose and finalizes his movement to it, this acts as an immediate concrete reinforcement to the rehabilitation exercise, increases the patient's self-esteem and its active reproduction in daily life.
- The intensity of training and the repeated request of the functions are key elements to achieve the best rehabilitation efficacy.

Their common mechanism of action aims to modulate plasticity starting from experience. Motivation and attention are vital modulators of neuroplasticity and if a specific training is rewarding and enjoyable for children, then they are stimulating to produce spontaneous movements outside the therapeutic setting too.

For an in-depth study on the most effective rehabilitation strategies for fragile children and the clinical practice guideline, we recommend reading the article by Jackman et al. [18].

Among the rehabilitation interventions with the greatest scientific evidence of effectiveness we have

- Bimanual training and Constraint Induced Motor Therapy (CIMT): specific to recover the function of upper limbs in hemiplegia and in bimanual integration deficits.
- Mobility training, treadmill training: specific for mobility and for the acquisition of correct gait patterns using treadmills or robotic exoskeletons linked to virtual reality.
- Robotic systems: devices developed in recent decades, used to enhance residual capacity and develop upper arm mobility, standing, balance and locomotion; these devices facilitate cortical reorganization through intensive, controlled, repetitive, task-oriented training and motor learning.
- Action observation training: exploits a neurophysiological mechanism based on the correspondence between observed and performed actions.
- Occupational therapy: in which strategies are sought to increase the patient's autonomy in daily life, having as a starting point the strengthening of his residual abilities.
- Dysphagia training: specifically to overcome the chewing difficulties of children and to promote autonomy in nutrition.

The environment in which the child lives, and the one where he carries out the rehabilitation treatments, must be full of stimuli. It is vital to adapt the environment in which the patient is inserted, in order to enhance his residual skills as much as possible and allow the execution of the activity through therapy focused on the context.

The motor deficit negatively impacts the cognitive development of the fragile child, delaying the acquisition of the normal stages of psychic development and the ability to experience reality, even in the absence of specific cognitive deficits. It has been shown that early motor rehabilitation intervention, based on learning ability, may be able to improve the child's cognitive abilities and sustain them over time. Similarly, early cognitive and psychomotor rehabilitation may be able to support and enhance the children's residual abilities, promote their language development, functional and social skills.

Therefore, it is necessary that all children with frailty, in the course of their development, receive a complete neuropsychological assessment, including an evaluation of cognitive level, executive functions and academic skills, in order to give useful suggestions for the school care through an individualized educational plan, shared with parents and rehabilitation figures and tailored to the child. It is also useful to monitor aspects relating to the self-esteem of fragile children over time because they have more difficulty than their peers. It is beneficial, to develop a correct image of oneself related to one's disability, and to support the fragile child by a psychological rehabilitation intervention, capable of strengthening and supporting self-esteem over time, especially in the adolescent period and in the transition phase towards adulthood.

There are numerous rehabilitation interventions focused on the development of the cognitive abilities of the fragile patient. It is important to consider early schooling (insertion in the nursery, support of social integration and interactions in a group of peers) and carry out rehabilitation as early as possible through an intensive and holistic intervention. Communication is a priority goal, linguistic understanding, meta-phonological aspects of discourse, communicative exchange using, if necessary, appropriate alternative augmentative communication devices to support language even in non-verbal form.

In support of psychomotor treatment, the GAME method can be considered: it is described in the article of Morgan et al. [19]. It is a combination of motor training, environmental enrichment and family educational therapy.

It is also useful to consider the Cognitive Orientation-Occupational Performance methodology (CO-OP; Novak and Honan [20]): initially designed for the population with coordination disorders and dyspraxia, to date, there is also evidence of efficacy in the population with CP. Patients set personalized goals and experience them in their daily life, through personalized Problem-Solving strategies.

The global care of a child with frailty must include family support too, essential both to optimize the development of the child and to reduce the risk of psychological stress in parents.

Among the various psychological support options for parents, the following should be noted:

- Triple P stepping stone: focused on improving parenting skills, setting realistic goals with the therapist based on the emerging needs of the moment, gradually achieving goals and then setting others
- Acceptance and Commitment Therapy (ACT): focuses on increasing parental flexibility and improving a parent's ability to change according to the changing needs of the child

It is established that an early and therapeutic rehabilitation intervention also on the parental figures allows the child to have more chances of obtaining the best outcomes.

In conclusion, the child with frailty needs a rehabilitation intervention as early as possible, in order not to lose functional residual abilities and to support the child during development. The rehabilitative approach must be multidisciplinary, paying attention to the global care of fragile children and their families. Periodic follow-ups must be regularly performed, in order to update the personalised rehabilitative project. It is equally important the construction of a social and health care network, involving the rehabilitation team, the school and the family, to guarantee the best possible quality of life.

References

1. Dent E, Morley JE, Cruz-Jentoft AJ. Physical frailty: ICFSR international clinical practice guidelines for identification and management. J Nutr Health Aging. 2019;23(9):771–87.
2. World Health Organization. International classification of functioning, disability and health: ICF. Geneva: World Health Organization; 2001.
3. Raghavendra P, Bornman J, Granlund M, Björck-Akesson E. The World Health Organization's international classification of functioning, disability and health: implications for clinical and research practice in the field of augmentative and alternative communication. Augment Altern Commun. 2007;23:349–61.
4. Logemann JA. Evaluation and treatment of swallowing disorders. 2nd ed. Austin: Pro-Ed Inc.; 1998. p. 1–22.
5. McGeachan AJ, Mcdermott CJ. Management of oral secretions in neurological disease. Pract Neurol. 2017;17(2):96–03.
6. Barbero P, Busso M, Tinivella M, Artusi CA, De Mercanti S, Cucci A, Veltri A, Avagnina P, Calvo A, Chio' A, Durelli L, Clerico M. Long-term follow-up of ultrasound-guided botulinum toxin-A injections for sialorrhea in neurological dysphagia. J Neurol. 2015;262(12):2662–7.
7. Thomas-Stonell N, Greenberg J. Three treatment approaches and clinical factors in the reduction of drooling. Dysphagia. 1988;3(2):73–8.
8. Blasco PA. Surgical management of drooling. Dev Med Child Neurol. 1992;34:368–9.
9. Marik PE, Kaplan D. Aspiration pneumonia and dysphagia in the elderly. Chest. 2003;124:328–36.
10. Martino R, Foley N, Bhogal S, Diamant N, Speechley M, Teasell R. Dysphagia after stroke incidence,

diagnosis, and pulmonary complications. Stroke. 2005;36:2756–63.
11. Ramsey DJ, Smithard DG, Kalra L. Early assessments of dysphagia and aspiration risk in acute stroke patients. Stroke. 2003;34(5):1252–7.
12. Dziewas R, Warnecke T, Ölenberg S, Teismann I, Zimmermann J, Krämer C, Ritter M, Ringelstein EB, Schäbitz WR. Towards a basic endoscopic assessment of swallowing in acute stroke-development and evaluation of a simple dysphagia score. Cerebrovasc Dis. 2008;26:41–7.
13. Dennis M, Lewis S, Cranswick G, Forbes J, FOOD Trial Collaboration. FOOD: a multicentre randomised trial evaluating feeding policies in patients admitted to hospital with a recent stroke. Health Technol Assess. 2006;10(2):3–4.
14. Finestone HM, Greene-Finestone LS. Rehabilitation medicine: 2. Diagnosis of dysphagia and its nutritional management for stroke patients. CMAJ. 2003;169(10):1041–4.
15. Burkhead LM, Sapienza CM, Rosenbek JC. Strength-training exercise in dysphagia rehabilitation: principles, procedures, and directions for future research. Dysphagia. 2007;22:251–65.
16. Kramer P, Shein D, Napolitano J. Chap. 13: Rehabilitation of speech, language and swallowing disorders. In: Acquired brain injury. New York: Springer; 2007. p. 238–58.
17. Novak I, Morgan C, Fahey M, Finch-Edmondson M, Galea C, Hines A, Langdon K, McNamara M, Paton MC, Popat H, Shore B, Khamis A, Stanton E, Finemore OP, Tricks A, Velde AT, Dark L, Morton N, Badawi N. State of the evidence traffic lights 2019: systematic review of interventions for preventing and treating children with cerebral palsy. Curr Neurol Neurosci Rep. 2020;20(2):3.
18. Jackman M, Sakzewski L, Morgan C, Boyd R, Brennan SE, Langdon K, Toovey RAM, Greaves S, Thorley M, Novak I. Interventions to improve physical function for children and young people with cerebral palsy: international clinical practice guideline. Dev Med Child Neurol. 2021;64(5):536–49. https://doi.org/10.1111/dmcn.15055.
19. Morgana C, Novak I, Daleb RC, Guzzetta A, Badawi N. Single blind randomised controlled trial of GAME (Goals-Activity-Motor Enrichment) in infants at high risk of cerebral palsy. Res Dev Disabil. 2016;55:256–67.
20. Novak I, Honan I. Effectiveness of paediatric occupational therapy for children with disabilities: a systematic review. Aust Occup Ther J. 2019;66(3):258–73.

Operational Improvement in Psychology

15

Giovanna Perricone

15.1 Introduction

The promotion of mental health in the child and adolescent (C/A), as an indication of developmental well-being [1] is a priority for all healthcare professions and others, and all fields and disciplines of the healthcare sector involved in the treatment of any given pathology, syndrome, disorder and, in particular, during the preparatory, operative and post-surgical recovery stages of surgery.

Mental health can be substantially affected by the fragility of the child/adolescent [2]. Fragility, (defined, according to the leading literature in the field of psychology, as the unusual sensitivity of the individual towards stress) leads to limitations in the management of daily life. It fosters a deterioration in the psycho-physical health of the patient, and, more importantly, in the correct functioning of life skills [3]. It is a mental state which can produce negative outcomes in terms of confusion, lack of stability, overlapping, etc.; a dissociation of Internal Working Models [4, 5] with which the child/adolescent has built relationships with the outside world and, therefore, with the surgical procedure. It describes a dissociation which, in some cases, can lead to the development of "disorganized attachment" [6, 7].

The paediatric perioperative period is undoubtedly considered to be a healthcare situation in which fragility is elemental in hindering successful support, listening and accompaniment aiming to moderate stress that this very perioperative period can create, especially in such a complex moment in this stage of life. It is a developmental stage which would seem to characterize psychic functioning, particularly active from birth to puberty and with specific emotional and cognitive changes during adolescence.

Perioperative period seems to compromise psychic functions which constitute the child's/adolescent's 'inner world' [8] and which are usually decisive for the typical development. In this sense, we refer to motivations, attachment, curiosity, the desire for relationships and communication and the construction of an effective mental model which allows the C/A to attribute mental states to the adult [9–11]. This is how the child/adolescent develops a "secure attachment" to the caregiver concerned in this developmental stage.

In this developmental condition during the perioperative period, these psychic functions in the C/A are put at risk, leading to "disorganized attachment". This is the type of attachment which becomes a predictor of psychological disorders and pathological dissociation as an adult [12, 13]. The

G. Perricone (✉)
Società Italiana di Psicologia Pediatrica (SIPPed), Department of Psychology, Educational Science and Human Movement, University of Palermo, Palermo, Italy

Guarantor Authority for The Laws of Childhood and Adolescence, Palermo, Italy
e-mail: giovanna.perricone@unipa.it

M. Lima, M. C. Mondardini (eds.), *Frailty in Children*,
https://doi.org/10.1007/978-3-031-24307-3_15

experience of the perioperative period, in fact, can lead to mentalization of experiences by the C/A which are not always coherent with the needs and emotional tendencies typical of the developmental stage in that moment. These experiences are disorganized and unstable, eliciting "disorganized attachment". These are mentalizations which also characterize dissociative disorders [14, 15]. This form of attachment can begin to manifest in the perioperative period, through internalized and externalized symptoms which evolve into developmental trauma [16].

These alterations and disorders affecting the developmental trajectory during the perioperative period are the object of study and intervention by paediatric psychology, a field of study which also specifically focuses on supporting the C/A in conditions of risk during the developmental process [17, 18]; conditions which appear to be determined or, however, present during the perioperative period [19].

Scientific literature on this subject ([17, 20–24], op. cit.) has provided a specific multisystemic model for psychological treatment, in consideration of paediatric assessment ([18, 25], op. cit.) of the child's condition. Specific attention is given to fragility, as a variable in functioning, this latter defined as lying between cognition and emotion, and between the biological and cultural, from an epigenetic perspective [26, 27]. We refer here to treatment based on strengthening ([22, 28, 29], op. cit.), which allows the child/adolescent to cope with a stressful event (surgical procedure) through emotional and cognitive coping skills, such as creative adaptation to the perioperative period [30] and the development of self-protection mechanisms, or further still, the strengthening a sense of agency [31, 32].

Paediatric psychology views this treatment as a multi-systemic "field", involving the caregiving system together with that of the family, school, rehabilitation, etc.

15.2 Fragility Between Nature and Nurture

When determining a condition of fragility in the C/A in situations of biological and psychological difficulty, healthcare professionals (surgeons, paediatricians, psychologists, child and adolescent neuropsychiatrists) do not always take into consideration the full complexity of this fragility. This simplified approach hinders the identification of those aspects (emotions, representations, etc.) which lead to distortions in perception, to problems with self-regulation and to perpetually active arousal processes, and which deter adaptive and adaptational functioning of the child during the perioperative period. These are the aspects which all those involved should take into consideration for more successful outcomes regarding clinical or surgical procedures.

In order to successfully provide support to the C/A in the perioperative period, it is fundamental to be aware that fragility (which characterizes the psychological functioning of the patient before, during and after the surgical procedure) constitutes a dysfunctional state of the various dimensions of development and relative developmental 'domains' (cognitive, emotional, social, perceptual, etc.) ([18], op. cit.). These domains are considered as organization systems which contain both representations and specializations of knowledge and experience (which help adapt instrumental skills to mental functioning), and facilitate the development of skills, itineraries, strategies, etc. [33, 34]. The latter ensure instrumental skills are operative and are considered functional to the relationship which each C/A builds with the self and with the surrounding reality (established through spacetime and people) during the perioperative period.

Each domain, therefore, is a complex plurality of conceptual categories (i.e. certain emotions: fear, sense of guilt; certain perceptions: sense of danger, etc.) and their relative significance (i.e. the type of script) (Macchi Cassia et al. op. cit.) concerning the degree of preparation for the surgical event. Thus, the script constitutes a model with which the child/adolescent represents the surgical situation and the roles of the people involved, well before the single events occur.

We refer here to meanings that the different categories assume in the development of the single domain. Each of these categories (cognitive, emotive, etc.) refers to individual specializations (associations, comparisons, principal connections of each domain) which are contextualized in the functioning of the mind (for example, choosing to adopt social roles on the ward; i.e. during rounds, the child externalizes the fear of being operated on, on behalf of all children on the ward, or the C/A adopts certain *routines* during treatment).

It is functioning represented within the complexity of thought and the function of orientation which thought itself adopts when guiding actions and when identifying behaviours, fixed within the complex workings of the C/A's mind. The contribution provided by these categories (together with their functions in terms of personal development) and the production which they activate in terms of products related to the specific domain (social, cognitive … domains), characterize the condition of fragility both in biological, psychological and social terms, thereby attributing the characteristic of *nature and nurture* to fragility.

This characteristic ensures that the different 'domains' foster specific forms of understanding and classification of the reality constituted by hospitalization, therapies and treatments linked to the surgical procedure, together with the factual and virtual reality which forms the individual nature of the fragility. Domains guide both the choice of means through which the fragile subject operates and relates to the event, and the search for solutions to and the management of problems posed by the surgery. Therefore, to talk of fragility in the perioperative period, when considering single domains, means to refer to the importance and relevance of schemas, representations, categories and classifications of the surgical procedure and its variables, but also to take into consideration conscious choice, or not, in relation to services, regulations which need to be observed, conduct, and behaviours attributable to the specific nature of all the child/adolescent's developmental aspects [35].

They are all elements which form a type of conceptual and emotional 'filter' (dysfunctional or functional), through which relationships between the C/A and the surgical procedure are defined. It is important to remember, however, that the cognitive element is always a fundamental factor in this 'filter', that is, in the interconnections between the different developmental aspects.

This approach 'filter' proves to be the origin of "cellular memory" transformation, through which a specific mentalization/interiorization of the surgical procedure (deposited, integrated in the complete archive of all experiences surrounding this event) is integrated with the child's mentalizations of the here and now during the perioperative period [36, 37].

Every cell provides not only inherited information (fear of the unknown which the surgery represents), but at the same time information integrated with data acquired through the mentalization of that same personal experience, developed during the perioperative period.

Taking into consideration the contribution neuroscience has made [38], it is important to note that these mentalizations, thanks to the activation of chemical substances produced by emotions (neuropeptides), become thoughts or ideas transformed into matter [39]. In this sense, emotions which are at the base of fragility (fear, sense of guilt …) seem to be present physically in the body, establishing a connection with tissues and cells [40, 41]. The body (that body which is preparing itself for surgery, or which has just undergone surgery) is a body which thinks, elaborates emotions, in graining and influencing its own feelings and those in the surrounding 'field' systems, through these thoughts or emotional elaborations [42].

These transformations brought about by the body, however, can be further modified based on the contribution of the amygdala. This region of the brain acts as a sentinel, sending danger signals which produce anxiety in the C/A. The signals contribute to characterizing the relationship with the various 'field' systems, for example, the healthcare system, which the child does not easily trust. Mirror neurons generate further fragility in the C/A by transmitting dysfunctional models which develop from this condition of anxiety.

Fragility, and any developmental disorders caused by it, interpreted in this way is the object of many international studies ([21, 25], op. cit.; [22]; Roberts et al. op. cit..; [18, 24], op. cit.) by a number of experts in paediatric psychology. It is a disciplinary sector which today constitutes a field of epistemology with related expertise, and which is considered particularly effective not only as regards fostering the process of growth (between psychological development and maturity) but also as regards its ability to contribute to a theoretical discussion on various professional practices in the area of paediatrics and maternal-child hospital and local community caregiving.

15.3 The Paediatric Condition in the Perioperative Period

The epistemological development of this field of study prefers to consider each C/A affected by a morbid event as a "condition of the field", rather than as a "case" (see Fig. 15.1). This "condition" is defined by the relationships that the child (as an ontosystem, affected both by resources and developmental disorders) creates between systems of reference [43].

In this sense, fragility is set within the context of psychological and biological disorders, and vulnerabilities, etc., which define the child/adolescent in the perioperative period, further influencing relationships between these factors. The perioperative period is part of the 'condition of the field'; a chronosystem defined as a specific, dysfunctional spacetime related to the developmental process. It is influenced by the developmental stage of the C/A, and, therefore, by age and by how or in what sense the child has mentalized experiences connected to preparation for the surgical procedure, to the procedure itself or to

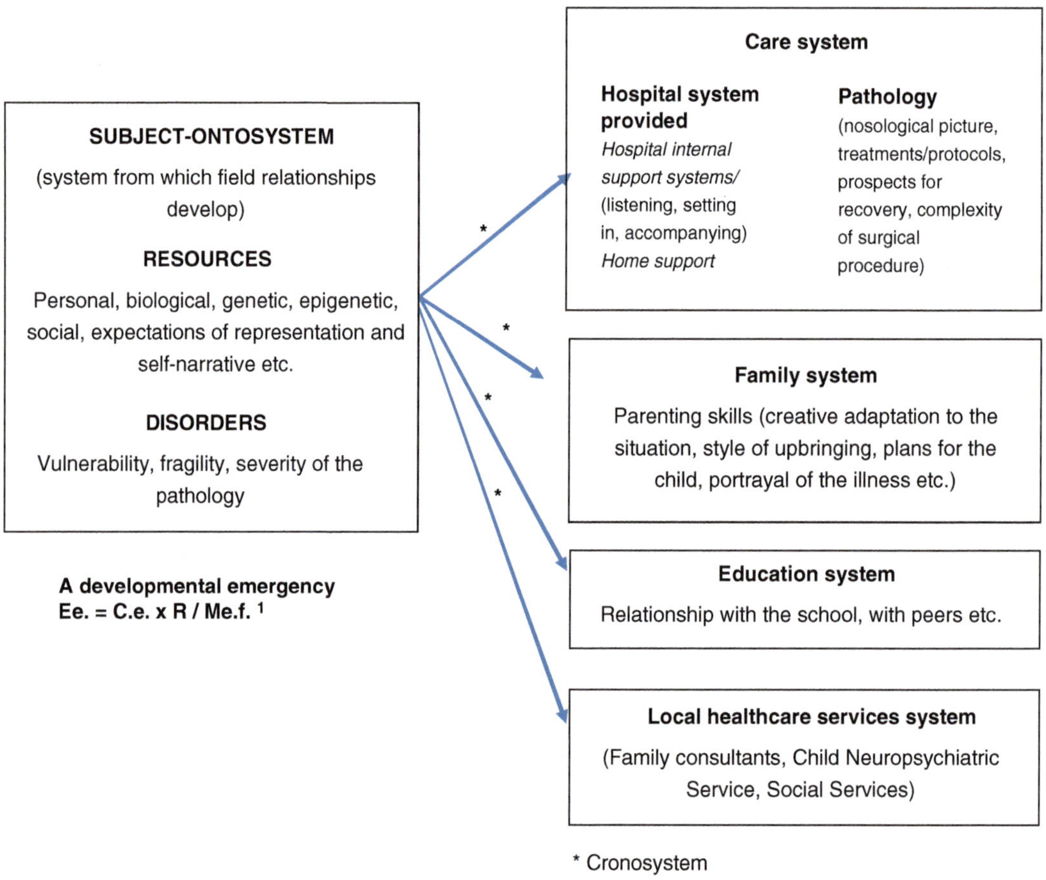

Fig. 15.1 Child/adolescent as a "condition of the field" in the perioperative period. [a]It is a formula which defines the Developmental emergency (Ee.) as a ratio between developmental impairments (C.e.) and resources (R.) and the relationship between this ratio and the C/A's functional mentalizations (Me.f.) in the management of the perioperative period. (Adapted from [17], op. cit., with permission)

the post-operative stay, etc. The type of disorder, the surgical procedure and the relationship the C/A has with various systems also affect this chronosystem; clearly each "field condition" is influenced by specific chronosystems.

We must also consider a twofold "epigenetic standpoint" when interpreting this field condition. Exposure of the ontosystem to the complexity of the field modifies the relationship the C/A (origin of the relationships) has with the surgical procedure in either a dysfunctional (parent who transmits anxiety in the relationship, doctor lacking confidence) and/or a functional way (trusting and entrusting her/himself to the surgeon), even though the C/A, origin of the field, is part of it.

At the same time, exposure of the "field condition" to the surgical procedure modifies relationships between the systems in this field; this modification has repercussions on the child's perception and behaviour in the perioperative period.

Therefore, accepting the paediatric psychology model means managing perioperative fragility not only regarding actions concerning the child directly but also actions and activities which involve relationships between the C/A and these systems. These are actions which manage both the representations which the C/A and the systems have of that fragility and the influence that the perception of fragility exerts. The influence of the experience of fragility, which the C/A attributes to him/herself and which the systems acknowledge, must also be taken into consideration. This becomes a deterrent to a possible sense of agency, and, therefore, to the possibility of overcoming the risk ([17, 29], op. cit.) that the perioperative period represents.

This perception of fragility and its outcomes proves to be integrated into cellular memory, both as deposits of representations, inherited emotions, and as a transformation of those deposits, (determined by the current relevance of the relations regarding the "field condition"). This memory will influence the C/A also in terms of weakening motivation and, therefore, will also affect her/his ability to create goals, experience a sense of self-sufficiency, self-realization, etc. It will heighten fragility and leave the C/A hostage to negative emotions, stress and anxiety. In this way, the perioperative period becomes an external riskiness factor; the combination of internal risk and external riskiness will produce a psychosocial risk [44] which can lead to a condition of cumulative stress caused by a series of traumas (amongst which the surgical procedure). In subsequent developmental stages, this stress can create Developmental Trauma Disorder [45].

15.4 Possible Dysfunctional or Functional Field Relationships in the Paediatric Perioperative Period

...in the relationship with the parents

Up to this point, considerations on the configuration of the field condition (which embraces the fragility of the child in the perioperative period), would seem to support the argument that this fragility is an aspect of the child/adolescent (origin of this field of relationships) but that evidently it can also be considered an emotional-cognitive aspect, caused and/or influenced by the type of relationship formed with systems.

One of the relationships to which the child/adolescent is exposed and that has the greatest influence is one which belongs to a dangerous configuration of parenting competence affected by a form of dysregulation, in the sense that it does not satisfy the needs of the C/A in the perioperative period.

Clinical and psychological evidence [46–48] has shown that spontaneous strategies adopted by parents, through parenting competence, within their relationship with the C/A, are heavily compromised. By this we mean that their incapacity to practice *scaffolding* [49, 50] (intended as a framework or a guide for the C/A in the perioperative period), *coping* (intended as the ability to face or anticipate the surgical procedure, etc.) and *caregiving* [51, 52], (intended as the ability to manage the C/A during the specific perioperative period), leads to an inability to express positive feelings towards the child and a refusal to interact, so as to create a neglect sort of dysfunctional mirror image of the relationship.

The child feels confused, alone, with a strong sense of incomprehension, let down and driven to ask 'who am I'; and the parent is unable to pay attention or to be in the relationship. Both become factors leading to a sort of latency in the attribution of sense and meaning to their being the parents of a C/A who is experiencing a period in his/her life where he/she anticipates, experiences and manages in a dysfunctional way, the complex nature of the surgical procedure.

Research regarding this relationship [53–58] reports that the child, when on the inside of this type of relationship, when asked to describe his/her condition during hospitalization or as a patient waiting for surgery, seems to push the presence of a parent into the background or not to contemplate it at all. Conversely, the parent seems to use a narration which is based on antipathy [59, 60], and so based on a critical parenting [61], dominated by hostility, revenge and guilt, leading to behaviours such as rejection and the tendency to consider the child a scapegoat for other siblings. This behaviour would appear to be linked to low parent genuineness, high variability in personality with a subsequent lack of stability ([61], op. cit.).

Child neglect as a form of maltreatment takes the form of omissive behaviour on the part of the parent, rather than intercepting the needs of the child in that moment of the perioperative period and its various stages. This form of maltreatment is defined in terms of acts of omission (or judged as such in reference to European [62] and professional standards), as they highlight the inappropriateness and risk of actions carried out by parental figures; figures which are in a position of unequal power compared to the child, creating a child–parent relationship which renders the child vulnerable.

It is, therefore, a form of maltreatment based on negligence and omission to meet current needs which the perioperative period creates in the child during its various stages. This form of maltreatment, which we identify as child neglect (ibidem; Dubowitz et al. 2000; Hornor 2014; Blumenthal 2015) and which is traced to dysregulation in parenting competence ([18], op. cit.), is clearly evident during perioperative stages and in specific behaviour, such as the lack of self-control exhibited by the parent during the diagnosis period prior to surgery and poor emotional intelligence (in the sense that the parent is not conscious of the emotions they are feeling, and experiences disorientation as a result of these emotions). It becomes dysfunctional as it hinders the ability to provide encouragement to the child and clear information, which would provide content to the unknown and the unfamiliar created by the surgery.

Behaviours which show dysregulation in parenting competence include the incapacity to behave in a balanced manner, and so the tendency to move from moments of frustration to exaltation, and accentuation of their role; dysfunctional behaviours include an inability to predict the outcomes of this omissive relationship, or behaviours we refer to as heuristic and/or bias [63]. These latter comprise all those prejudices and preconceptions of the C/A which characterize the relationship in terms of clichés (incapacity, weakness, vulnerability, unreliability of the C/A in managing the post-operative stage).

In this sense, specific omissions can be identified ordinarily used by the parents for the functions of scaffolding, coping, caregiving.

Regarding behaviours governing the relationship with the C/A, they can be attributed to a model defining child neglect validated by scientific evidence (Bifulco et al., op. cit., Bifulco, op. cit., Hornor, op. cit.; [64]), and to a number of indicators which are defined as opposing and lie on a continuous line of three factors:

- *Stimulation*, including hypo and hyper stimulation; during hospitalization prior to surgery, the parent provides the C/A constantly with activities/tasks or the parent keeps the child away from any opportunity that might involve the child in carrying out a task.
- *Acknowledgement*, in the form of non-recognition and, therefore, the incapacity of the child to be able to take any responsibility in the post-operative stage. On the contrary, adulation (for example, giving the C/A all the

responsibility for therapeutic alliance regarding management of the pre-op stage: diet, control of physical activity, etc).
- *Care*, intended as hypo-care, parent who is careless about therapy appointments, misses follow-up appointments, does not provide the surgeon with the necessary information to ensure full knowledge of illness relapses. In contrast, we have hypercare, the parent puts pressure on the child to observe the most important aspects of daily life, during hospitalization, convalescence, etc.

This model for the definition of child neglect is supported by a study of the Italian Society of Paediatric Psychology (2012/2021) aimed at the design, construction and validation of an observation tool, supported also by a data collection sheet to detect the risk of child neglect. This form is useful during hospital stay to identify "clinical" couples in terms of child neglect. Following the administration of observation tool on these couples and the positive identification of child neglect, the data (condition of child neglect in a situation of dysregulation of parenting competence) can be used to activate protected hospital discharge, also during follow-ups.

Often added to this is the preconception of medical incompetence, inadequacy in the hospital care or even an overemphasis of their own knowledge, of information regarding the surgery or possible therapeutic alliance, and of possible consequences or side effects of the procedure.

... in the relationship with the rehabilitation system

In a number of paediatric conditions during the postoperative period, rehabilitation is required [65–68], for example, in children with disability, with disorders or suffering from neurodevelopmental disorders, in addition, clearly, to children suffering from certain cancers and from pre-existing mental disorders not always identified prior to the perioperative period.

All of these are conditions that can lead to clinical pictures of maladjustment, including attention and executive functions dysfunction, meta-cognitive sensitivity (if concerning pre-school age children, meta-cognition beyond this developmental stage, etc.) and disturbances in control, etc. Often it concerns disorders which appear either due to a state antecedent to surgery, or caused by the manifestation of specific biological disorders or by emotional and cognitive stress induced by the surgery itself. These are paediatric conditions for which psychological support, in terms of listening and accompaniment are not generally envisaged. The appearance of these disorders is often underestimated and only careful follow-up on progress made post-surgery is able to detect red flags indicating a dysfunctional psychic state. In this case, integrated rehabilitation is required ([18, 69, 70], op. cit.).

During post-operative period, children can experience a fall in energy levels [71]. This weakening leads to a condition of "fatigue" [72], which would seem to constitute a specific developmental risk condition and psycho-developmental blackouts, as outlined below:

- Selective attention: defined as the ability to focus on specific aspects or elements of the situation, with repercussions in terms of a poor sense of reality [73] (for example, concerning the organization of daily life in the hospital).
- Self-control: unable to manage the self-regulation process of behaviour and of changing activities due to rules and requirements related to the paediatric condition [74].
- Meta-cognitive sensitivity and/or meta-cognition: unable to identify strategies to understand the task assigned in treatment and therapy, and to locate dysfunctions in their own behaviour compared to the successful outcome of all the medical procedures "involved in the treatment process" [75].
- Problem-solving: unable to solve tasks assigned during caregiving and treatment, etc., with significant difficulty in identifying possible solutions [76].

Paediatric psychology, when viewed as complementary to child and adolescent psychiatry and integrated care, and as an ethical process of solidarity [77], promotes, on a national and international level, the significance of psychological rehabilitation models applied to the assessment and to the surgery, in child and adolescent disorders ([78]; Kazak and Noll 2015). It is, in fact, this complementary which allows the child and adolescent to develop the capacity for community life, the development of resources (often, consciousness of these resources), and the interruption of a vicious circle of chronicization of "disorders" in and of the developmental processes which form the various domains. In this sense, the pillar of psychological rehabilitation in paediatric psychology is managing all the components which create the domains in cognitive terms, and of the "specializations" ([18], op. cit.). This rehabilitation perspective also manages conflict in the relationship between needs in every paediatric condition, including needs arising from the developmental stage and needs caused by the pathology, or in our case, the post-operative state.

In paediatric psychology, a multidimensional rehabilitation model is evident [17, 79, 80]: psychiatric rehabilitation, which manages structural functions and processes [81], and psychological rehabilitation, or better described as psychosocial and educational rehabilitation [82], which focuses on the developmental processes of the domains (social, cognitive, etc.). It is through these that the structural processes related to functions are developed in everyday life (of psychiatric relevance) ([18], op. cit.), allowing the child and adolescent to organize the most important systems of that domain as a function of his/her mental health (ibidem).

Complementarity in psychiatric/psychosocial-educational rehabilitation means adopting an epigenetic perspective [83, 84]. It is a perspective which, during rehabilitation, promotes the importance of contexts seen not as a variable but as an epiphenomenon of mental health ([17, 85–87], op. cit.). It is worth noting here the importance that surgical follow-ups, together with the family paediatrician, assume whilst accompanying the rehabilitation period (part of the Child and Adolescent Neuropsychiatric Service) providing continuity through hospital and local community services.

Psychological rehabilitation thus becomes an integrated, psychosocial-educational type of rehabilitation, outlining, in the meantime, the development of a possible "alternative representation of the self" in the child or adolescent, oriented towards redefining their own skills and reinforcing functional resources, to enable reinsertion into their context in a different way. It is important to note that in all types of psychological support, including and above all rehabilitation, the C/A must be given support in the development of an experiential self [88], that is, a self which is constantly in transformation as it assimilates the various experiences and, in particular, the mentalizations of those experiences. These latter include experiences connected to the surgery during the perioperative period.

Integrated rehabilitation, thus, describes, in particular, a supplementary model and professional practices relating to the two directions indicated (psychiatric/psychosocial-educational), and, more specifically, the direction linked to the psychological intervention is defined according to the following:

- A psychological perspective aimed at promoting developmental alternatives regarding the "mentalization"/interiorization of experiences linked to the child's own conditions, and, thus, of themselves and relationships with the systems connected to their conditions. It is further aimed at promoting alternatives regarding behaviours, relationships, the transformation of their emotions and "attachment ties", and finally, the possible recovery of those abilities and skills compromised within the various domains, together with the reactivation (restoration, start-up) of the conditions typical of mental health, and, thus of well-being of the developmental process. Furthermore, this perspective allows us to emphasize the importance of identifying boundaries in terms of development (cognitive, motor, social, etc.), relating to damage and to the possibility of planning an itinerary for possible transformation.

Regarding rehabilitation perspectives identified by paediatric psychology and applicable to the post-operative stage, in cases of stress, an educational perspective is indicated [70], aimed at modifying behaviour through the promotion of learning. This form of rehabilitation uses specific types of education, amongst which psychoeducation [89]. Finally, regarding rehabilitation perspectives in the post-operative stage, the social perspective should be taken into consideration, aiming towards "social healing" in such a way that the C/A recontextualizes her/himself within roles, relationships, tasks, actions, activities belonging to the everyday social routine.

One of the most used rehabilitation models in paediatric psychology is that of the developmental crisis ([17, 64, 90–94] op. cit.) and crisis readapted to child and adolescent disorders. An example is the condition in which, compared to a critical event (represented by post-operative stress disorder and a state of fragility), the child and/or adolescent, with greater or lesser awareness, experiences distress when thinking and "feeling" that the skills used up to that moment to relate to the world in everyday life, are no longer adequate to manage the event [95, 96].

Integrated rehabilitation, when managing the C/A during the post-operative stage, must carry out certain developmental tasks which constitute a turning point in the rehabilitation process, in as much as the C/A is seen to have a sense of agency within a significant stage of the life cycle (the perioperative period) in addition to the development stages involved in growth. These transformation tasks must include as a priority

- Redefining an understanding of the self, the concept of self and the image of the self
- Managing an experiential self in the here and now of the disorder
- Mentalizing the experience of the surgical procedure as part of the self
- Building integrated mapping to represent his/herself
- Recognizing his/her own resources
- Redefining meanings of those resources
- Projecting his/herself in regard to the C/A's own paediatric condition [93, 97].

Psychosocial-educational rehabilitation in paediatric psychology assumes three directions when managing processes (disorders and resources); *an assessment direction,* which allows us to guide the intervention; *a support direction* when seeking to provide answers to the developmental tasks posed by the crisis; and the *rehabilitation intervention* for disturbed domain processes. The development of these processes constitutes specific outcomes relating to effective rehabilitation. This is an orientation supported by the strengthening perspective ([28, 29], op. cit.), used in paediatric psychology when guiding rehabilitation in an attempt to strengthen skills and abilities. These latter, in the form of present and developed resources, can ensure the child or adolescent passes through the risk or developmental blackout, doubtless caused by the perioperative period, and which constitutes a very real "developmental emergency" ([17], op. cit.).

It is an emergency whose profile depends on the relationship between developmental process disorders and resources in the various domains in relation to interiorizations that the child/adolescent has developed concerning experiences linked to the condition and other connected variables. All of this must also take into consideration the fact that the perioperative period informs the trend of the developmental trajectory both in terms of dimension/domain (cognitive, social, etc.) and in terms of evolution (and so of mentalization, as an interiorization of the experience).

15.5 Integrated Working Within the *System* to Provide Support During the Perioperative Period

Configuration of the "condition of the field", which can highlight the C/A's factors of functioning (fragility, vulnerability, etc.) as well as the possible dysregulation of parenting competence, the severity of the pathology, malformation, and the complexity of the surgical procedure, etc., inevitably poses a number of questions concerning time, space and available resources for multi-professional, integrated working.

When referring to integrated working in the hospital and local community healthcare *system*, obviously we indicate an inclusive model that the *system* itself can promote using an integrated, inclusive model which needs to be contextualized in the surgical unit, by means of "approved" hospital procedures. The model which paediatric psychology proposes for this type of work is based on knowhow and refers to a shared concept [98, 99], that the professional figures involved (psychologist, surgeon anaesthetist, nurses, etc.) can consider when working together and in their own practices whilst managing the C/A.

This concept, which goes beyond the aim, becomes the backdrop for each procedure in the care taking process during the various stages of the perioperative period, and, therefore, within the different hospital and local community services and home care. The clarity of concept should be supported by equal clarity in criteria which can guide integrated working, and which include managing the involvement of the psychologist in everyday routines and not only consultancy based. This is an aspect which not only provides accompaniment of the child and parent throughout the most difficult moments of preparation for surgery, but also affects time management of the nursing staff. It avoids pulling this staff away from other duties due to the fact that, in the absence of specific professions such as the psychologist, it is the nursing staff that is required to deal with issues related to a lack of regulation, poor therapeutic alliance, difficult relations between family and doctors, etc.

Regarding criteria for integrated working, joint, transversal accompaniment is suggested—psychologist/surgeon—during the different stages of treatment, in addition to bearing in mind the patient's quality of life (also in the case of surgery for serious pathologies, which in some cases includes a poor prognosis), the inseparability of 'cure' and 'care,' and managing the C/A not as a "case" but as a condition of the field [100]. This concept and the criteria indicated refer to specific perspectives of inclusive, integrated working and can be identified in the complete contextualization of the figure and psychological intervention, in the functional organization of the "connections" ([17], op. cit.) between surgery and other units, services, clinics and paediatric emergency units. These are "connections" which lead to better quality healthcare. Finally, amongst the perspectives, there is also the identification of the psychological intervention as promotion of well-being and development of the cycle of life.

The "connections" indicated translate into certain directions: *connection,* in terms of the ability to connect information and transmit it; *ties*, in terms of commitments between figures, departments; *sequences,* intended as connections which define a common theme, a logical-operational framework governing relationships between the various professional practices. A concluding remark on the management of the perioperative period in terms of integrated working, brings to the forefront three dynamic factors which affect the *system* and which should be considered if the *system* wishes to embrace an integrated working ethos successfully. These three factors include *Energy* [101], which constitutes the efficiency of the functioning (i.e. support shift work), but also the efficacy of the healthcare provided (i.e. encourage trust in clinics/day hospitals); *Strength* and *Solidarity* [102], which represent a defensive barrier and scaffolding (set of aspects of reference); and *Communication* [103, 104] defined as a structural system action, both in terms of institutional communication [105] and in terms of dissemination/awareness raising [106].

Regarding the functionality of communication, it is important to remember that integrated working means (Ravioli, op. cit; Ferro and Tosco, op. cit.; [107–113])

- Creating space for others [114]
- Listening
- Satisfying demand, based on both explicit and implicit needs [115]
- Ensuring an image of "health"
- Creating engagement
- Intercepting the emotional world of the patient

- Giving functional messages to the adaptative behaviours and processes of the C/A, family and staff
- "Playing" the game of closeness, distance, security, limits [116, 117]
- Rejecting the fear-appeal, and, therefore, not eliciting fear when providing information, directives [118]
- Rejecting the idea of always opposing whatever
- Rejecting the idea of astounding/shocking however

It is clear that communication needs to focus on a specific aim, that of promoting a condition of well-being in all of the subjects involved in the perioperative period of a child, taking into consideration that the quality of management of a surgical procedure also depends on the conditions of well-being of the healthcare workers. This is especially so as regards life in the department, clinic and local community services.

The complex nature of the perioperative period, in terms of time and planning specific medical procedures, necessitates an integrated, inclusive type working culture [119, 120]. This implicates the use of a specific "language" shared by the healthcare workers involved; a "language" which should be developed in terms of reciprocity, sharing, pooling of ideas [121, 122] and stability of each professional identity. Based on this working culture, which characterizes the relationship between the various professional figures, adaptive behaviours can be developed; not only adaptive (healthcare workers already take a holistic approach to the child or adolescent undergoing an operation, within the "field" of each single patient), but also adaptational, knowing how to build an integrated working system between professional figures.

This is developed using: *acknowledgement* of the importance of the role of the other professional (also in front of the C/A and family), recognizing the efficacy of the contribution of the other professional, and, finally, activating problem-solving in the search for situations and tools which will allow professionals to receive feedback regarding the results of their actions and those of others. This "adaptational nature" leads to the protection and safeguard of all subjects involved (patients/visitors, surgeons, anaesthetists, psychologist, nurses, etc). Furthermore, the healthcare system and the specific professional practice of the single patient are also safeguarded, defeating the need for defensive medicine [123]. This also contributes to preventing work-related stress (Balducci, Fraccaroli, op. cit.).

There are minimum integrated working conditions based on the following

- Joint training
- Creation of a pact of shared responsibility with a deliberate and approved framework governing integrated working
- Constant involvement of the administration offices, with tailored awareness-raising training, defined in terms of place and time
- Creation of synergies between various itineraries/projects and relative financial resources involving the Department (projects connected to various national funding programmes PSN-National Health Framework), conventions, voluntary organizations and community services, which are advised to create synergic planning as a single organizing body, whilst maintaining each contributor's specificity (*Art. 5 of the S.I.P.U.Ò Convention.*)
- Executive plan for integrated working
- Monitoring of patient management through integrated working and the deliberate, executive plan, with specific tools and dissemination of the data obtained

The choice to adopt integrated working is certainly not the sole responsibility of the doctors and nurses, etc.; it needs to be facilitated and supported by positions created specifically to assist and accompany not only the single subjects (C/A, family, healthcare workers) but also the *system* itself. These figures can be paediatric psychologists specifically trained nationally for this position (masters, specialized training) and internationally (training programmes proposed by the 54th Division, in Roberts' works).

15.6 Trauma in the Perioperative Period; A Multidimensional Approach

During the perioperative period, the specific paediatric condition can develop into a traumatic condition for the C/A. The psychological trauma, which certainly is not an illness and, therefore, the characteristics cannot be standardized, does not produce the same symptoms and reactions [124] and leads to a complex configuration. Obviously here we are referring to a condition based on the contemporary nature of a biological, physical event and a psychological state. This distinction helps us to define the trauma of our C/A as a dynamic relationship between the psyche and the body, which creates a dysfunctional holistic nucleus, restorative and dissipative in nature. This migrates towards an interconnection which can create a psychic mental functioning that helps the child to transform emotions and representations, and in which the body is no longer considered separate from the mind. This functioning, however, can be managed, can be "confronted", transforming it into an "opening" for new possibilities; psychological intervention can foster this on a cognitive, emotive, perceptive level.

In this sense, the psychological intervention follows an itinerary leading to a more complex reconfiguration of the developmental resources than the C/A possessed before the trauma [125]. This allows the management of this condition of "displacement" that the child experiences as an annihilation of thought and emotions, and thus of ties or connections to the "body wound" [126]; the absence of a "social hook". The child has distanced her/himself in mental and perceptional terms. However, they contextualize themselves in a distant mental space where they feel an indistinct sense of "draining" of their resources [57] and, finally, displacement activates a lack of engagement with the body [127].

It is important to remember that the C/A lives in a traumatic state, this state is the result of dysfunctional relationships which form the specific "condition of the field", and are not attributable exclusively to the fragility of the child, to the severity of the pathology or to the malformation, etc., which he/she has. When we refer to trauma, we are indicating a psychic event resulting from a breach in mental balance, mental functioning and emotional regulation. It is often accompanied by a distortion in perception, dissociation and the inconceivability of the event, otherwise risking fragmentation of the sense of identity, of relationships and emotions.

When referring to trauma in the C/A, during the perioperative period, we refer to a catastrophic event in a condition of chaos; it is a cognitive and emotional "leap" forcefully undermining the dynamic balance of the domains which preside over functioning. This renders the surgery, invasive treatments, medications and "inconceivable mental contents" something either to flee from or to succumb to [127].

Trauma in the perioperative period can evolve into psychopathogenetic dissociative processes (Farina and Liotti, op. cit.), which produce symptoms of dissociation and create a specific clinical picture (dissociative disorders). Alternatively, it can be linked to nosographic classifications regarding various psychopathologies. Self-regulation domains (emotions, identity, relations) seem to be particularly affected [128], more precisely: concerning the *emotional domain*, we witness excessive emotional reactivity, outbursts of aggression, imprudent and destructive behaviour, a tendency to experience dissociative states prolonged under stress, an inability to feel pleasure and positive emotions. Concerning *dysregulation of the identity,* the concept of the self is disturbed, together with denigration, low self-esteem, and a sense of guilt. Finally, regarding *interpersonal dysregulation,* we detect difficulty in maintaining relationships, difficulty feeling close to others, avoidance with little interest in relationships, and a general social withdrawal, in addition to occasional very close or intense relationships but with difficulty in maintaining involvement.

Careful consideration of trauma during the perioperative period also implies an analysis of the impact that this has on executive systems of the brain [129]. Regarding the impact of the trauma on the primitive executive system, and, thus, on the neural networks surrounding the amygdala (mainly involving the right subcortical structure and the corpus callosum), high reactivity and significant use of the right of veto are seen, in addition to the tendency to impose yourself on others. Regarding impact on the second executive system, and, therefore, on the frontoparietal networks and the hippocampus (responsible for spacetime sequencing of experience and behaviour) the presence of a trauma inhibits cognitive elaboration and memory. In addition, the learning process seems to be inhibited and damaged by the multiple consequences of chronic activation [130–132]. As regards the third executive system, and, therefore, pertaining to the medial structures in the brain associated with attachment, self-awareness and empathy towards others, Default Mode Network [133], inhibitions in affections and syntonization, compassion and empathy are detected, together with decreased development of self-awareness and the capacity for insight [134, 135].

It is important to note that in this developmental condition determined by the trauma, a substantial deterrent can be established by the capacity for mind-mindedness in the parents. As correlated to parental sensitivity, it can promote secure attachment, with the relative resources in terms of domain development.

This mapping of the impact of trauma, from a bio-psychosocial perspective, should also take into consideration repercussions on the health of the C/A's developmental process during the perioperative period, highlighting the fact that, apart from post-traumatic stress disorder, recent studies have produced consensus criteria relating to Developmental trauma disorder ([45, 136], op. cit.) and, at the same time, Adjustment disorder [137]. The aforementioned criteria provide meanings, explanatory models to define the objectivization of the psychic disorder, demonstrating that cumulative stress created by overlapping of macro and micro traumas during childhood and adolescence leads to very real distress conditions, or even disorders due to an impact on the executive systems, and, therefore, disorders pertaining to forms and types of dysregulation in adulthood.

15.7 Closing Considerations

Paediatric psychology embraces these two directions in caregiving theory, starting from a model of C/A Health in paediatric treatment, which recognizes an "adaptive and adaptational personality" ([17], op. cit.). It delineates, as the central nucleus of functioning, the interconnection (fundamental for the well-being of the developmental trajectory of the child affected by the pathology), between regulation processes which cut across the various domains, executive systems and field relations.

The perioperative period thus becomes a longitudinal itinerary in which, managing the risk of the child and adolescent adopting dysregulation (as a "reason for being" in their everyday life) as a perverse antidote to the fragility which defines them. In this way, it is not feasible to contemplate accompaniment and support as being provided only by a paediatric psychologist within specific dedicated spaces (clinics, departments, home); we need to focus our attention, rather, on creating a multi-professional model which is able to direct intervention to focus on prevention from a bio-psychosocial perspective. It is prevention which, on the one hand, can contrast the patient's dysregulated behaviour, even during the treatment process with the surgeon, and, on the other hand, can enhance their life skills.

References

1. Ventola M. Promuovere la cultura del benessere psicologico nei giovani. Analisi e sviluppo di buone pratiche nelprogetto "Guadagnaresalute in adolescenza". Rome: Università Sapienza di Roma; 2011.
2. Benzoni S. Figli fragili. Bari: Laterza; 2017.
3. World Health Organization. Life skills education in schools. Geneva: World Health Organization; 1993.
4. Albasi C. Il conoscere relazionale implicito e il concetto di Modelli Operativi Interni Dissociati (MOID). A E R: Abilitazione E Riabilitazione. 2005;14(2):25–40.
5. Albasi, C. (2011). Modelli operativi interni dissociati e attaccamenti traumatici. In P. Di Benedetto, La dissociazione. Prospettive teoriche ed esperienze cliniche (pp. 11–30). Milan, CIS Editore.
6. Speranza AM. Disorganizzazione dell'attaccamento e processi dissociativi: il contributo di liotti allo

studio delle traiettorie di sviluppo. Cognitivismo Clinico. 2018;15(2):217–20.
7. Tani F. I legami di attaccamento fra normalità e patologia: aspetti teorici e d'intervento. Psicoanalisi Neofreudiana. 2011;1:1–31.
8. Epstein J. Comprendere il mondo del bambino. Roma: Armando; 2011.
9. Baldoni F. Modelli operativi interni e relazioni di attaccamento in preadolescenza. In: Crocetti G, Agosta R, editors. Preadolescenza. Il bambino caduto dalle fiabe. Teoria della clinica e prassi psicoterapeutica. Bologna: Pendragon; 2007. p. 57–77.
10. Engel S. Children's need to know: curiosity in schools. Harv Educ Rev. 2011;81(4):625–45.
11. Ensink K, Mayes LC. The development of mentalisation in children from a theory of mind perspective. Psychoanal Inq. 2010;30(4):301–37.
12. Crugnola CR. Relazioni precoci, esperienze avverse e attaccamento: traiettorie evolutive e psicopatologiche. Riv Psicoanal. 2017;63(3):645–58.
13. Stovall-McClough KC, Dozier M. Attachment states of mind and psychopathology in adulthood. In: Handbook of attachment: theory, research, and clinical applications. New York: Guilford Press; 2016. p. 715–38.
14. Barone L, Lionetti F. Quando l'attaccamento si disorganizza. Indicatori e fattori di rischio dell'esperienza traumatica nel ciclo di vita. Psicol Clin Svilupp. 2013;17(1):3–26.
15. Farina B, Liotti G. Dimensione dissociativa e trauma dello sviluppo. Psicobiettivo: rivista quadrimestrale di psicoterapie a confronto, XXXVIII. 2018;3(2018):183–95.
16. Muzi S, Pace CS. Relazioni tra sintomi internalizzanti ed esternalizzanti, attaccamento, regolazione emotiva e alessitimia in adolescenti in comunità residenziale. Psicol Clin Svilupp. 2020;24(1):117–26.
17. Perricone Briulotta G. Il vento della psicologia pediatrica: l'esperienza di un know how oltre la psicologia applicata in pediatria. Milan: McGraw-Hill; 2019.
18. Perricone G, Polizzi C, Morales R, Carollo A, Fontana V, Rotolo I, Burgio S. Corso di psicologia dello sviluppo e dell'educazione con elementi di psicologia pediatrica. Milan: McGraw Hill; 2021.
19. Caprilli S, Vagnoli L. Il bambino ed i genitori di fronte all'intervento chirurgico: analisi qualitativa di interviste al caregiver. In: Terapia familiare: rivista interdisciplinare di ricerca ed intervento relazionale. Rome: Accademia di Psicoterapia della Famiglia; 2009. p. 1000–27.
20. Aylward BS, Lee JL. Historical developments and trends in pediatric psychology. In: Roberts MC, Steele RG, editors. Handbook of pediatric psychology. 5th ed. New York: Guilford Press; 2017. p. 3–13.
21. Kazak AE, Schneider S, Kassam-Adams N. Pediatric medical traumatic stress. In: Roberts MC, Steele RG, editors. Handbook of pediatric psychology. New York: The Guilford Press; 2009a. p. 205–15.
22. Perricone Briulotta G. Psicologia pediatrica: dalla teoria alla pratica evolutiva-clinica. Milan: McGraw-Hill; 2012.
23. Roberts MC, Aylward BS, Wu YP. Clinical practice of pediatric psychology. New York: Guilford Press; 2014.
24. Roberts MC, Steele RG. Handbook of pediatric psychology. 5th ed. New York: The Guilford Press; 2017.
25. Polizzi C. Pensarsi psicologo pediatrico. Modelli, percorsi e strategie di una formazione. Milan: Franco Angeli; 2011.
26. Gottlieb G. Normally occurring environmental and behavioral influences on gene activity: from central dogma to probabilistic epigenesis. Psychol Rev. 1998;105:792–802.
27. Hofer M. La nuova" biologia evoluzionistica dello sviluppo": da Freud all'epigenetica. Psicoterapia e Scienze Umane. 2014;3:395–408.
28. Grotberg EH. A guide to promoting resilience in children: strengthening the human spirit. In: Early childhood development: practice and reflections, vol. 8. The Hague: Bernard Van Leer Foundation; 1995. p. 1–43.
29. Rutter M. Resilience as a dynamic concept. Dev Psychopathol. 2012;24(2):335–44.
30. Latal B, Helfricht S, Fischer JE, Bauersfeld U, Landolt MA. Psychological adjustment and quality of life in children and adolescents following open-heart surgery for congenital heart disease: a systematic review. BMC Pediatr. 2009;9(1):1–10.
31. Isokääntä S, Koivula K, Honkalampi K, Kokki H. Resilience in children and their parents during pediatric medical traumatic stress. Paediatr Anaesth. 2019;29(3):218–25.
32. Rutter M. Nature, nurture, and development: from evangelism through science toward policy and practice. Child Dev. 2002;73(1):1–21.
33. Gervasi P. Critica della mente. Una rassegna di studi su letteratura e Scienze cognitive. Nuova informazione bibliografica. 2015;12(1):69–102.
34. Macchi Cassia V, Valenza E, Simion F. Lo sviluppo della mente. Dalle teorie classiche ai nuovi orientamenti. Bologna: il Mulino; 2012.
35. Halford GS, Andrews G. Information-processing models of cognitive development. In: Goswami U, editor. The Wiley–Blackwell handbook of childhood cognitive development. Hoboken: Wiley-Blackwell; 2011. p. 697–721.
36. Foer J. L' arte di ricordare tutto. In: Storia, scienza e miracoli della memoria. Milan: TEA; 2019.
37. Marchetti A, Intra FS. Mentalizzazione e tempo. La comprensione della mente attraverso le età e le relazioni. Rivista internazionale di Filosofia e Psicologia. 2015;6(2):198–211.
38. Luyten P, Fonagy P. The neurobiology of mentalizing. Pers Disord Theory Res Treat. 2015;6(4):366–79.
39. Kim S. The mind in the making: developmental and neurobiological origins of mentalizing. Pers Disord Theory Res Treat. 2015;6(4):356–65.

40. Lipton BH. La biologia delle credenze. Come il pensiero influenza il DNA e ogni cellula. Cesena: Macro Edizioni; 2020.
41. Pert CB. Molecole di emozioni. Il perché delle emozioni che proviamo. Milan: TEA; 2016.
42. Damasio AR. The somatic marker hypothesis and the possible functions of the prefrontal cortex. Philos Trans R Soc Lond Biol Sci. 1996;351(1346):1413–20.
43. Kazak A, Rourke M, Navsaria N. Families and other systems in pediatric psychology. In: Roberts M, Steele R, editors. Handbook of pediatric psychology. New York: The Guilford Press; 2009b. p. 159–75.
44. Bucci N, Luna M, Viloria A, García JH, Parody A, Varela N, López LAB. Factor analysis of the psychosocial risk assessment instrument. In: International conference on data mining and big data. Cham: Springer; 2018. p. 149–58.
45. Van Der Kolk BA. Developmental trauma disorder: towards a rational diagnosis for chronically traumatized children. Praxis der Kinderpsychologie Und Kinder psychiatric. 2009;58(8):572–86.
46. Franck LS, Mcquillan A, Wray J, Grocott MP, Goldman A. Parent stress levels during children's hospital recovery after congenital heart surgery. Pediatr Cardiol. 2010;31(7):961–8.
47. Nelson PA, Caress AL, Glenny AM, Kirk SA. 'Doing the "right" thing': how parents experience and manage decision-making for children's 'normalising' surgeries. Soc Sci Med. 2012;74(5):796–804.
48. Scrimin S, Haynes M, Altoè G, Bornstein MH, Axia G. Anxiety and stress in mothers and fathers in the 24 h after their child's surgery. Child Care Health Dev. 2009;35(2):227–33.
49. Axia V, Capello F. La comunicazione. Elementi di psico-oncologia pediatrica. Roma: Carocci; 2004.
50. Carr A, Pike A. Maternal scaffolding behavior: links with parenting style and maternal education. Dev Psychol. 2012;48(2):543–51.
51. George C, Solomon J. The caregiving system: a behavioral systems approach to parenting. In: Handbook of attachment: theory, research, and clinical applications, vol. 2. New York: Guilford Press; 2008. p. 833–56.
52. Malagoli Togliatti M, Zavattini GC. Relazioni genitori-figli e promozione della genitorialità. Presentazione Psicologia clinica dello sviluppo. 2000;4(2):259–66.
53. Bongiovanni M, Travagliante P. La medicina narrativa strumento trasversale di azione, compliance e empowerment. Milan: Franco Angeli; 2017.
54. Caso R. Storie bambine: vivere e raccontare la malattia e l'ospedalizzazione attraverso le fiabe. Ricerche di pedagogia e didattica. 2012;7:123–55.
55. Farneti A, Tschiesner R. L'ospedale come bene comune. Padova: libreria universitaria. it Edizioni; 2018.
56. Longaretti R, Cirillo S, Sacchi L, Baldoli C. «In viaggio nello spazio»: accompagnare bambini e genitori durante gli esami neuroradiologici. Psicol Clin Svilupp. 2015;19(3):545–52.
57. Schivalocchi E, Pozzi C. Favorire nel bambino il riconoscimento delle emozioni attraverso lo stimolo alla narrazione in occasione dell'intervento chirurgico. In: Psiba: Quaderno dell'Istituto di Psicoterapia del bambino e dell'adolescente. Milan: Mimesis Edizioni; 2014. p. 73–87.
58. Smorti A, Bartoli E. Raccontare la malattia del bambino. In: Farneti A, Tschiesner R, editors. L'ospedale come bene comune. Padua: edizioni; 2017. p. 57–88.
59. Bifulco A. The long-term effects of childhood neglect or abuse. Implications for child and family services in the UK. Pap Soc Pedagogy. 2019;12(2):57–78.
60. Maggiolini A. Psicopatologia del ciclo di vita. Milan: Franco Angeli; 2017.
61. Bifulco A, Moran P, Jacobs C, Bunn A. Problem partners and parenting: exploring linkages with maternal insecure attachment style and adolescent offspring internalizing disorder. Attach Hum Dev. 2009;11(1):69–85.
62. Sethi D, Bellis M, Hughes K, Gilbert R, Mitis F, Galea G. European report on preventing child maltreatment. Geneva: World Health Organization; 2013.
63. Gagliardi F. La naturalizzazione dei concetti: aspetti computazionali e cognitivi. Sistemiintelligenti. 2014;26(2):283–98.
64. Perricone G, Polizzi C, Morales MR, Carollo A, Rotolo I, Caldarella R. Corso di Psicologia dello Sviluppo e dell'Educazione con elementi di Psicologia pediatrica. Milan: McGraw-Hill; 2018.
65. Adduci A, Poggi G. I bambini e il tumore. Strategie di supporto in ambito clinico, familiare e scolastico. Milan: Franco Angeli; 2011.
66. Lerman J. Perioperative management of the paediatric patient with coexisting neuromuscular disease. Br J Anaesth. 2011;107(S1):i79–89.
67. Martin E, Renouil M, Lombard C, Ruzic JC, Poinsot E. Malattie neuromuscolari nel bambino e nell'adolescente: screening, valutazioni mirate, priorità e trattamenti rieducativi e chirurgici. EMC Medicina Riabilitativa. 2015;22(4):1–14.
68. Pruneti C. Psicologia clinica e malattia organica: i disturbi neurologici. Bologna: Società Editrice Esculapio; 2018.
69. Maki DR, Riggar TF. Concepts and paradigms. In: Handbook of rehabilitation counseling. New York: Springer; 2004. p. 1–24.
70. Vaccaro AG, Guerrini A. Abilitazione e riabilitazione: dall'assistenza all'autodeterminazione. Milan: McGraw-Hill; 2003.
71. Jankovic M, Loiacono NB, Spinetta JJ, Riva L, Conter V, Masera C. Telling young children with leukemia their diagnosis: he flower garden as analogy. Pediatr Hematol Oncol. 1994;11(1):75–81.
72. Bogdanov S, Brookes N, Epps A, Naismith SL, Teng A, Lah S. Fatigue in children with moderate or severe

traumatic brain injury compared with children with orthopedic injury: characteristics and associated factors. J Head Trauma Rehabil. 2021;36(2):E108–17.
73. Marzocchi GM, Portolan S, Usilla A. Autoregolare l'attenzione. Trento: Edizioni Erickson; 2006.
74. Del Giudice M, Colle L. Differences between children and adults in the recognition of enjoyment smiles. Dev Psychol. 2007;43(3):796–803.
75. De Beni R, Moè A, Cornoldi C. AMOS. In: Abilità e motivazione allo studio: Prove di valutazione e orientamento, vol. 30. Trento: Edizioni Erickson; 2003.
76. Marzocchi GM, Valagussa S. Le funzioni esecutive in età evolutiva. Franco Angeli: Milan; 2011.
77. Lavanco G, Novara C, Romano F. Relazionarsi nella comunità: quale formazione per un'etica della solidarietà. In: La Rosa S, editor. La qualità delle relazioni umane nell'Università. Milan: Franco Angeli; 2010. p. 95–110.
78. Harrison LE, Pate JW, Richardson PA, Ickmans K, Wicksell RK, Simons LE. Best-evidence for the rehabilitation of chronic pain part 1: pediatric pain. J Clin Med. 2019;8(9):1267.
79. Kaufman JN, Lahey S, Slomine BS. Pediatric rehabilitation psychology: rehabilitating a moving target. Rehabil Psychol. 2017;62(3):223–6.
80. Maynard CS, Amari A, Wieczorek B, Christensen JR, Slifer KJ. Interdisciplinary behavioral rehabilitation of pediatric pain-associated disability: retrospective review of an inpatient treatment protocol. J Pediatr Psychol. 2010;35(2):128–37.
81. Lah S, Phillips NL, Palermo TM, Bartlett D, Epps A, Teng A, et al. A feasibility and acceptability study of cognitive behavioural treatment for insomnia in adolescents with traumatic brain injury: A–B with follow up design, randomized baseline, and replication across participants. Neuropsychol Rehabil. 2021;31(3):345–68.
82. Frank RG, Rosenthal M, Caplan B. Handbook of rehabilitation psychology. Washington DC: American Psychological Association; 2010.
83. Basso M, Sleiman S, Ratan RR. Looking above but not beyond the genome for therapeutics in neurology and psychiatry: epigenetic proteins and RNAs find a new focus. Neurotherapeutics. 2013;10(4):551–5.
84. Bhattacharya D, Pomeroy SL, Pomeranz Krummel DA, Sengupta S. Epigenetics and survivorship in pediatric brain tumor patients. J Neuro-Oncol. 2020;150:77–83.
85. Braibanti P, Strappa V, Zunino A. Psicologia sociale e promozione della salute. In: Volume I: Fondamenti psicologici e riflessioni critiche. Milan: Franco Angeli; 2009.
86. Goldbeck L, Vitiello B. Reporting clinical trials of psychosocial interventions in child and adolescent psychiatry and mental health. Child Adolesc Psychiatry Ment Health. 2011;5:4.
87. Saita E. Pensare alla salute e alla malattia: legami tra mente, corpo e contesto di appartenenza. Milan: EDU-Catt; 2014.
88. Simoncini A. Un "sé privo di sé": l'identità relazionale. Complexity Insitute. Testo disponibile al sito. 2013. http://www.complexityinstitute.it/?p=4406.
89. Di Pietro M, Bassi E. L'intervento cognitivo-comportamentale per l'età evolutiva: Strumenti di valutazione e tecniche per il trattamento. Trento: Edizioni Centro Studi Erickson; 2013.
90. Hicks M, Davitt K. Chronic illness and rehabilitation. In: Thompson RH, editor. The handbook of child life: a guide for pediatric psychosocial care. Springfield: Charles C Thomas Publisher, Ltd; 2018. p. 446–91.
91. Lattuada P. Oltre la mente: teoria e pratica della psicologia transpersonale. Milan: Franco Angeli; 2018.
92. Perricone Briulotta G. Manuale di psicologia dell'educazione. Una prospettiva ecologica per lo studio e per lo studio e l'intervento sul processo educativo. Milan: McGraw-Hill; 2005.
93. Perricone G, Polizzi C, De Luca F. Self-representation of children suffering from congenital heart disease and maternal competence. Pediatr Rep. 2013;5(1):1–7.
94. Marcoli A. Passaggi di vita. Le crisi che ci spingono a crescere. Milan: Edizioni Mondadori; 2004.
95. Kazak AE, Derosa BW, Schwartz LA, Hobbie W, Carlson C, Ittenbach RF, Mao JJ, Ginsberg JP. Psychological outcomes and health beliefs in adolescent and young adult survivors of childhood cancer and controls. J Clin Oncol. 2010;28(12):2002–7.
96. Righetti PL, Santoro L, Sinatora F, Ricca M, editors. Psicologia e pediatria. Strumenti per le professioni socio-sanitarie: Strumenti per le professioni socio-sanitarie. Milan: Franco Angeli; 2013.
97. Polizzi C, Fontana V, Perricone G, D'Angelo P, Jankovic M, Taormina C, Nichelli F, Burgio S. Coping strategies and locus of control in childhood leukemia: a multi-center research. Pediatr Rep. 2015;7(2):22–7.
98. Daft RL. Organizzazione aziendale. 7th ed. Santarcangelo: Maggioli Editore; 2004.
99. Lechner C, Floyd S. Attività di influenza del gruppo e realizzazione di iniziative strategiche. Giornale di gestionestrategica. 2012;33(5):478–95.
100. Wilson DK, Lawman HG, Roberts MC, Steele R. Health promotion in children and adolescents: an integration of the biopsychosocial model and ecological approaches to behavior change. In: Handbook of pediatric psychology, vol. 4. New York: Guilford Press; 2009. p. 603–17.
101. Bricolo MG, Bellamoli E, Serpelloni G. Rassegna dei modelli teorici di interpretazione della dipendenza da sostanze stupefacenti. Elementi di Neuroscienze e Dipendenze. 2010;2:8.

102. Kaitz JE, Ray S. Psychologist and physician interprofessional collaborative experiences in primary care integration. J Clin Psychol Med Settings. 2021;28(3):436–46.
103. Foronda C, MacWilliams B, McArthur E. Interprofessional communication in healthcare: an integrative review. Nurse Educ Pract. 2016;19:36–40.
104. Pirnejad H, Niazkhani Z, Berg M, Bal R. Intra-organizational communication in healthcare. Methods Inf Med. 2008;47(04):336–45.
105. Ravioli S. Verso una comunicazione istituzionale al servizio dell'inclusione sociale. Libertà civili. 2011;2:63–9.
106. Ferro E, Tosco E. Stili e strategie per comunicare la salute. In: Cucco E, Pagani R, Pasquali M, Soggia A, editors. Secondo Rapporto sulla comunicazione sociale in Italia. Carocci Editore: Rome; 2011.
107. Balducci C, Fraccaroli F. Stress lavoro-correlato: Questioni aperte e direzionifuture. G Ital Psicol. 2019;46(1–2):39–66.
108. De Carlo NA, Falco A, Capozza D. Stress, benessere organizzativo e performance. Valutazione e intervento per l'azienda positiva. Milan: Franco Angeli; 2013.
109. Radeva S. Communication problems in a medical organization. Knowl Int J. 2020;38(4):1005–10.
110. Schiavo R. Health communication: from theory to practice. Hoboken: Wiley; 2013.
111. Varvogli L, Darviri C. Stress management techniques: evidence-based procedures that reduce stress and promote health. Health Sci J. 2011;5(2):74–89.
112. World Health Organization. Guidelines for the management of conditions that are specifically related to stress. Geneva: World Health Organization; 2013.
113. World Health Organization. Communicating risk in public health emergencies: a WHO guideline for emergency risk communication (ERC) policy and practice. Geneva: World Health Organization; 2017.
114. Anolli L. Psicologia della comunicazione. Bologna: Il Mulino; 2006.
115. Carli R, Paniccia RM. Analisi della domanda: Teoria e tecnica dell'intervento in psicologia clinica. Bologna: Il Mulino; 2003.
116. Caramaschi G. I confini della comunicazione: discorsi, immagini, pratiche nella società dell'informazione. Bologna: CLUEB; 2008.
117. Rossi S, Travaglini R. I confini nei contesti relazionali. Dalla fusionalità alla temporalità. Milan: Franco Angeli; 2011.
118. Romani G. Fear appeal e message framing: strategie persuasive in interazione per la promozione della salute. Firenze: Firenze University Press; 2013.
119. Bianco F. Lo psicologo nelle cure primarie: dall'utenza alla realizzazione. Tesi di dottorato. Padua: Università degli Studi di Padova; 2018.
120. Vlasveld MC, Anema JR, Beekman AT, van Mechelen W, Hoedeman R, van Marwijk HW, et al. Multidisciplinary collaborative care for depressive disorder in the occupational health setting: design of a randomised controlled trial and cost-effectiveness study. BMC Health Serv Res. 2008;8(1):1–12.
121. Ashforth BE, Harrison SH, Corley KG. Identification in organizations: an examination of four fundamental questions. J Manag. 2008;34(3):325–74.
122. Schuman H, Presser S. Questions and answers in attitude surveys: experiments on question form, wording, and context. Thousand Oaks: Sage; 1996.
123. Rizzo ML. Modelli e strumenti di supporto alla scelta informata del paziente: unargine alla medicinadifensiva. Bologna: Università di Bologna; 2015.
124. Di Cori R, Fedeli N, Sabatello U. Traiettorie evolutive e possibili destini del trauma nell'infanzia. Dal minore vittima al giovane autore di reati sessuali. Rassegna italiana di criminologia VI. 2012;4:259–71.
125. Facchini R. I più comuni traumi nel pronto soccorso pediatrico. In: Scritti medici in onore e memoria di Vincenzo Pietrogrande. Milan: Keyword Europa; 2006. p. 145–54.
126. Hopper JW, Frewen PA, van der Kolk BA, Lanius RA. Neural correlates of reexperiencing, avoidance, and dissociation in PTSD: symptom dimensions and emotion dysregulation in responses to script-driven trauma imagery. J Trauma Stress. 2007;20(5):713–25.
127. Van Der Kolk BA. Il corpo accusa il colpo. Mente, corpo e cervello nell'elaborazione della memoria traumatica. Milan: Raffaello Cortina; 2015.
128. Matar M, Van der Hart O. Amnesia dissociativa e trauma: una prospettiva secondo la teoria della dissociazione strutturale. Rivista Sperimentale Freniatria. 2012;2007:121–35.
129. Clerici CA, Giacon B, Veneroni L, Ferrari A, Luksch R, Meazza C, et al. Disturbi psico-organici in bambini e adolescenti affetti da neoplasie pediatriche. Minerva Pediatr. 2013;65:651–67.
130. De Cillis S, Mauro M, Romagnoni A. Il disturbo specifico dell'apprendimento come conseguenza di un evento traumatico complesso e di un attaccamento insicuro. Psiba: Quaderno dell'Istituto di Psicoterapia del bambino e dell'adolescente. 2017;46(2):97–109.
131. Panti M. Difficoltà Di Apprendimento Come Sintomo. Legami, Trauma E Identità Psiba: Quaderno dell'Istituto di Psicoterapia del bambino e dell'adolescente. 2018;47:1.
132. Simonetta E. Il corpo che apprende: per una nuova teoria dei DSA. Milan: Mimesis Edizioni; 2014. p. 1–110.
133. Raichle ME. The brain's default mode network. Annu Rev Neurosci. 2015;38:433–47.

134. Muetzel RL, Blanken LM, Thijssen S, van derLugt A, Jaddoe VW, Verhulst FC, et al. Resting-state networks in 6-to-10 year old children. Hum Brain Mapp. 2016;37(12):4286–300.
135. Patriat R, Birn RM, Keding TJ, Herringa RJ. Default-mode network abnormalities in pediatric posttraumatic stress disorder. J Am Acad Child Adolesc Psychiatry. 2016;55(4):319–27.
136. Van der Kolk BA, D'Andrea W. Verso una diagnosi di disturbo traumatico dello sviluppo per il trauma interpersonale infantile. In: Lanius RA, Vermetten E, Pain C, editors. L'impatto del trauma infantile sulla salute e sulla malattia. L'epidemia nascosta. Rome: Fioriti Editore; 2010. p. 57–68.
137. Carati MA, Dell'Erba GL. I disturbi dell'adattamento. Un modello di concettualizzazione. Cognitivismo clinico. 2014;11(2):207–26.

Part V

Conclusions

Follow-Up to Ensure Continuity of Care and Support Preventive Care

16

Giuliana Ferrante, Vincenzo Antona, Mario Giuffrè, Ettore Piro, Gregorio Serra, and Giovanni Corsello

16.1 Introduction

Over the last decades, the prevalence of chronic health conditions and disabilities among children rose steadily, thanks to medical advances in both treating the primary condition and managing its complications. The improved long-term survival rates led to persistently high rates of pediatric chronic health conditions [1], which are often burdened with limitation in daily activity and dependence on medication, special diets, medical technology, assistive devices, and specialized staff. Therefore, children with complex chronic conditions are a frail population who generally need healthcare services beyond what is usual for healthy children [2]. Indeed, their health issues often require specialized and continuing care. Such specificities expose this population to become highly vulnerable. The healthcare services are generally poorly efficient in delivering continuity of care for chronic health conditions. As a matter of fact, healthcare services are mainly focused on delivering urgent care, whereas the management of children with chronic health problems is still suboptimal. Poor and disadvantaged children are at even greater risk, with an increased need for hospitalization and high costs for the healthcare system as a whole.

Children and adolescents with chronic health conditions have special needs in each stage of the disease that should be managed in a proactive way [3]. Indeed, many of them require complex care plans with long-term treatments and assistance imposing a high economic burden on the healthcare system. Thus, the progressive change in the pediatric morbidity profile implies an urgent remodeling of healthcare systems in order to meet the special needs of frail children, overcoming the organization of existing care models aimed at treating acute conditions. Noteworthy, planning for healthcare services directed to children with complex chronic diseases must take into account relevant differences in the needs of this population compared with adults [4, 5]. In particular, their developmental status and the key role played by parents/caregivers in the interaction between the child and the healthcare services and providers [6] should be considered along with the relevant role of the school environment in shaping the social development of schoolchildren and adolescents.

Continuity of care is directed toward those subjects who need to access healthcare services over time [7] and is crucial for children with special healthcare needs. Continuity of care of such

G. Ferrante · V. Antona · M. Giuffrè · E. Piro · G. Serra · G. Corsello (✉)
Department of Health Promotion, Mother and Child Care, Internal Medicine and Medical Specialties "G. D'Alessandro", University Hospital "P. Giaccone", Palermo, Italy
e-mail: giuliana.ferrante@unipa.it; mario.giuffre@unipa.it; ettore.piro@unipa.it; gregorio.serra@unipa.it; giovanni.corsello@unipa.it

M. Lima, M. C. Mondardini (eds.), *Frailty in Children*,
https://doi.org/10.1007/978-3-031-24307-3_16

children should be oriented to a comprehensive and tailored approach toward each individual. According to the American Academy of Pediatrics, comprehensive health care should ensure continuity, providing care over an extended period of time, and organizing transitions both to other pediatric providers and into the adult healthcare system [8]. Three types of continuity of care were identified across healthcare settings: relational, informational, and management. Relational continuity refers to an ongoing relationship between a patient and one or more healthcare providers; informational continuity is defined as "the use of information from prior events and circumstances to make current care appropriate for the individual and his or her condition"; management continuity is defined as the prompt provision of complementary services delivered by a variety of providers within a shared management plan [9, 10].

In pediatrics, some studies have demonstrated that high continuity of care is associated to decreased emergency department (ED) visits [11, 12], increased therapeutic adherence [13], and improved receipt of preventive screening [14]. Nearly 1 in 7 pediatric ED visits may be preventable and thus associated with continuity [15]. In addition, a positive association between continuity of care in childhood and improved preventive care has been observed [14]. Providers who are more familiar with their patients may have more time to address preventive screening topics. Moreover, higher continuity is associated with higher parental knowledge of anticipatory guidance topics [16]. Discussing the benefits of continuity with parents may also improve continuity itself. Furthermore, continuity influences parental trust and perceptions about the quality of care and coordination of healthcare services [17–19]. Therefore, assuring continuity is the key to high-quality pediatric primary care [20]. Otherwise, limitations in the continuity of care may contribute to the suboptimal clinical management of children and adolescents with chronic diseases, leading to unnecessary hospital admissions. Parents of children with complex care needs frequently attend pediatric EDs, with a study from England showing that 77% of children with four or more ED admissions over 12 months had a chronic disease [21]. The provision of fragmented care and the poor coordination between healthcare services underline the need for identifying efficient strategies to improve this network. The clinical follow-up of frail children should include high-quality care programs with enough patient volume to support both clinical expertise and ancillary services to address their special needs. Subspecialty units and primary care providers may collaborate on many aspects of care. Such organization would facilitate data gathering, enabling comparisons among centers, and rapid translation of new research findings into clinical practice [22]. Recognizing the relevance of ensuring the quality of subspecialty care, several organizations have set training programs to support healthcare professionals in delivering the most appropriate care for children with complex needs. Studies reported heterogeneous experiences of accessing subspecialty care by families of children with complex conditions [23], especially in children's hospitals. Some issues that families have identified were a lack of awareness of community resources, fragmented services delivery, and inconstant ability to meet linguistic and cultural needs [24, 25].

16.2 Models of Care Delivery for Children with Complex Conditions

The need for obtaining substantial improvements in care delivery for children with complex conditions led to the rapid proliferation in the creation of new models of care [26] aimed at delivering a set of services provided by a defined team, assessment-driven, and designed to address the needs of patients and their family. Continuity, familiarity, accessibility, and partnership are key elements in enhancing care coordination. Models of care can be divided into three categories: primary care-centered (PCC) models, consultative- or co-management-centered (CC) models, and episode-based (EB) models (Table 16.1). **PCC** models of care function as a single location for comprehensive primary care and care coordination services. They may be community- or tertiary care-based and rely on the strength of long-term relationships

Table 16.1 Main characteristics of the three categories of models of care for children with complex conditions

Model	PCC	CC	EB
Examples	Community-based; tertiary care center	Ambulatory; tertiary care center	Inpatient service; transitional facility
Services provided	Comprehensive primary care; preventive care/anticipatory guidance; care coordination services	Co-management of medical issues; subspecialties visits; care coordination services	Management of acute medical issues; bedside care; care coordination services
Target population	Local patients	Patients with rare diseases who need frequent subspecialties visits and high levels of technology for assistance	Patients with frequent/prolonged hospitalizations; patients using new medical technologies; patients undergoing surgery

Modified by *Pordes E, Gordon J, Sanders LM, Cohen E. Models of Care Delivery for Children With Medical Complexity. Pediatrics. 2018; 141 (Suppl 3): S212–S223*

between primary care practitioners, families, and their local communities. Advantages include the proximity to a patient's home, an understanding of the local context and cultures, an ability to provide care for family members [27]. Barriers to delivering care within these models may include costs and time needed to provide services, lack of communication and coordination, inadequate knowledge to address complex acute illness, and limited personnel and community resources [28]. Interventions to overcome these issues may include the involvement of nonphysician care coordinators and external case managers, longer and more frequent visits, parental advisory groups, and telemedicine. **CC** models are those in which providers in subspecialty programs, or more general complex care programs at tertiary care centers, deliver care services, often in partnership with primary care practitioners. CC models are commonly focused on care coordination services and co-management of medical issues, providing a link between the tertiary care center and the community [29]. Providers involved in these models are well trained to care for frail children who need frequent subspecialties visits and high levels of technology for assistance. However, it should be pointed out that the centralization of resources and expertise in tertiary care centers possibly makes difficult the remote management of acute illness and communication with local services. **EB** models of care deliver location-limited interventions for a specific illness episode or for a defined period. The main advantage is the ability of trained staff to deliver care when children and their families are most vulnerable. Nonetheless, there is a risk that chronic needs are not met because acute health issues are prioritized. To improve care within this model, hospital staff could be involved in a child's care beyond the period of hospitalization [30]. Transitional facilities also represent an emerging strategy to improve continuity. These facilities can be used when the child is stabilized but cannot come back to the community for a variety of reasons. Children, and sometimes their families, can reside for a period of time at these locations where caregivers acquire the skills for home management and children receive therapies.

There is evidence that several gaps in care are common across models. Integrating information and services from a variety of sources (e.g., schools, the home, social, and medical services) is complex. The inclusion of social workers in care teams and the implementation of novel technologies enabling communication between social and medical services [31], may link medical and community services with the aim to develop the ideal "patient-centered medical neighborhood". Moreover, few care delivery systems are targeted for children with primary mental health issues, and few models integrate mental health services. Additionally, there are few standards of practice for transitioning children to adult health care and few adult care providers are appropriately trained and/or interested in caring for complex childhood-onset diseases. Ideal models of care include partnerships with adult medical providers to ensure the continuation of coordinated care services and structured planning for care transition [32]. Moreover, an ideal care delivery model for children with complex conditions should include proactive plans based on family and children's requirements, ensuring prompt treatment of acute health issues and shared decision-making to address comprehensive needs [33]. An ideal care delivery system for children with medical complexity should also ease parental financial, time, and emotional burdens through support strategies such as in-home care, access to respite facilities, increased financial resources, and adult mental and physical healthcare services. There is currently a lack of studies comparing different models of care for children with medical complexity. Given the heterogeneous needs across a child's life, probably no one-size-fits-all approach exists in facilitating optimum care for this population. Ongoing research to develop standardized outcome measures and evaluate existing care delivery systems is essential to ensure the delivery of high-value care for children with complex conditions [34].

16.3 Assuring High Quality of Care and Best Outcomes for Children with Complex Conditions

There is no simple solution for achieving an efficient system of care delivery for chronic conditions [35]. Advances in the care strategies for people with chronic conditions are required, as it is recognized that the biomedical model approach, merely based on the prescriptive act, is not thoroughly efficient nowadays. Successful experiences indicate the need for the coordination of all healthcare sectors to overcome the possible practice gaps in providing continuity of care [36]. The adoption of a comprehensive approach by policymakers, managers, and healthcare providers is necessary to recognize the needs of frail children and their families.

Key aspects in the follow-up of children with chronic conditions are: the collaborative care between the general practitioner and the specialist, the shared care, in addition to supported self-management. The collaboration among professionals improves the efficiency and the continuity of care. Children with complex care needs have to access multiple points of care to treat their conditions as well as to monitor their psychophysical development [37]. This requires a coordination of efforts to guarantee a continuum of preventive, curative, and rehabilitation care delivery. The general value of various specialized treatments such as speech and language therapy, physical therapy, and respiratory care is well recognized. Nonetheless, efforts should also address both primary and secondary prevention, that is, preventing the onset of a condition and preventing the consequences of a condition, respectively. In frail children, improved outcomes also may result from the prevention of serious disability in adulthood [38]. Through the limited available evidence, integrated care models have the potential to improve care processes, health outcomes, and patient experience [39, 40]. The communication between professionals could be facilitated by the use of shared medical records. This is particularly relevant when the monitoring process after discharge involves primary care professionals and hospital specialists. Family pediatricians are key persons playing a mediating and coordinating role in the network of clinicians and service providers. However, a study investigating the willingness and ability of pediatricians to accept children with special healthcare needs into their practice reported that they do not feel adequate to care for all types of conditions and this reduces the ability to implement effective medical home care [41].

The shared care ensures the development of expanded partnerships among healthcare professionals and between the professionals and the population and could increase co-responsibility and an acknowledged positive evaluation of users [42]. Shared decision-making should be individualized according to the preferences of patients/families [7].

Self-management and the empowerment process aiming to provide skills to manage the child both during hospitalization and at home is another issue of extreme relevance from the parents' perspective [43]. Providing caregivers with specific tools about the medical care of their children and referrals for social services during the transition to home and thereafter may empower families and improve health outcomes [44]. Special efforts should be made to reach an effective alliance between healthcare providers and families in order to sustain and ameliorate children's care. A personalized written plan enabling the identification of the procedures to be adopted in case of acute illness can be considered a useful strategy to support parent engagement and strengthen the partnership between parents and clinicians.

Evaluating the team composition along with the activities performed can be useful in order to identify possible solutions to achieve the best integrated care models [45], such as phone services to support primary care physicians for questions about treatment or diagnosis, and nonphysician care coordinators to ensure access to social services [46]. Another solution can be the dissemination of emerging technologies, including mobile applications, telemedicine, patient portals, video chat, and other web-based resources, which can facilitate the monitoring of symptoms, increase adherence to treatments, and connect patients with each other. Implementation of telehealth into pediatric patient-centered care is suitable for managing safely and effectively some pediatric conditions. In particular, during a state of emergency, such as the COVID-19 pandemic, telemedicine can play a central role in supporting physicians with the management of children with complex medical conditions. Telemedicine involves the use of information and communication technologies to improve patient outcomes by increasing access to care and medical information [47] and might provide an additional resource, replacing in-person visits [48, 49]. Moreover, it offers the opportunity to bridge many divides, including geographical and logistical challenges. Implementing a combined model using both in-person and remote visits can help integrate face-to-face evaluation with the need to ensure continuity of care [50]. Although socioeconomic status may influence access to the Internet and other technologies, these tools hold the potential to improve the delivery of care for chronic conditions, enabling follow-up in a more flexible manner. This may be relevant for minority and low-income families who often have to face additional barriers related to transportation, language, and cultural issues [34]. Parents could provide information about their child's status daily or weekly, allowing the medical staff to review the data in real time, decide about treatment changes, and evaluate the actual need for clinical visits [51]. Lastly, investment in the training of healthcare professionals, along with investment in adequate therapeutic projects, network services, and care resources is urgent. With adequate training, community healthcare professionals can acquire the skills and knowledge necessary to provide appropriate care. Through such an approach, the savings from high-cost urgent visits will balance the costs of strengthening continuity [42].

A set of benchmarks for implementation of integrated care for children with complex diseases is shown in Fig. 16.1. These benchmarks

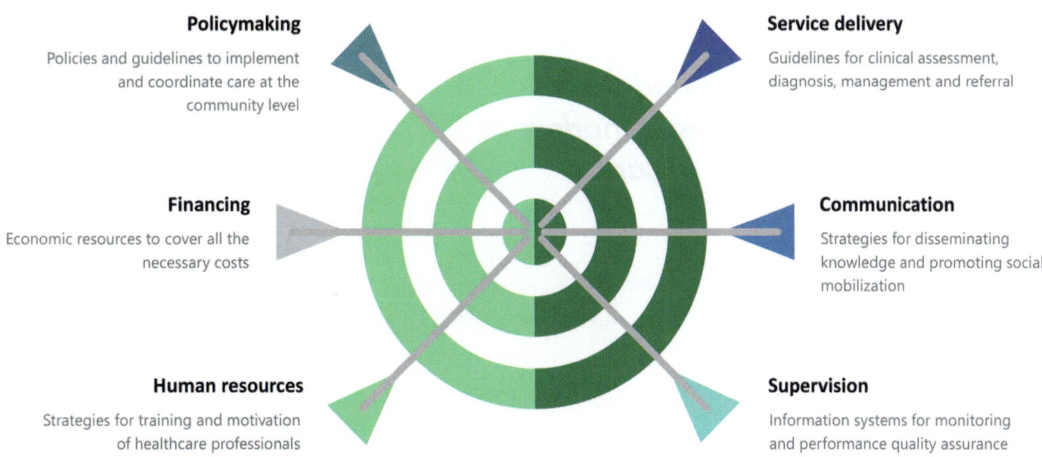

Fig. 16.1 Benchmarks for implementation of integrated care for children with complex diseases

will help to define the support for operational activities, identify research priorities, and disseminate good practices implementation [52].

16.4 Promoting Integrated, Coordinated, and Child-and-Family-Centered Models of Care

The UN Convention on the Rights of the Child states that the highest attainable standard of healthcare is a fundamental right of every child [53]. In real life, achieving an optimal health status means taking into account the child's subjective well-being as well as the ability to perform daily activities and participate socially at home, school, and in the community [54]. To reach this goal, frail children require a variety of services encompassing medical and nursing assistance, rehabilitation, educational, social, and family support services (Fig. 16.2) [55, 56]. The connection between different kinds of services and different providers is a prerequisite for the healthcare system to help children and families cope with chronic illness and disability. Hence, efforts are needed in order to set new models of care that emphasize coordinated services focused on child and family needs [46, 55, 57].

The care of children with chronic conditions can be highly demanding and interfere with everyday family life. Nowadays, many needs (e.g., care coordination, medication management, mental health) frequently go unmet [58], and families are often burdened with the responsibility of providing medical and/or nursing assistance and ensuring care coordination for their children. Parents of frail children often report increased stress, decreased sleep quality, and a sense of frustration since they are fully absorbed by care coordination, administration, and advocacy activities [59]. The need for care at home after discharge from the hospital usually generates anxiety, insecurity, and scare. This underline how could be important, in the period preceding hospital discharge, preparing the fam-

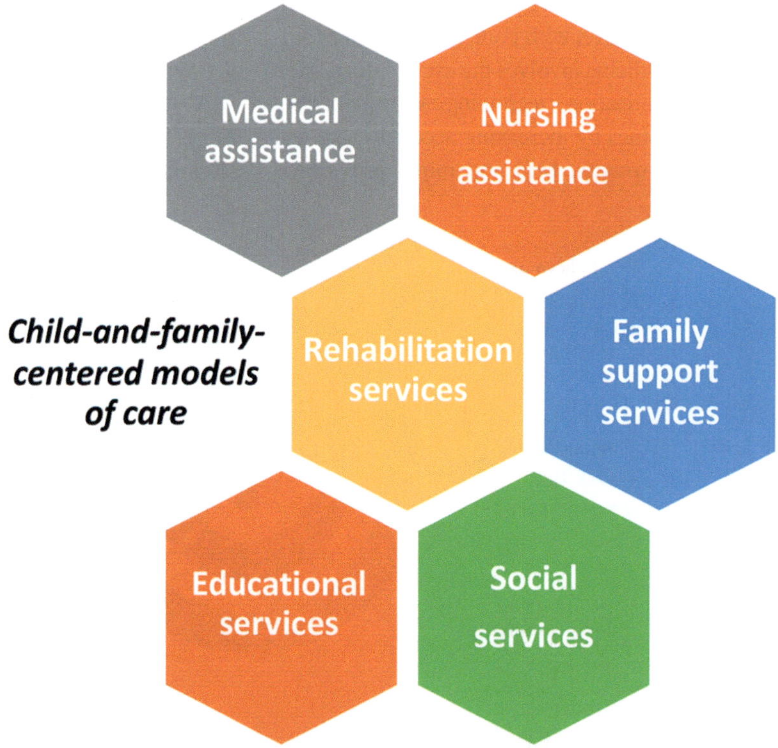

Fig. 16.2 Variety of services in child-and-family-centered care

ily for home care, considering the social context and that each caregiver may experience the child's condition in a different way. Therefore, professionals should be inserted into the family context in order to know its structure and functioning, identify the specific needs, and provide comprehensive care to all members [60]. A smooth organization of care would imply a reduced burden for the parents caring for children with chronic diseases. On the contrary, the lack of patient/parent acceptance may exacerbate the vulnerability of these families by creating a sense of insecurity and doubts about their competence in care [61]. The presence of a social worker either in the hospital or in the primary care setting may help to embrace the social component in order to identify and accomplish the child and family needs.

16.5 The Models of Child Health Appraised (MOCHA) Project

The complex care needs of children with chronic conditions pose great challenges for healthcare systems, due to many reasons: they require medical and social care over a long period as well as coordinated delivery services; minor illnesses must be addressed in the context of the primary complex health condition; the clinical presentation can be rare, thereby challenging diagnosis and care management. Special healthcare needs in children are a field of interest of the Models of Child Health Appraised (MOCHA) project [61]. MOCHA is the first systematic study evaluating how different systems of primary care for children in Europe address the needs of children and their families. Results from the MOCHA project showed that countries across Europe have few systems for identifying all the healthcare providers who deliver care to children with complex needs. In particular, less than half of the 30 countries involved in the project have adopted policies to support integrated healthcare services for children with complex diseases. Integration of care is at different stages of progress for different clinical situations. Primary care physicians are generally little involved in care planning for children before their discharge from the hospital. There is poor parental participation in policy development; nonetheless, non-governmental organizations have been increasingly involved in communicating family issues to government representatives. Common barriers to integration of care across Europe include poor care coordination, lack of standards of care, inadequate clinical expertise and specialist training, geographical heterogeneity in care delivery, limited resources for service development and insufficient implementation of electronic health records, and scarce access to psychosocial services [62]. As part of the MOCHA project, core principles and standards for the effective, personalized care of children with special healthcare needs were established with the aim to improve the quality of care and support parents/caregivers. The core principles include access to care, co-creation of care, and effective integrated governance. **Access to care** refers to high-quality, prompt, and accessible care services that are equitably available to all groups within the population to meet their needs and improve their health status. **Co-creation of care** refers to the ability to design, develop, deliver, and evaluate health and social care-related support. Specifically, this principle focuses on transitioning to home as well as transitioning to adult services, supporting a partnership approach to prepare the family to care for the child at home, and the development of a plan of care for facilitating the transition to adult services. **Effective integrated governance** refers to the governance necessary to enhance and support the delivery of integrated, equitable, accessible, and responsive care services to children with complex health conditions. The MOCHA principles rely on a child-centric approach to the delivery of care. The application of these principles is obviously influenced by each individual child's needs, stage of development, and age, in the context of the family and socioeconomic background. Nonetheless, these principles offer a means to press policy in relation to service delivery for children with special health needs, to evaluate existing services, and to function as indicators to guide future service development in this field [63].

16.6 Conclusions

The increased prevalence of multidisciplinary and multiprofessional health conditions in childhood over the last decades, requires urgent efforts to improve the care of affected children. The economic and social burden of childhood disability involves both the present and the future, through growing demands on support for healthcare and social needs. Meeting the needs of frail children will require targeting clinical, developmental, functional, and quality of life outcomes. Promising results could arise from the spread of condition-specific networks that gather patients and scientists in order to enhance the quality of care. Critical will be translating research findings into specific interventions to improve outcomes in real life. Major changes will also require investment in community and social services to make children and their families less dependent on the healthcare sector.

Comprehensive and integrated systems of care will ensure that frail children receive all those services that can improve their daily activities and their ability to take part in social and educational activities. Through this, integrated care should include health services as part of a whole system of prevention and care in both primary care and subspecialty units that is coordinated, comprehensive, team-based, and multidisciplinary. Information systems to support monitoring and communication among levels of care and with parents and children will be therefore fundamental. It will be also crucial to focus on key areas of child and adolescent short- and long-term functioning and development, as well as to better assess their physical and social environment. If these actions are not taken, the growing number of children with chronic conditions and associated disabilities will pose a substantial burden on healthcare and social services; in addition to this, childhood disability is expected to lead to major health and social impairments among a large number of young adults in the next decade [64]. Hence, it is time for an inter-governmental strategy to help ensure that policies dedicated to the rights and needs of children with chronic health conditions receive the attention and budget they urgently deserve [65], with equity and homogeneous distribution. Indeed, even though the prevalence of complex medical conditions has increased overall, the burden disproportionately affects vulnerable populations. Disparities by ethnicity and language may limit access to healthcare services. Therefore, barriers faced by racial/ethnic minority groups or those of low socioeconomic status and poor health literacy should be addressed to avoid that social disparities could leave out children and their families who traditionally have poor access to care.

References

1. Tommiska V, Heinonen K, Lehtonen L, Renlund M, Saarela T, Tammela O, Virtanen M, Fellman V. No improvement in outcome of nationwide extremely low birth weight infant populations between 1996–1997 and 1999–2000. Pediatrics. 2007;119(1):29–36. https://doi.org/10.1542/peds.2006-1472.
2. Stein RE, Bauman LJ, Westbrook LE, Coupey SM, Ireys HT. Framework for identifying children who have chronic conditions: the case for a new definition. J Pediatr. 1993;122(3):342–7. https://doi.org/10.1016/s0022-3476(05)83414-6.
3. Nóbrega VMD, Silva MEA, Fernandes LTB, Viera CS, Reichert APDS, Collet N. Chronic disease in childhood and adolescence: continuity of care in the health care network. Rev Esc Enferm USP. 2017;51:e03226. https://doi.org/10.1590/S1980-220X2016042503226.
4. Miller AR, Recsky MA, Armstrong RW. Responding to the needs of children with chronic health conditions in an era of health services reform. CMAJ. 2004;171:1366–7. https://doi.org/10.1503/cmaj.1040019.
5. Forrest CB, Simpson L, Clancy C. Child health services research. Challenges and opportunities. JAMA. 1997;277:1787–93.
6. Miller AR, Condin CJ, McKellin WH, Shaw N, Klassen AF, Sheps S. Continuity of care for children with complex chronic health conditions: parents' perspectives. BMC Health Serv Res. 2009;9:242. https://doi.org/10.1186/1472-6963-9-242.
7. Zanello E, Calugi S, Rucci P, Pieri G, Vandini S, Faldella G, Fantini MP. Continuity of care in children with special healthcare needs: a qualitative study of family's perspectives. Ital J Pediatr. 2015;41:7. https://doi.org/10.1186/s13052-015-0114-x.
8. American Academy of Pediatrics. Medical home initiatives for children with special needs project advisory committee. The medical home. Pediatrics. 2002;110(1 Pt 1):184–6.
9. Haggerty JL, Reid RJ, Freeman GK, Starfield BH, Adair CE, McKendry R. Continuity of care: a multi-

disciplinary review. BMJ. 2003;327:1219–21. https://doi.org/10.1136/bmj.327.7425.1219.
10. Reid R, Haggerty J, McKendry R. Defusing the confusion: concepts and measures of continuity of healthcare. Ottawa: Canadian Health Services Research Foundation (CHSRF); 2002.
11. Christakis DA, Mell L, Koepsell TD, Zimmerman FJ, Connell FA. Association of lower continuity of care with greater risk of emergency department use and hospitalization in children. Pediatrics. 2001;107(3):524–9. https://doi.org/10.1542/peds.107.3.524.
12. Brousseau DC, Meurer JR, Isenberg ML, Kuhn EM, Gorelick MH. Association between infant continuity of care and pediatric emergency department utilization. Pediatrics. 2004;113(4):738–41. https://doi.org/10.1542/peds.107.3.524.
13. D'Agostino JA, Passarella M, Saynisch P, Martin AE, Macheras M, Lorch SA. Preterm infant attendance at health supervision visits. Pediatrics. 2015;136(4):e794–802. https://doi.org/10.1542/peds.2015-0745.
14. Flores AI, Bilker WB, Alessandrini EA. Effects of continuity of care in infancy on receipt of lead, anemia, and tuberculosis screening. Pediatrics. 2008;121(3):e399–406. https://doi.org/10.1542/peds.2007-1497.
15. Jaeger MW, Ambadwar PB, King AJ, Onukwube JI, Robbins JM. Emergency care of children with ambulatory care sensitive conditions in the United States. J Emerg Med. 2015;49(5):729–39. https://doi.org/10.1016/j.jemermed.2015.03.001.
16. Bradford WD, Kaste LM, Nietert PJ. Continuity of medical care, health insurance, and nonmedical advice in the first 3 years of life. Med Care. 2004;42(1):91–8. https://doi.org/10.1097/01.mlr.0000102368.39193.5a.
17. Christakis DA, Wright JA, Zimmerman FJ, Bassett AL, Connell FA. Continuity of care is associated with high-quality care by parental report. Pediatrics. 2002;109(4):e54. https://doi.org/10.1542/peds.109.4.e54.
18. Christakis DA, Wright JA, Zimmerman FJ, Bassett AL, Connell FA. Continuity of care is associated with well coordinated care. Ambul Pediatr. 2003;3(2):82–6. https://doi.org/10.1367/1539-4409(2003)003<0082:cociaw>2.0.co;2.
19. Horn IB, Mitchell SJ, Wang J, Joseph JG, Wissow LS. African-American parents' trust in their child's primary care provider. Acad Pediatr. 2012;12(5):399–404. https://doi.org/10.1016/j.acap.2012.06.003.
20. Enlow E, Passarella M, Lorch SA. Continuity of care in infancy and early childhood health outcomes. Pediatrics. 2017;140(1):e20170339. https://doi.org/10.1542/peds.2017-0339.
21. Wiljaars LP, Gilbert R, Hardelid P. Chronic conditions in children and young people: learning from administrative data. Arch Dis Child. 2016;101:881–5. https://doi.org/10.1136/archdischild-2016-310716.
22. Cooley WC, Kemper AR, Medical Home Workgroup of the National Coordinating Center for the Regional Genetic and Newborn Screening Service Collaboratives. An approach to family-centered coordinated co-management for individuals with conditions identified through newborn screening. Genet Med. 2013;15(3):174–7. https://doi.org/10.1038/gim.2012.122.
23. Cohen E, Jovcevska V, Kuo DZ, Mahant S. Hospital-based comprehensive care programs for children with special health care needs: a systematic review. Arch Pediatr Adolesc Med. 2011;165(6):554–61. https://doi.org/10.1001/archpediatrics.2011.74.
24. Zuckerman KE, Chavez AE, Reeder JA. Decreasing disparities in child development assessment: identifying and discussing possible delays in the special supplemental nutrition program for women, infants, and children (WIC). J Dev Behav Pediatr. 2017;38(5):301–9. https://doi.org/10.1097/DBP.0000000000000446.
25. Lakshmanan A, Kubicek K, Williams R, Robles M, Vanderbilt DL, Mirzaian CB, Friedlich PS, Kipke M. Viewpoints from families for improving transition from NICU-to-home for infants with medical complexity at a safety net hospital: a qualitative study. BMC Pediatr. 2019;19(1):223. https://doi.org/10.1186/s12887-019-1604-6.
26. Mosquera RA, Avritscher EB, Samuels CL, Harris TS, Pedroza C, Evans P, Navarro F, Wootton SH, Pacheco S, Clifton G, Moody S, Franzini L, Zupancic J, Tyson JE. Effect of an enhanced medical home on serious illness and cost of care among high-risk children with chronic illness: a randomized clinical trial. JAMA. 2014;312(24):2640–8. https://doi.org/10.1001/jama.2014.16419.
27. Morin MJ, Alvery J, Murphy N, Glader L. Models of care for children with medical complexity. In: Rubin L, Merrick J, Greydanus DE, Patel DR, editors. Health care for people with intellectual and developmental disabilities across the lifespan. 3rd ed. Cham: Springer; 2016. p. 195–208.
28. Van Cleave J, Okumura MJ, Swigonski N, O'Connor KG, Mann M, Lail JL. Medical homes for children with special health care needs: primary care or subspecialty service? Acad Pediatr. 2016;16(4):366–72. https://doi.org/10.1016/j.acap.2015.10.009.
29. Cohen E, Lacombe-Duncan A, Spalding K, MacInnis J, Nicholas D, Narayanan UG, Gordon M, Margolis I, Friedman JN. Integrated complex care coordination for children with medical complexity: a mixed-methods evaluation of tertiary care-community collaboration. BMC Health Serv Res. 2012;12:366. https://doi.org/10.1186/1472-6963-12-366.
30. Simon TD, Mahant S, Cohen E. Pediatric hospital medicine and children with medical complexity: past, present, and future. Curr Probl Pediatr Adolesc Health Care. 2012;42(5):113–9. https://doi.org/10.1016/j.cppeds.2012.01.002.
31. Nguyen OK, Chan CV, Makam A, Stieglitz H, Amarasingham R. Envisioning a social-health information exchange as a platform to support a patient-centered medical neighborhood: a feasibility study. J Gen Intern Med. 2015;30(1):60–7. https://doi.org/10.1007/s11606-014-2969-8.

32. Schor EL. Transition: changing old habits. Pediatrics. 2015;135(6):958–60.
33. Berry JG, Agrawal RK, Cohen E, Kuo DZ. The landscape of medical care for children with medical complexity. Lenexa: Children's Hospital Association; 2013.
34. Pordes E, Gordon J, Sanders LM, Cohen E. Models of care delivery for children with medical complexity. Pediatrics. 2018;141(Suppl 3):S212–23. https://doi.org/10.1542/peds.2017-1284F.
35. Lima RAG. Chronic conditions and the challenges for knowledge production in health. Rev Latino Am Enfermagem. 2013;21(5):1011–2.
36. Rosenthal MP. Childhood asthma: considerations for primary care practice and chronic disease management in the village of care. Prim Care. 2012;39(2):381–91. https://doi.org/10.1016/j.pop.2012.04.001.
37. Brenner M, Kidston C, Hilliard C, Coyne I, Eustace-Cook J, Doyle C, Begley T, Barrett MJ. Children's complex care needs: a systematic concept analysis of multidisciplinary language. Eur J Pediatr. 2018;177(11):1641–52. https://doi.org/10.1007/s00431-018-3216-9.
38. Guyer B, Ma S, Grason H, Frick KD, Perry DF, Sharkey A, McIntosh J. Early childhood health promotion and its life course health consequences. Acad Pediatr. 2009;9(3):142–149.e1. https://doi.org/10.1016/j.acap.2008.12.007.
39. Wolfe I. Health services for children with long-term conditions and non-communicable diseases. In: Wolfe I, McKee M, editors. European child health services and systems: lessons without borders. Maidenhead: Open University Press; 2013. p. 63–93.
40. Asarnow JR, Rozenman M, Wiblin J, Zeltzer L. Integrated medical-behavioral care compared with usual primary care for child and adolescent behavioral health: a meta-analysis. JAMA Pediatr. 2015;169(10):929–37. https://doi.org/10.1001/jamapediatrics.2015.1141.
41. Agrawal R, Shah P, Zebracki K, Sanabria K, Kohrman C, Kohrman AF. The capacity of primary care pediatricians to care for children with special health care needs. Clin Pediatr (Phila). 2013;52(4):310–4. https://doi.org/10.1177/0009922813476572.
42. Duarte ED, Silva KL, Tavares TS, Nishimoto CLJ, Silva PM, Sena RR. Care of children with a chronic condition in primary care: challenges to the healthcare model. Texto Contexto Enferm. 2015;24(4):1009–17.
43. Souza JMOD, Magro MCS. Supported self-management as a tool to combat chronic conditions in Brazilian primary health care context. Nurse Care Open Access J. 2017;4(1):00100.
44. Fleegler EW, Lieu TA, Wise PH, Muret-Wagstaff S. Families' health-related social problems and missed referral opportunities. Pediatrics. 2007;119(6):e1332–41. https://doi.org/10.1542/peds.2006-1505.
45. Luzi D, Pecoraro F, Tamburis O, O'Shea M, Larkin P, Berry J, Brenner M. Modelling collaboration of primary and secondary care for children with complex care needs: long-term ventilation as an example. Eur J Pediatr. 2019;178(6):891–901. https://doi.org/10.1007/s00431-019-03367-y.
46. Antonelli RC, McAllister JW, Popp J. Making care coordination a critical component of the pediatric health care system: a multidisciplinary framework. New York: Commonwealth Fund; 2009.
47. Telemedicine—World Health Organization. https://www.who.int/goe/publications/goe_telemedicine_2010.pdf.
48. Orozco-Beltran D, Sánchez-Molla M, Sanchez JJ, Mira JJ, ValCrònic Research Group. Telemedicine in primary care for patients with chronic conditions: the ValCrònic quasi-experimental study. J Med Internet Res. 2017;19(12):e400. https://doi.org/10.2196/jmir.7677.
49. Brophy PD. Overview on the challenges and benefits of using telehealth tools in a pediatric population. Adv Chronic Kidney Dis. 2017;24:17–21. https://doi.org/10.1053/j.ackd.2016.12.003.
50. Milne Wenderlich A, Herendeen N. Telehealth in pediatric primary care. Curr Probl Pediatr Adolesc Health Care. 2021;51(1):100951. https://doi.org/10.1016/j.cppeds.2021.100951.
51. Perrin JM, Anderson LE, Van Cleave J. The rise in chronic conditions among infants, children, and youth can be met with continued health system innovations. Health Aff (Millwood). 2014;33(12):2099–105. https://doi.org/10.1377/hlthaff.2014.0832.
52. Young M, Wolfheim C, Marsh DR, Hammamy D. World Health Organization/United Nations Children's Fund joint statement on integrated community case management: an equity-focused strategy to improve access to essential treatment services for children. Am J Trop Med Hyg. 2012;87(5 Suppl):6–10. https://doi.org/10.4269/ajtmh.2012.12-0221.
53. United Nations. Convention on the rights of the child. Treaty Series. 1989;1577:3.
54. National Research Council and Institute of Medicine. National Research Council and Institute of Medicine: children's health, the nation's wealth: assessing and improving child health. Washington, DC: The National Academies Press; 2004.
55. Perrin JM, Romm D, Bloom SR, Homer CJ, Kuhlthau KA, Cooley C, Duncan P, Roberts R, Sloyer P, Wells N, Newacheck P. A family-centered, community-based system of services for children and youth with special health care needs. Arch Pediatr Adolesc Med. 2007;161(10):933–6. https://doi.org/10.1001/archpedi.161.10.933.
56. Stein RE. Challenges in long-term health care for children. Ambul Pediatr. 2001;1:280–8.
57. American Academy of Pediatrics Council on Children with Disabilities. Care coordination in the medical home: integrating health and related systems of care for children with special health care needs. Pediatrics. 2005;116(5):1238–44. https://doi.org/10.1542/peds.2005-2070.
58. Aboneh EA, Chui MA. Care coordination, medical complexity, and unmet need for prescription medications among children with special health care needs.

Res Soc Adm Pharm. 2017;13(3):524–9. https://doi.org/10.1016/j.sapharm.2016.05.043.

59. Kuo DZ, Cohen E, Agrawal R, Berry JG, Casey PH. A national profile of caregiver challenges among more medically complex children with special health care needs. Arch Pediatr Adolesc Med. 2011;165(11):1020–6. https://doi.org/10.1001/archpediatrics.2011.172.
60. Nishimoto CLJ, Duarte ED. Family organization for the care of children with chronic conditions, discharged from the neonatal intensive care unit. Texto Contexto-Enfermagem. 2014;23(2):318–27.
61. World Health Organization Regional Office for Europe. Meeting on child health redesign in the WHO European Region. Copenhagen, Denmark, 31st October–2nd November, 2017. http://www.euro.who.int/__data/assets/pdf_file/0003/364530/child-health-redesign-meeting-eng.pdf.
62. Brenner M, O'Shea MP, Larkin P, Luzi D, Pecoraro F, Tamburis O, Berry J, Alexander D, Rigby M, Blair M. Management and integration of care for children living with complex care needs at the acute-community interface in Europe. Lancet Child Adolesc Health. 2018;2(11):822–31. https://doi.org/10.1016/S2352-4642(18)30272-4.
63. Brenner M, O'Shea MP, McHugh R, Clancy A, Larkin P, Luzi D, Pecoraro F, Olaso EM, Lignou S, Alma M, Satherley RM, Tamburis O, Warters A, Wolfe I, Hilliard C, Berry J, Alexander D, Rigby M, Blair M. Principles for provision of integrated complex care for children across the acute-community interface in Europe. Lancet Child Adolesc Health. 2018;2(11):832–8. https://doi.org/10.1016/S2352-4642(18)30270-0.
64. Perrin JM. How can quality improvement enhance the lives of children with disabilities? Futur Child. 2012;22(1):149–68. https://doi.org/10.1353/foc.2012.0005.
65. Wolfe I, Lemer C, Cass H. Integrated care: a solution for improving children's health? Arch Dis Child. 2016;101(11):992–7. https://doi.org/10.1136/archdischild-2013-304442.

17 Social Aspects: Sustainability for the Patient, the Family, and the Healthcare System

Chiara Gibertoni and Alessandra De Palma

Abbreviations

DALY	Disability-Adjusted Life Year
GDP	Gross Domestic Product
ICT	Information and Communication Technology
NHS	National Health Service
QALY	Quality Adjusted Life Years
WHO	World Health Organization

17.1 Introduction

The Italian National Health Service guarantees by law the uniform provision of care throughout the country. The fifth Title V of the Constitution assess that the responsibility for healthcare is shared between the central government and the Regions and the Autonomous Provinces. However, enormous differences in the organization and delivery of regional health services are still present.

Public health spending has absorbed a relatively small share of gross domestic product, although it has consistently exceeded central government forecasts over the past 40 years. Changes in payment systems, in particular for hospital care, have encouraged containment of expenditure, as the tax sources used to finance the National Health Service (NHS) have progressively regressed. Limited evidence on vertical equity suggests that the NHS guarantees equal access to primary care; however, low-income groups still face obstacles when they require specialist cares. The health status of Italians has progressively improved (up to the SARS-CoV-2 pandemic) and compares favorably with that of other countries, even if regional disparities remain [1].

Unfortunately, given the economic crisis that has persisted for many years, cost containment has been and is a central issue for the NHS. Health authorities require evidence of the economic and clinical value of each health interventions. In this context, the integration and evolution of techniques to measure the economic sustainability of new technologies is essential. The *Disability-Adjusted Life Year* (DALY) and the *Quality Adjusted Life Years* (QALY) are two measurements tools used in the evaluation of the quality of health interventions. DALY is an impartial measure of sustainability. It can exceed the limit of using arbitrary economic threshold values, since it is a benchmark directly comparable with the per cap*ita* Gross Domestic Product (GDP).

C. Gibertoni
Sant'Orsola Hospital, IRCSS, University of Bologna, Bologna, BO, Italy

A. De Palma (✉)
Legal Medicine and Integrated Risk Management Unit, Sant'Orsola Hospital, IRCSS, University of Bologna, Bologna, BO, Italy
e-mail: alessandra.depalma@aosp.bo.it

M. Lima, M. C. Mondardini (eds.), *Frailty in Children*,
https://doi.org/10.1007/978-3-031-24307-3_17

Indeed, in 2002, the World Health Organization (WHO) suggested that interventions costing less than three times the per capita GDP per avoided DALY could be considered profitable.

The expected value of information and the estimated contribution to GDP (social costs due to presence and absenteeism) should be implemented, together with divestment decisions based on health technology assessment and the generation of a complete set of health data (analyzing data using artificial intelligence). These procedures can improve the effectiveness of health governance and improve the quality of health services [2].

The European Union also believes that the Italian NHS should be strengthened, starting with the staff. The indications of the EU Commission in Italy suggest a substantial increase in public investments in health care and in the adoption of policies aimed at enhancing health personnel. The aim is removing impediments to training, hiring and maintaining human and professionals resources which are becoming difficult to find in the European panorama.

Following the economic consequences related to SARS-CoV-2 epidemic, the European Commission has published several recommendations to reform policies of each member country. First of all, improve the coordination between the State and the Regions. In fact, the Commission underlines that, in our country, healthcare spending is below the EU average and that the response to the pandemic was essentially based on an extraordinary mobilization that offset the limitations of infrastructure, the number of healthcare workers and limited investments of the past years.

The pandemic has imposed new models of organization, work, and life to respond to the health emergency and has given further importance to values such as trust, freedom, care, giving more importance to the so-called soft skills among health professionals.

Furthermore, a wide gap between the different territories in Italy (consequence of the NHS reform—Constitutional Law 3/2001) has emerged. Differences between the regions have been observed as consequences of the constraint of regional budget (a new tool for controlling health expenditure).

Tensions have occurred in institutional relations as a result of the "regionalization" of the NHS, to which conflicts have been added to redefine the financial, institutional, and political relations between the national government and the regions.

During crises, the main objective is to maintain the balance over time between the contribution required to health care to favor fiscal consolidation and to maintain the primary function of protecting health by responding to increasing demand deriving from the new needs induced by the crisis and the spread of chronic and degenerative diseases.

The addition of new problems puts a strain on the sustainability of the NHS, strongly underlining the need for appropriateness in the provision of services also in compliance with ethics in the allocation of the resources assigned.

To get an idea of the extent of the low funding of the Health System, it is enough to recall that public health expenditure in 2017 was just $ 2622 per capita in Italy, against—at purchasing power parity—France's $ 4068 and $ 4986 of Germany.

A systematic contraction in the last 20 years: an annual growth rate passed from 7.1% in the period 2001–2006 to just 1% from 2007 to 2015, during which the main contribution came from the reduction of expenditure for employee income category: it is easy to understand on which shoulders the effort for the survival of the NHS has weighed.

There are three fundamental issues that have characterized a new health policy

1. The need to configure a multilevel governance of the NHS: Law 833/78 was clear in giving responsibility for epidemics to the state. During the COVID-19 pandemic, we witnessed a deployment of separation strategies and actions to hoarding of health goods by the Regions, which have generated tensions between them and the national government. Health protection is a complex function and requires a multilevel government, as it is expressed in both local, regional (for example networks for complex pathologies and high-tech treatments for which Hub centers are set

up), supra-regional (the national IRCCS network), and worldwide. The defeat of the re-centralization at the Constitutional Referendum then opened a new season to regionalism which, at present, in health care is a knot to be solved if the meaning of a National Health Service is to be recovered.

2. Extent, and costs of universalism, that is, selectivity or conditionality of the global coverage and free healthcare services. Over the years, the cut in public spending has gradually increased citizens' share in the cost of services, with an increase in the output to private producers or abandonment of care, with estimates ranging from 12.2 million people according to the survey Census to four million people communicated by ISTAT at the hearing in the Chamber on the 2010 budget law, giving space to the traditional arguments in favor of the need to develop a second and third pillar for the population with the highest income. There are about 11 million policyholders, of which eight million through category funds or contractual/corporate welfare policies negotiated with employers who can transfer the burden to the community according to the classic scheme of discounts and tax breaks.
3. The governance of the effects of re-organization: In all the regions there has been the phenomenon of the merger of Healthcare Companies in recent years, but the gigantism of the companies could only become a shortcut with respect to the longer and more difficult processes of true integration. There is no need to erase the boundaries between companies, but only to improve skills and services. In the future, it will be of strategic importance to do this through new technologies, and making political and functional boundaries soft and permeable. The ability to create integration will pass through the expansion of the relationship to ensure the development of research on the themes of the predominantly territorial levels of assistance and to train the new generations of health professionals through the extension of teaching and training to aspects and territorial dynamics, not stopping at the hospital.

The sustainability of this system model also depends by economic equity and good relationships between professional communities involved.

17.1.1 Innovations for Healthcare System

COVID-19 today remains still an urgency and a series of questions must be addressed: what synergy is possible between hospital and territorial services (which has proved the keystone in the management of the epidemic), what solutions could be adopted for a flexible, intensive care system capable of being activated when needed and, above all, how to cope with the sudden loss of availability of beds that necessarily requires effective management of hospitalizations to prevent the virus from spreading?

It is necessary to invest in the training of the staff of the District (Directors) and of the interlocutors closely linked to them, to equip the Districts with the skills, tools (Information and Communication Technology—ICT), and the resources to have governance of part of the production chain (health, social and health care, social), able to monitor

- The appropriateness, quality, and timing of delivery of services
- The needs of citizens and inconsistent responses to needs (to identify and combat areas of inadequacy)
- The quality of the relationship with citizens and/or patients
- The quality of the paths and processes of health promotion and prevention, community co-planning, integrated participation with the external interlocutors of associations and the third sector, integrated work with the social and socio-health network, health promotion, and community building
- To attribute to the Districts the competences regarding the definition and implementation of integrated assistance paths for taking care of people with chronic diseases and frailties

- To make the role of the Districts really effective
- A new definition of the Company Staff to move toward organizing the activities more in support of the Districts.

In health services there is a need to evaluate and develop tools and health and social interventions to support the care pathways of subjects with multimorbidity and fragility. A critical moment in the management of health services is the transition between the hospital and the territory, which must be supervised in a bidirectional sense. On the one hand, favoring the return home after an acute episode, and on the other, also by guaranteeing easy access to emergency care for people, with a well-defined management plan. Therefore, it is essential to define the organizational infrastructure, establish roles and responsibilities of services and professionals, share criteria and methods for managing cases and implement the model by focusing on the training of professionals and on the evaluation of processes and outcomes.

In this context, the development of inter-company models, the enhancement of the Integration Department, the definition of the areas of competence and responsibility with respect to the Primary Care Department and the strengthening of collaboration with the Mental Health and Social Services of the Municipality represent aspects relevant to be supervised.

The introduction of these innovations represents an opportunity to develop research projects to assess the impact of the interventions introduced on the processes and outcomes for patients.

On the basis of this priority, some essential actions are identified to be implemented

- Redesign the collaboration between the Companies of the Regional Health Service, General Medicine, the Accredited Private and the territorial Social Services for the management of more complex cases
  - Define a transverse organization to ensure linear care pathways between the various companies in the region
  - Identify/review the roles and professional skills to be involved in hospital-territory transition models, in particular by defining the role and relationships between the different Departments (hospital, primary care, Integration, Mental Health, etc.)
  - Identify useful tools to ensure patient care at all stages of the care path (acute, chronic, end of life); build facilitated pathways that provide a rapid response to the needs of care in the worsening phase of the patients' clinical conditions (e.g., direct referrals by the care provider to specialists/multidisciplinary teams/technical beds to avoid hospitalization)

17.2 Disability Assessment

The need to share with parents a clinical-assistance path that, in compliance with the regulatory provisions, can be experienced in the less traumatic possible way. In this perspective, the specialist who is in charge of a minor with disabilities, in addition to agreeing to a therapeutic path with family members, must also inform the family in detail about the therapeutic possibility. In Italy, disability assessment by law is crucial (Law 104/92 and subsequent amendments), in order to be able to exercise the rights contemplated as a consequence of this situation of need and vulnerability. It is not easy for parents to take this step, because it means certifying—quite possibly—the unamendability of disease conditions and functional deficits, together with the fear that certified disability means increasing stigma and marginalization. The process for the accreditation of disability is very difficult and stressful for both children and their family. In order to simplify and humanize this path, sessions dedicated only to minors would be indispensable. Commissions integrated by the reference specialists for the prevalent pathology, competent to contribute to the expression of a judgment formulated also in the light of all the existing health documentation and of the aspects of social inclusion in the child's life spheres (school, family, etc.), considering all the useful elements to be evaluated. In the case of pathologies that can be modified over time, the Commission may deem it necessary to revise it and establish a date in which to carry out a new forensic examination and the process is repeated. In the initial phase of assessing the disability, the main aim is the development of the network of social and health services, including both hospital and local services. Today these objectives must be combined with the need to guarantee at the same time an ever-increasing qualification of operators and their technical-professional specialization for a correct care of people with disabilities and their families. For several years, the WHO itself has proposed through the ICF (international classification system) a biopsychosocial model that overcomes the contradictions between traditional models of an exclusively "medical" or "social" nature.

For many years now, the medico-legal activity, aimed at protecting the so-called "Weak groups", was carried out in a way that is no longer adequate to the real needs of people.

The "Consolidated Law", which has been hoped for for a very long time, should bring order to the mass of laws, legislative decrees, ministerial and circular decrees that make, in daily practice, almost unmanageable and complicated a matter which, to be applied, constitutes a real obstacle for people with disabilities and their families.

The application of the legislation still currently represents a very hard process and often the laws are inadequate to answer to the real needs of families. The first definition of civil invalidity (legge 30 marzo 1971, n. 118) was based on the only assumption of the "loss of working capacity" (for individuals aged 18–65; from 15 years for minors for whom a placement aimed at work is assumed) and "persistent difficulties in perform the acts and functions proper to age". Over the years, new laws have been introduced and actually an economic support is guaranteed for those who have been certified as invalid. In this framework, the primary task is to develop integrated pathways and concerted policies between institutions (ASL, Municipalities, Metropolitan Cities, and Provinces), families, and associative representatives, to promote synergies that are crucial for people with disabilities. First of all, the true state of implementation of Law 104/92 should be verified. Often the assessment of the handicap ends up being a duplication of the assessment of the state of civil invalidity, not so much because the assessment is carried out in a single session (in some Regions for years already; in others, hopefully in implementation of L. 80/2006), as well as because the social worker cannot fully carry out his function (the preliminary social investigation is missing, mainly due to a lack of resources). On this topic, many Associations have also been showing the need to introduce a truly multidisciplinary assessment (with the active participation of all the members of the Commission and a social investigation), and therefore allow a global takeover for all the social, health, and socioeducational interventions really necessary.

Different strategies have been proposed to simplify the process of recognition of invalidity. First of all, since many people who belong to the Assessment Commissions have already undertaken treatment paths, it would be enough to network and be able to share the health documentation already available. In fact, it is sufficient to think, for example, of minors followed by Child Neuropsychiatry Services or with rare diseases: for all of them the specialists have already performed visits and/or instrumental and/or laboratory tests, etc. Further investigations, carried out for the sole medical-legal purpose, must be considered inappropriate and sometimes vitiated ab initio: a specialist and/or instrumental examination performed for clinical purposes is much more reliable than that carried out for the medico-legal evaluation, because the degree of collaboration of the user who can do it is certainly much higher if the purpose is that of treatment and the execution setting is a clinical one.

The use and networking of existing documentation in an "institutionalized" manner (always delivering at least a copy to the interested party in order to safeguard privacy) create computer links between the various services that contribute to the evaluation activities and between the various bodies involved (for example, between the Services/Operating Units of Forensic Medicine of the ASL and branches of INPS), allow to reduce waiting times, inconvenience for citizens, and duplication of investigations.

In order to carry out adequate assessments to the needs of the individual concrete case, a high degree of integration between health and social services must be developed. A synergic collaboration between social and health assistance is essential to achieve the best possible result. The assessment to which the Commissions for assessing the state of civil invalidity are obliged by the legislation currently in force, contemplates the assessment of the health requirement only. An integrated assessment, always conducted with a view to health, but also from a social point of view, is undoubtedly able to quantify the services and benefits to the real needs of the person. A new evaluation methodology aims to evaluate the potential and resources for each person based on the ICF.

It is necessary to build a network that improves human and material resources, avoiding multiplication in the assessments.

It would be innovative to envisage a multidisciplinary Commission, composed of a specialist in forensic medicine, a specialist, in the prevalent pathology from which the person is affected, and a social operator, which could be a professional educator for minors, simplifying the complex and cumbersome national legislation that determines the Commissions operating at the Health Authorities (with verification of the operated by INPS) for the Commissions for assessing the state of invalidity with a legislative act that reforms and simplifies the composition of the collegial bodies. Equally, by making the Regions responsible for the necessary quality control, it could be envisaged a sample control only by INPS (although significant) and not systematic, but with re-evaluation of the cases (not simple practices) and with the appropriate rigor. With the law of March 3, 2009, n. 18, bearing the "Ratification and execution of the United Nations Convention on the Rights of Persons with Disabilities, with optional protocol, made in New York on 13 December 2006 and establishment of the National Observatory on the condition of people with disabilities", Italy had made a commitment to the international community.

In fact, with the ratification of the UN Convention on the Rights of Persons with Disabilities (Law 18/2009), the definitive transition from a vision of people with disabilities "as sick and handicapped" to a vision of the condition of disability based on respect of human rights, aimed at enhancing human diversity—gender, sexual orientation, culture, language, psycho-physical conditions, etc.—and to consider the condition of disability not as deriving from subjective qualities of people but from the interaction between people and the environment, that is, between individual characteristics and the ways in which society as a whole provides access and enjoyment of the rights of persons with disabilities, goods, and services.

As required by the law, the National Observatory on the Condition of Persons with Disabilities was established, inspired by the same principles

(a) Respect for intrinsic dignity, individual autonomy with the freedom to make one's own choices and independence
(b) Non-discrimination
(c) Full and effective participation and social inclusion
(d) Respect for difference and acceptance of persons with disabilities as part of diversity and humanity
(e) Equal opportunities
(f) Accessibility
(g) Respect for the development of the capacities of minors with disabilities and their right to preserve their identity

The mandatory call for the equality of people with disabilities with the rest of the population, affirmed by the UN Convention, requires limiting all forms of inequality.

17.3 Disability Certification

The need of a broad and structural reform of the current system of certification of the condition of disability has been current for many years. The system is obsolete, complex, and cause of potential inequalities of treatment and far from the spirit and letter of the UN Convention.

The matter needs a global reform, which goes beyond the rules on civil disability that have repeatedly been repeated in fragments in the years and on the condition of disability and instead lays the foundations for a synergy between the national level—which would maintain the responsibility for recognizing disability—and the regional one, to which the specific evaluative action would remain.

The regions and their operational divisions should be entrusted, with greater clarity and incisiveness, the role of accompanying people with disabilities in the development and implementation of a "personalized project" of intervention with the joining of all the supports necessary for social inclusion and to exercise rights, obviously also through the ASLs, Municipalities, and Metropolitan Cities.

17.3.1 Policies, Services, and Organizational Models for Independent Living and Inclusion in Society

The main aim of a new approach to the condition of disability is the reorientation of services toward social inclusion and the contrast to the institutionalization and segregation of the person with disabilities. This could be reached by promoting independent life and support for self-determination, through innovation and training of operators, proposing new quality and accreditation criteria for services, adoption of guidelines to encourage independent living processes, and a review of the service and performance nomenclatures. This last point aims to accommodate a new generation of interventions for the promotion participation and equality of people with disabilities.

17.3.2 Health, Right to Life, and Rehabilitation

The protection of the health of people with disabilities is crucial, consistent with a biopsychosocial vision of disability. However, the National Health Service is not yet able to guarantee full access to care, quality of interventions, respect for fragile people.

Specific actions need to be implemented to enrich and consolidate the Essential Levels of Assistance and social and health integration.

Other critical issues of the current scenario are configured in

(a) The overlap of two systems of assessment "handicap" and "disability, deafness and blindness".
(b) The "tabular" methods of assessing civil disabilities, which are based on generic work incapacity. This is inadequate to design a proper management plan to support for the full and effective social participation of people with disabilities.
(c) The adoption by the Regions of differentiated criteria that often include further multidisciplinary and multidimensional assessments for access to regional and local services.
(d) The lack of separation and specialization of assessment paths for minors.
(e) The lack of an adequate information feedback system on the results of clinical results and on the sharing of data deriving from investigations.
(f) The absence of criteria of access to the system of services and benefits, for multidimensional assessment to define a customized project.
(g) The lack of introduction of the International Classification of the Functioning of Health and Disability (ICF) and the International Statistical Classification of Diseases and Related Health Problems—tenth revision (ICD10).

17.3.3 The Best Interests of the Child and Parental Responsibility: A Delicate Balance

One more critical aspect is the will of the minor person who turns to the NHS, linked to their decision-making competence and the legal validity of the decisions to be taken.

As is known, until reaching the age of majority, the minor's capacity to act is limited, as it is acquired—pursuant to the civil code—upon reaching the age of majority; from a strictly legal point of view, there is no doubt that the approval of the parents or, failing that, of the guardian is always required.

With respect to the choices related to health treatments, this ability is understood as the ability to self-determine and fully understand the consequences of one's choices and decisions. Therefore, even if the minor must always be involved in information activities and involved in the decision-making process, based on his age and degree of maturity, legally the parents are the holders and exercisers of parental responsibility, in the name and in the exclusive interest of the minor (even if sometimes the interests of the parents and the minor do not coincide).

Based on Article 337 of the Italian Civil Code "Parental responsibility is exercised by both parents. The decisions of greatest interest to children relating to education, upbringing, health and the choice of the child's habitual residence are taken by mutual agreement taking into account the abilities, natural inclination and aspirations of the children".

The law expressly recognizes (art 315-bis, 336-bis of the civil code) the right of the minor to be heard in all matters concerning them, at the age of 12, or even at a younger age if they are capable of discernment: the hearing is conducted by the judge who, in advance, informs the minor of the nature of the procedure and the effects of the hearing.

Many years ago, the National Committee for Bioethics, invited to take into account the participation in the decision-making process of the child over the age of seven and the need to seek his consent and yet "to consider the consent or dissent of the adolescent starting from the age of 14 as mandatory and priority [...] (because) it is certain that children and adolescents are subjects of knowledge, more or less evolved and with infinite nuances in the continuity of his evolve, and always require deep respect".

The Code of Medical Ethics also suggests the professional to guarantee "useful elements for the minor to understand his health condition and the programmed diagnostic-therapeutic interventions, in order to involve him in the decision-making process".

Our legal system does not yet contemplate specific provisions governing the matter relating to the right of the minor to autonomously take decisions with respect to his or her moral personality, body and health, but includes general rules contained in the civil code on parental responsibility, on representation and various sector laws.

Instead, an international and constitutional system of principles has been gradually created to protect human rights expressed mainly within various regulatory texts

- The Italian Constitution in art. 32 qualifies health as a fundamental right of the individual and establishes—Article 13—the freedom of self-determination of the person as basically inviolable.
- The Charter of Fundamental Rights of the European Union makes any medical or biological intervention subject to the free and informed consent of the interested party (Article 3).
- Article 12 of the UN Convention on the Rights of the Child establishes the right of the child to be heard in any proceedings concerning him, to express his opinion and to be informed of the consequences that may derive from the implementation of his opinion and the decisions that concern him.
- The Oviedo Convention (European Convention on Human Rights and Biomedicine, 4 April 1997), despite not being formally in force, although ratified by the Italian State with Law no. 145, is often referred to and the principles

expressed on informed consent (Articles 5–9) are considered to be immanent in the international and constitutional system of protection of human rights.

Today, with reference to the decision-making possibility of minors, during the pandemic emergency and in the midst of the vaccination campaign, the Grand Chamber of the European Court of Human Rights ruled on the vaccination obligation, examining the issue in the particular prospective context of parental refusal to submit their minor children to the vaccinations required by law. This decision turns out to be very interesting both with regard to the question of the correct determination of the best interest of the child, and with regard to the possible contrast between compulsory vaccinations and religious freedom, dealt with in the Vavřička and Others v. the Czech Republic, of April 8, 2021, in which the Court has assessed the alleged violation of Articles 8 and 9 of the European Convention by state laws that impose an obligation to vaccinate minors, when the parents of the children are against vaccines for reasons of conscience. In the appeal, the Strasbourg judges were asked to consider the claims for exemption from the vaccination obligation as an expression of a form of secular conscientious objection, a request that makes it necessary to establish whether personal opinions contrary to vaccines can be included in the context of the exercise of the right to freedom of conscience and religion. After reviewing the different legal events (six) gathered in the examination before the Grand Chamber, and reporting the conclusions reached by the Czech constitutional jurisprudence, the Vavřička judgment examined the decisions of other European constitutional courts, which show unanimous recognition of the lawfulness of the vaccination obligation, including the Italian one. Our legal system has repeatedly addressed the question of the legitimacy of compulsory vaccinations, establishing the need for the law to provide for compensation for those who may suffer damage following the administration of a vaccine. The Consult pointed out that the opposition to vaccinations is based on theories not supported by scientific evidence: science agrees in supporting the need for vaccines to protect individuals and society as a whole, from the spread of serious diseases.

Therefore, the problems emerging in facing difficult choices are increasing, especially with regard to the will of the minor to consent or not to the treatment, given his/her right to be involved in the formation of the consent that authorizes the intervention, especially when risky and invasive.

Recently, it has been accepted that "the opinion of the minor is taken into consideration as an increasingly determining factor, depending on his age and his degree of maturity" (art. 6 of the Oviedo Convention) and similar principles are contained in the Code of Medical Ethics and in the Code of Ethics for Nurses (2019), in mind of which "*The nurse, taking into account the age and of the degree of maturity found, endeavors to ensure that the minor's opinion is duly taken into consideration with respect to curative, welfare and experimental choices, in order to allow him to express his will. The nurse, when the minor consciously opposes the choice of care, takes steps to overcome the conflict.*" (Article 23, Will of the minor). The need to involve the minor capable of discernment in the process that leads to the manifestation of consent by the representative is a fact by now acquired in living law, not only in Italy.

However, the legal texts lack a general rule that establishes the level of self-determination due to minors with particular regard to the freedom to manage their own bodies.

As long as the minor is considered a subject devoid of discernment, his opinion is irrelevant, while starting from the moment he is capable, he must first of all be listened to to understand his psychological conditions and provide him with the necessary information.

The capacity for discernment is not linked to a specific age, but differs from person to person: it is described as the capacity of one who is able to understand the meaning of his actions.

Health treatment cannot be imposed on a person with the capacity of discernment who consciously opposes it, thus recognizing in the minor a real power of veto, a right not to undergo any form of coercive execution on his body.

The decisions of the parents must be made with regard to the interests of the minor: they are therefore decisions that have a prognostic nature, inherent to issues of fundamental importance.

However, in Italy, many laws still entrust the choices exclusively to parents: just think of the legislation on organ and tissue removal and transplants, in which the legislator has chosen to substitute the will of the parents for that of the minor. In the delicate choice regarding the removal of organs after death, even if more recent laws show small openings (for example, the Law 219/2005 allows the child giving birth to arrange the donation of hematopoietic stem cells, placenta, and umbilical cord blood).

The discipline of informed consent and advance treatment provisions is finally clear, according to which "The informed consent to the health treatment of the minor is expressed or refused by the exercisers of parental responsibility or by the guardian, taking into account the will of the minor person, in relation to his age and degree of maturity, and having as its purpose the protection of the psycho-physical health and life of the minor in full respect of his or her dignity".

A different issue is that of adequate information, necessary for the minor to build up his own opinion, even in the case of the minor not yet capable of discernment. The duty to provide information rests on parents, in the correct exercise of their responsibility, and on doctors as an ethical duty. We reiterate that the minor's decision-making competence, correlated to his ability to discern, does not depend exclusively on the mere personal data, but on the degree of psychological maturity, understood as the ability to adequately understand the consequential effects of the choices made on the future life, with a sufficient sense of reality.

Health professionals are required to acquire specific skills and competences, given that as a patient, the child is not a "small adult", but represents an "other world", equally their training must also include skills related to his involvement in the care, the relational aspects and the ability to put him at the center of the relationship, together with the parents.

17.3.4 The Clinical Ethics Committees

Professionals should be supported by committees "for ethics of care" or "for ethics in the clinic", multidisciplinary and that in particularly complex situations could support them in the difficult choices they are called to make.

It is true that the Decree of 8 February 2013 states: "if not already attributed to specific bodies, the ethics committees can carry out a consultative function in relation to ethical issues connected with scientific welfare activities in order to protect and promote the values of the person; the ethics committees can also propose training initiatives for health professionals in relation to bioethical issues", but it is true that they carry out almost exclusively evaluations for clinical pharmacological trials. Instead, clinical practice poses increasingly complex problems to healthcare professionals in the light of new technologies that open up new scenarios with the consequent questions; moreover, the increased awareness of citizens (patients and legal representatives) with respect to the right to self-determination, to autonomy of choice, they may require different skills than those generally provided for in the ethics committees. Evaluations on pharmacological trials privilege the procedural aspects and methodological rigor of the study designed by the researchers, while clinical ethics, on the other hand, focuses on the individual and existential conditions of patients and on the care relationship. The ethics committees in the clinic must not overlap, replace, or interfere in the relationship between doctor, health team, and patient, but strengthen this relationship when, in the opinion of the doctor or at the request of the patient, it seems necessary to acquire further elements of evaluation and to broaden the horizons of dialogue. In such cases, the Clinical Ethics Committee can provide a non-binding opinion without taking away from the professionals the autonomy and decision-making responsibility.

The painful pandemic experience highlighted that the Clinical Ethics Committees could have supported professionals at times when there were many people to be treated—especially in high-intensity care settings—and the availability was not adequate, because they would have avoided exacerbating loneliness, of health workers in the face of dramatic decisions, which must not be based on abstract criteria considered objectively valid, but contextualized and individualized with respect to concrete cases, at the "sick bed".

The ethical dilemma that arises when deciding whether to "cure" or "take care" of a patient is faced almost daily in some clinical contexts and, in particular, in intensive care units, where, under normal conditions, we proceed on the basis of consolidated experience and accredited guidelines, in compliance with the provisions of the law 219/2017 on informed consent, advance treatment provisions, and shared care planning. Unfortunately, in a period in which a disease that is in some ways still unknown, sometimes serious and fatal, which simultaneously involves many people, has spread ubiquitously, professionals are forced to make decisions in a short time without the possibility of sharing choices. And they are answers to crucial questions: who to transfer to an intensive care unit to start intubation? Who should you suspend assisted ventilation for? How to distribute limited health resources equally? That similar problems could arise was an awareness even previously: in our Polyclinic, years ago there was the birth of two Siamese twins, whose separation would have meant the certain death of one of the two, if not both. In order to decide which treatment path to take (invasive surgical or accompanying palliative), several interdisciplinary consultations were carried out, the opinion of the University Bioethics Committee was sought and the Cardinal was involved. Instead of providing extemporaneously, it is believed, at present, to have to provide for a stable body, which can be used in case of need.

17.4 Conclusions

Recently, the National Agency for Regional Health Services, indicated how to organize various services, especially territorial, stressing the importance of interaction and integration between hospital and territory.

There are very important services for the developmental age, just think of those for mental health, for pathological addictions, in particular for child neuropsychiatry and adolescence that are part of the integrated network for mental health present in all Local Health Authorities. This area is one of the most complex because its pursuit requires a close integration of the health system with social services, the relational network of the person concerned and society, as well as extensive coordination between the network of related health services to the integrated network for mental health, having to value various dimensions at the same time: general, personal, proximal, and primary in the basic levels, the specialist and departmental dimensions in the higher levels. Equally for the services dedicated to the health of women and children, with counseling activities and in-hospital and inter-service care paths. The declinations formulated repeatedly in the last 18 months, also in the light of the lessons learned from the COVID-19 pandemic, lead to the conclusion that there is still a long way to go, but that by innovating and dedicating resources to research, even organizational, it is possible to maintain and enhance an effective health care, still sustainable, equitable, and provided by a public National Health Service—capable of communicating with the private sector—and universalistic.

17.5 Frail Children—Specific Considerations

Any kind of hospital admission involves risk to this vulnerable population once it is a break from home routine medication and medical care, exposure to the hospital environment, rotating providers not familiarized with the patient and generation of stress and anxiety [2, 3]. Frail children are at higher risk for prolonged length of stay compared to the general population, as they have more postoperative complications such as slow return of bowel function, hemodynamic instability, and respiratory insufficiency. Also they have higher rates of readmissions, medical errors, as well as in-hospital mortality [2, 3]. Heterogeneity among this population, specific medication requirements, different anatomy or physiology, uncertainty about the best treatment protocol for the underlying conditions, and developmental needs can make perioperative management challenging. Anatomic abnormalities such as micrognathia, muscular contractures, excessive adipose tissue can make common procedures difficult (airway management, vascular access, positioning of the patient, etc). Previous surgery history is associated with postoperative adhesions which can hamper surgical approach. Malnutrition can delay wound healing. Past hospital admissions and infectious disease history increases the risk for antimicrobial resistance raising concerns on deciding prophylactic antibiotics and dealing with possible postoperative infection. Baseline organ dysfunction can require modifications in treatment algorithms as the threshold for starting treatment may be lower. Developmental or behavioral disabilities can make communicating pain and other symptoms difficult [2]. Familiar socioeconomical insufficiencies may hamper the best clinical contacts and treatment adherence. There will be frail children that, due to their physical or clinical condition, do not arouse compassion. Eventually we come across the ethical question that some of these patients require a lot more of us than we could possibly give in return, either emotionally, materialistically, and professionally.

17.6 Operational Improvement

The spectrum of frailty in children extends through all ages, originating from congenital and acquired conditions, with a range of static, potentially resolving, and progressive declining trajectories. Such heterogeneity presents challenges for categorization, prediction modeling, research, bedside care, and support of families. Nonetheless, we intend to establish some strategies in pre-operative evaluation, coordination of care, post-operative planning, and expectation to respond to these special needs children.

17.6.1 Referencing and Multidisciplinary Team

First of all, frail children should receive surgical care at institutions that offer multidisciplinary, pediatric-centered care, involving Pediatric Surgery, Pediatrics, Pediatric Anesthesiology, Physiatry, Psychology and Social Service, making an extensive preoperative planning possible. The team should be trained for complex special health care, meaning they should have experienced specialists, continuing education of healthcare providers, and guidelines for the management of these children [4]. It is essential that effective communication exists between all involved specialists of the team in order to have an organized, high-quality plan that fulfills the child's needs. It is useful to have a central practitioner coordinating care, which is usually the child's general pediatrician or family physician. The role would be to make the bond between every specialist and also the family, providing organized and updated data [5]. When there is a planned surgery, the involved in-hospital specialists should stay informed of each other's plans.

Families or primary care providers always play an important role as they can provide invaluable patient-specific details, including health summaries, interpretation of the symptoms, rare disease-specific expertise. Specialists and generalists must always involve families in decision-making, preoperative planning, and postoperative management, and should be educated on successful means of interaction and communication.

17.6.2 Surgical Indication and Conservatism

The principles upon which medical decisions are made for frail children are the same as for any other child: autonomy, beneficence justice, nonmaleficence, veracity, and fidelity [6]. Toward a potentially surgical problem, the decision making is not always easy and should be part of a multidisciplinary consensus. Discussions can be improved by engaging the family and the primary care team as shared decision-making promotes co-operation, with ultimate goals of improved health and satisfaction [7]. When cognitively competent, children should also be involved in decisions about their care, on the basis of developmental age. This can help them understand the condition and treatments, reduce fear, enhance self-confidence and acceptance, and improve collaboration with treatment decisions [6].

Nevertheless, a surgical procedure is a physical aggression, and it is well known that frail children have increased risk of prolonged length of stay due to pre-procedural optimization, overnight respiratory optimization, general uncertainty of response to procedural stress, and possible postoperative complications. There is also a higher rate of medical errors and even in-hospital death. The anxiety around the surgery and the disruption it causes to the family dynamics is also important to take into account. Surgical indication should be a decision made after careful consideration of risks and benefits, keeping in mind that good outcomes likely reflect a conservative approach [1]. The surgeon must consider the natural history, the risks of surgery for mortality and morbidity, namely, postoperative complications, and decide if there is an absolute need to perform surgery or if the child would be able to have an acceptable quality of life with conservative treatment.

For hopelessly ill children, or who have a progressive degenerative neurologic disease, it is important to understand what are the parents' expectations and determine precociously if parents want care to be limited. Patients in palliative care may obviously benefit from surgical procedures as long as it is to provide relief and/or prevention of pain and discomfort. If parents request do not resuscitate (DNR) status for their child, it should be documented in the medical record for clarity and legal protection of the team. This does not mean they are not eligible for surgical procedures. Some patients with DNR status may have significant benefit with a surgical intervention, even though the procedure may not change the natural history of the underlying disease. The surgeon plays an important role to discern if the procedure is important or a futility for the purpose of prolonging life. If there is a disagreement between parents and physicians' decision, a second opinion from another specialist is recommended [8].

17.6.3 Day-Case Surgery and Early Discharge

The longer the length of hospital stay, the higher the risk of nosocomial infections, medical errors, stress, and anxiety. There should always be an attempt to keep the admission as soon as possible. Therefore whenever it is feasible, the procedure should be on a day-case basis. This will only be possible if the underlying condition is stabilized, time of surgery is not very long (<120 min), postoperative pain can presumably be controlled (regional anesthesia, use of minimally invasive techniques), and there is no high risk of postoperative bleeding or alimentary intolerance [9].

When the procedure is not suitable for a day-case surgery, efforts should be made to reduce the length of stay as much as possible. Enhanced recovery after surgery (ERAS) has been a hot theme for adult surgeons lately, as it have been found to decrease hospital length of stay and complications in diverse adult surgical populations. These interventions theoretically maintain physiological homeostasis and minimize surgical stress, thus facilitating a quicker return to baseline. There is a paucity of literature assessing enhanced recovery protocols in the pediatric population, let alone in frail children, although there have been numerous pediatric studies demonstrating improved outcomes with isolated elements of ERAS (perioperative counseling, limited perioperative fasting, non-routine bowel preparation, antibiotic prophylaxis, use of short-acting anesthetics, epidural anesthesia/analgesia, limited use of narcotics, nausea and vomiting prophylaxis, early enteral intake and mobilization, and nonroutine use of surgical drains and tubes) [10]. Some of them have included frail children as oncologic patients and transplant recipients [11]. The creation of ERAS protocols in these populations must be an area of research as it seems to have a lot of potential in minimizing stress, complications, and length of stay. In fact, some elements of ERAS will be mentioned beneath as strategies for operational improvement, such as perioperative counseling, minimally invasive techniques, avoiding prolonged fasting, and postoperative pain management.

17.6.4 Pre-operative Planning

17.6.4.1 Patient and Family Preparation

The preoperative evaluation of frail children should comprehend common concerns that may impact perioperative decision-making. The surgeon must anticipate the unique intraoperative and postoperative potential challenges.

Preparing the child and family to face the surgery is important on a basis of good communication methods and promptness to answer doubts and questions. Adaptation to the hospital environment is a basic condition for a smooth uneventful stay. Some non-pharmacological adjuvant interventions proved to have a positive role on pediatric patients' outcomes, such as hospital decorations, facilities to play, and participation in team games, miniature cars for children to play with while waiting for surgery and to drive them to the operating room (OR). The presence of hospital clowns help in reducing stress and anxiety in children during medical procedures, induction of anesthesia, and as part of routine care. It might contribute to improve the psychological well-being and emotional responses in frail children and adolescents [12]. Also, while contributing to reduce parents' stress and anxiety, they can contribute for their respite by providing some distraction and entertainment for their child. Music has also potential in reducing pain, anxiety, and distress in children undergoing surgery [13]. If possible, it brings calmness to the child to make a preparation visit to the actual OR where all the stages of surgery are explained. Right before surgery, the presence of parents provides comfort and assurance.

For hopelessly ill children with a DNR order, after a decision to undergo surgery, the team should always have a discussion with the family on their options. Cardiopulmonary resuscitation in the OR carries a much better medical prognosis than when performed in other hospital scenarios (around 50–80% of patients resuscitated in the OR return to their former level of functioning). At the OR, the event is always witnessed allowing rapid and effective intervention. Also, the adjacent cause is usually known, often reversible effects of anesthesia or hemorrhage and not usually due to the patient's underlying disease. So the family should decide whether to suspend the DNR order during surgery and the perioperative period, keeping the original DNR order, or modifying the DNR order [8].

17.6.4.2 Medical Optimization

Whenever possible, frail children should be brought to their individual optimum level of health before undergoing a surgical procedure. Malnourished children (or at risk of malnourishment) should have a nutrition plan prior to surgery, either by optimizing oral intakes or by tube feedings. Prolonged fasting should be avoided so clear liquids should be emphasized until 1–2 h before surgery. Although with some limitations, serum albumin is generally considered a useful index of nutritional status and the target serum level should be 4 g/dL [14]. Dehydration is common and frequently underdiagnosed in malnourished children who are affected by several kinds of disability, so it should be considered and treated before surgery [15]. Children with chronic disorders or renal disease often have associated anemia with usual hemoglobin concentrations of 6–9 g/dL. Target preoperative hemoglobin values should be individualized to the type of procedure planned and pointed after a discussion with the anesthesiologist. Coagulopathies and electrolyte imbalances must be corrected before surgery. Patients receiving corticosteroids for extended periods may not be able to support a natural stress response because of chronic suppression of the hypothalamic–pituitary–adrenal axis, so they should receive perioperative supplementation. Patients taking antihypertensive drugs should not suspend it but must be closely monitored for intraoperative hypotension. Other drugs that should be continued in the perioperative period include antiepileptics, drugs for asthma, and immunosuppressants. Drugs that should be discontinued before surgery include anticoagulants, anti-thrombotic, nonsteroidal anti-inflammatory drugs, and diuretics. Patients with chronic lung disease should be preoperatively asymptomatic and for that pharmacologic, environmental, or dietary control may be necessary. Medications should not be suspended during perioperative period. In some difficult cases, such as in cystic fibrosis the pneumologist's cooperation is essential to optimize the patient before surgery to minimize the surgical risk. In patients with chronic kidney disease, renal function and electrolyte monitoring is important in the preoperative period, and any acid–base imbalances and electrolyte disturbances must be corrected. Careful attention must be paid to the patient's intake and output. The fasting period should not be prolonged before surgery because they can become dehydrated quickly. In such patients, securing peripheral intravenous access is always sensible, even before surgery. When prescribing drugs that are metabolized and excreted by the kidney, monitoring of serum drug levels is essential. In patients with chronic liver disease, edema or ascites should be treated preoperatively with diuretics and sodium-restricted diet. Liver enzyme levels and coagulation should be accessed before surgery. If coagulopathy is present, vitamin K and fresh frozen plasma should be ensured in the preoperative period as well as during surgery. When prescribing drugs that are metabolized and excreted by the liver, monitoring of serum drug levels is essential. Patients with neurological disease and seizure disorder are often considered at high risk of seizures occurring during or shortly after the procedure. There should be an appropriate plan for continued use of antiepileptic drugs throughout pre and immediate postoperative periods. In patients with obesity, measures should be taken to prevent deep-vein thrombosis and pulmonary embolism, such as postoperative enoxaparin, elastic compression stockings, and/or intermittent compression devices. Also, additional measures to prevent surgical site infection should be considered.

17.6.4.3 Anesthesia Plan

Frail children should always have an observation by an anesthesiology specialist prior to an elective surgery. The pediatric surgeon must communicate to the pediatric anesthesiologist the surgical plan so that together they can anticipate problems or concerns, especially for complex or uncommon procedures. The anesthesia team should be aware if the patient has a history of complications with anesthetics, malignant hyperthermia, coagulation disorders, or if the patient has symptoms of an upper respiratory tract illness that increases the risk of postintubation laryngotracheal edema. Preoperatively, the anesthesia team must have a plan, according to the surgical intervention, for postoperative pain control as caudal injection, epidural catheter insertion, or peripheral nerve block.

17.6.5 The Surgery

17.6.5.1 Positioning and Surgical Approach

Planning a surgical approach anticipatedly is very important considering these patients may have altered anatomy or surgical implanted devices that restrict standard surgical steps. In patients with neurological or neuromuscular diseases, the body habitus may hamper surgical positioning and access. For instance, in a patient with severe lower extremity contractures, a laparoscopic operation may not be feasible if there is no adequate extracorporeal clearance of laparoscopic instrumentation, unless there is an alternative for port sites position. Surgical implanted devices such as ventriculoperitoneal shunts or venous catheters, digestive or urinary stomas, previous scars may limit surgical approach like surgical incision site. Every detail must be considered when deciding what technique to perform, if any modification will be required, and what to do in case of a difficulty or complication.

17.6.5.2 Minimally Invasive Surgery (MIS)

Minimally invasive surgery revolutionized pediatric surgery since it has been proven to be feasible in a great proportion of pediatric surgery procedures. Advantages of minimally invasive surgery are unquestionable and well known throughout the fields of abdominal, thoracic, and urologic conditions. Of interest in this population, MIS is associated with decreased risk of infection, decreased recovery time and length of stay, greater surgical visualization and precision [16]. If surgery is inevitably a physical aggression, MIS tends to minimize it, as it is possible to make smaller incisions and limited mobilization of structures when trying to achieve an adequate exposure. Greater visualization, magnification, and precision might prove to be an advantage in children who have altered anatomy. MIS should always be considered a first-line approach after disclosing any kind of cardiopulmonary contra-indication.

17.6.5.3 Preoperative Simulation

Whenever there is a high-complexity surgical case, experience and competency are expected of the team. In pediatric surgery and specifically in frail children, there are some conditions that are rare, and the team will not have experienced significant case volume. Even if there is considerable volume of similar cases, each case might have particularities in this population. Frail children will be frequently complex cases on their altered anatomy and physiology, increased risk of complications, and less tolerability to minor errors and distractions. That is why preoperative simulation can improve safety and effectiveness of surgical procedures. Significant advances in diagnostic imaging modalities and image processing software enable surgeons to obtain detailed anatomical information preoperatively for each patient and incorporate this data in surgical simulation. A surgical simulator based on radiological images from an individual patient using three-dimensional visualization techniques may greatly assist surgeons to preoperatively rehearse an operation and facilitate sharing of information among the operative team [17, 18]. Surgeons should have the means to achieve the best preparation they possibly may have and we must always offer the best of our knowledge and competence to treat a child.

17.6.6 Postoperative Management

Together with the anesthesia team, a plan must be accomplished to minimize postoperative pain and analgesics requirement, which can involve epidural anesthesia/analgesia or a peripheral nerve block. These can be performed prior or immediately after surgery. Nausea and vomits prophylaxis should also be considered according to each surgical procedure and in high-risk patients. Oral/enteral feedings and physical mobilization should be started as early as possible. Tubes and catheters should be avoided or removed precociously. Every effort should be made so the child can have a safe and early discharge. Family support should be guaranteed during the admission and after discharge, reassuring they will have response to all of their concerns.

17.7 Conclusion

Optimal treatment for frail children may be challenging and requires an experienced pediatric-centered multidisciplinary team. The surgeon, together with the rest of the team and family, must bear in mind associated disorders, possible altered anatomy and physiology, and potential complications that may occur. Whenever there is a potentially surgical condition, the surgical indication must be analyzed considering risks and benefits. After the decision has been made, the team should carefully plan the procedure and implement individual pre-, peri-, and postoperative care for the child's best interest.

References

1. France G, Taroni F, Donatini A. The Italian health-care system. Health Econ. 2005;14(Suppl 1):S187–202.
2. Capone A. Towards an effective assessment of the sustainability of health interventions. Ig Sanita Pubbl. 2019;75(3):189–99.
3. Murphy Salem S, Graham RJ. Chronic illness in pediatric critical care. Front Pediatr. 2021;9:686206. https://doi.org/10.3389/fped.2021.686206.
4. Sacchetti A, Sacchetti C, Carraccio C, Gerardi M. The potential for errors in children with special health care needs. Acad Emerg Med. 2000;7(11):1330–3.
5. McAteer JP, LaRiviere CA, Drugas GT, Abdullah F, Oldham KT, Goldin AB. Influence of surgeon experience, hospital volume, and specialty designation on outcomes in pediatric surgery. JAMA Pediatr. 2013;167(5):468–75. https://doi.org/10.1001/jamapediatrics.2013.25.
6. Hamonet-Torny J, Le Bellego D, Jasper E, Suc A-L, Fourcade L. Regional consensus on the health care pathway of disabled children in surgery. Ann Phys Rehabil Med. 2016;59:e47. https://doi.org/10.1016/j.rehab.2016.07.109.
7. Okun A. Children who have special health-care needs: ethical issues. Pediatr Rev. 2010;31(12):514–7. https://doi.org/10.1542/pir.31-12-514.
8. Adams RC, Levy SE. Shared decision-making and children with disabilities: pathways to consensus. Pediatrics. 2017;139(6):956. https://doi.org/10.1542/peds.2017-0956.
9. Calkins CM, Oldham KT. Surgical problems of children with physical disabilities. In: Pediatric surgery. Cham: Springer Nature; 2020. p. 541–58. https://doi.org/10.1007/978-3-662-43588-5_36.
10. De Luca U, Mangia G, Tesoro S, Martino A, Sammartino M, Calisti A. Guidelines on pediatric day surgery of the Italian Societies of Pediatric Surgery (SICP) and Pediatric Anesthesiology (SARNePI). Ital J Pediatr. 2018;44(1):1–10. https://doi.org/10.1186/s13052-018-0473-1.
11. Shinnick JK, Short HL, Heiss KF, Santore MT, Blakely ML, Raval MV. Enhancing recovery in pediatric surgery: a review of the literature. J Surg Res. 2016;202(1):165–76. https://doi.org/10.1016/j.jss.2015.12.051.
12. Reismann M, von Kampen M, Laupichler B, Suempelmann R, Schmidt AI, Ure BM. Fast-track surgery in infants and children. J Pediatr Surg. 2007;42(1):234–8. https://doi.org/10.1016/j.jpedsurg.2006.09.022.
13. Lopes-júnior LC, Bomfim E, Olson K, et al. Effectiveness of hospital clowns for symptom management in paediatrics: systematic review of randomised and non-randomised controlled trials. Br Med J. 2020;371:m4290. https://doi.org/10.1136/bmj.m4290.
14. Van Der Heijden MJE, Araghi SO, Van Dijk M, Jeekel J, Hunink MGM. The effects of perioperative music interventions in pediatric surgery: a systematic review and meta-analysis of randomized controlled trials. PLoS One. 2015;10(8):1–11. https://doi.org/10.1371/journal.pone.0133608.
15. Viani K, Trehan A, Manzoli B, Schoeman J. Assessment of nutritional status in children with cancer: a narrative review. Pediatr Blood Cancer. 2020;67(S3):1–9. https://doi.org/10.1002/pbc.28211.
16. Calcaterra V, Cena H, Ruggieri A, et al. Metabolically unhealthy phenotype: a key factor in determining "pediatric" frailty. Pediatr Rep. 2021;13(3):340–6. https://doi.org/10.3390/PEDIATRIC13030042.
17. Schukfeh N, Kuebler JF, Dingemann J, Ure BM. Thirty years of minimally invasive surgery in children: analysis of meta-analyses. Eur J Pediatr Surg. 2020;30(5):420–8. https://doi.org/10.1055/s-0039-1687901.
18. Endo K, Sata N, Ishiguro Y, et al. A patient-specific surgical simulator using preoperative imaging data: an interactive simulator using a three-dimensional tactile mouse. J Comput Surg. 2014;1(1):2–9. https://doi.org/10.1186/s40244-014-0010-5.

Transitional Medicine, from Childhood to Adulthood

18

Andrea Pession

18.1 Definitions of Health Care Transition

Several definitions exist to describe Health care transition (HCT). In its simplest term, the transition is defined as "the planned process of chronically ill adolescents from a child-centred to an adult-centred system of care" [1]. In a more detailed way, we could also define HCT as "a purposeful, planned process that addresses the medical, psychosocial, educational, and vocational needs of adolescents and young adults with chronic medical conditions, as they advance from a paediatric and family-centred to an adult, individually focused health care provider" [2], but for us, HCT is "the process of moving from a child/family-centred model of health care to an adult/patient-centred model of health care, with or without transferring to a new clinician."

Concerning the apparent contradiction of being able to carry out the HCT process without changing the reference clinic, this fact can be explained not so much by the existence of dedicated services capable of taking care of a specific pathology in all phases of life, but rather by the possibility that some pathological fragility conditions occur after the age of 10, that is, in an adolescent age group that can be taken care of by services dedicated to adult medicine. The latter, however, should not underestimate the need to structure HCT courses for the population thus taken care of.

It is clear, that even a healthy child would have the right to transition to adult medicine in a gradual and planned way, but this aspect is beyond the scope of this volume dedicated to frailty and therefore to HCT in the strict sense. However, it is essential to emphasize, especially here, that at present, transitional medicine still deals almost exclusively with the transition to adult medicine of a paediatric subject (10–18 years) suffering from a chronic disease and/or the long-term side effects of the treatment received for that disease.

I therefore feel it is useful to draw the reader's attention, first of all, to the subject of adolescence, since it is the lack of knowledge of the peculiarities of this complex age which causes the greatest difficulties in planning and realizing the transition.

18.2 Adolescence

Adolescence can be defined as the 'transition phase between childhood and adulthood'. This definition could be reductive if one considers that adolescence is a rather long and important period

A. Pession (✉)
Pediatrics Unit, IRCCS Azienda Ospedaliero Universitaria di Bologna, Bologna, BO, Italy
e-mail: andrea.pession@unibo.it

M. Lima, M. C. Mondardini (eds.), *Frailty in Children*,
https://doi.org/10.1007/978-3-031-24307-3_18

of life consisting of complex and specific dynamics with important physical and psychological changes that can be at the basis of organic and behavioural pathologies. It is not necessarily a 'difficult' period of life, but it certainly requires special attention, bringing into play elements that may affect the future development of the young person. It is recognized that many of the biological and neuropsychological characteristics of adolescents, as well as their main causes of morbidity and mortality, have their specificities, which differentiate them from both childhood and adult life [3, 4].

The many physical, sexual, cognitive, social, and emotional changes that occur during adolescence determine a profound reshaping of the boy's identity. These changes are rapid and often radical: the boy finds himself unconsciously passing, most of the time in an inadequate way, from a carefree phase, such as the childhood period, to a phase of growing uncertainties from which worries arise. So, we can say that adolescence is that phase of life during which the individual begins to acquire the skills and requirements necessary to assume the responsibilities typical of adulthood. In the process of transitioning to adulthood under normal health conditions, biological, psychological, and social factors come into play and interact with each other.

Classically, adolescence is the age between 10 and 18 years, although the American Society of Adolescent Medicine identifies the upper limit at 21 years … and beyond! This extension of the upper limit is because today's youth, due to a variety of social changes over time, require more time to educate themselves, access the world of work, and achieve economic independence later, as well as the responsibilities and roles of adult social life, such as marriage and parenthood.

Adolescence is generally divided into three phases

- Early adolescence (10–12 years). It is the phase characterized by rapid somatic growth and the beginning of pubertal development. Group life and the search for greater independence within the family begin. On a cognitive level, the capacity for abstraction and depth of thought increase, and on a behavioural level, the search for one's own identity predominates.
- Second adolescence (13–15 years). In this phase, somatic and pubertal development is completed. Group life is consolidated and risk behaviour begins (alcohol, smoking, early sex, eating disorders). There are the first sexual relationships, often with unstable partners. On a cognitive level, there is a greater definition of one's goals, and contrasts with the adult world begin.
- Third adolescence (16–18 years). At this stage, concerns about social inclusion and economic independence begin. Risk behaviours are reduced and couple ties become more stable. More mature and responsible behaviour is accompanied by a resumption of dialogue with the family.

We can consider adolescence as a change that can be considered a real rebirth, in which the individual is completely renewed in appearance and personality, with changes so rapid that it often makes it difficult to understand them, especially for educators distracted by the rhythms of life and values that in many societies of industrialized countries do not allow sufficiently dedicated parenting.

Physical change begins at a varying age, usually earlier for females (11–13 years) and later for males (12–14 years), and continues until reaching adulthood, that is, until about age 21. Full brain maturation occurs even later, completing at the age of 24. From the biological point of view, some processes—hormonal, metabolic, and neuronal—are typical of this time window and cannot be properly associated either with childhood or adulthood. The body changes quickly and in a disharmonious way, the adolescent sees his stature grow and increase. His physique matures, with the development of secondary sexual characteristics: there is an increase in the odour of body secretions, the oiliness of skin and hair, and the appearance of acne. It is clear, therefore, that this period presents complex dynamics and requires multidisciplinary attention. It goes towards a full somatic maturation and completion of sexual development. The adolescent is aware of this, of the progressive independence implemented primarily with the detachment from parental figures, as well as the search for his own identity and self-esteem, in relation to new guiding figures. As far as cognitive development is concerned, the adolescent reaches the operant-formal stage, can systematically organize knowledge and thinks in hypothetical-deductive terms, acquiring the ability to formulate abstract thought. With a new self-awareness, the adolescent is no longer intent on understanding the rules to accept them, but wants to understand, to know, to affirm his precise identity in the group as well as in society. It is the era of experimentation with one's own body: clothing, haircuts, tattoos, piercings. A recent survey shows that adolescents face their sexual life knowing the risks of HIV, but not of other sexually transmitted infections; they hardly orient themselves through a multitude of information, sometimes erroneous, and rarely practice contraception correctly. Changes from the physical sphere explode and involve the sphere of instincts and emotions, which are perceived more intensely, but confusedly. Adolescents are poised between the need for independence and the lack of autonomy, they are conceited and shy, selfish and generous at the same time, they enjoy going against traditions, they can't stand constraints, they demand their independence, they defend their ideas, the more vigorously they are hindered by parental authority. The adolescent is in an unstable mood, may have moments of verbal or physical rebellion and then suddenly turn in on himself, to the point of isolation. He may take extreme positions with the use of smoking, alcohol, and drugs and may manifest mood disorders, aggression towards his body, and eating disorders. All this generates confusion and bewilderment in those around him: the parents, astonished spectators of this metamorphosis, do not recognize in this "strange and alien" boy, the son who was until that moment. Being a parent of an adolescent imposes the fundamental task of reassuring, welcoming, understanding, transmitting trust and security, being ready to listen "on demand", to "walk beside", and to dialogue when possible. Adolescents, in fact, still need more and more to be recognized, to enjoy their rightful freedom, but also to have precise boundaries within which to stay and feel protected. In any case, everyone will have his or her personal path, but after a variable period, the unstable attitude of the adolescent will give way to the attainment of a maturation stage typical of the adult, in which the subject is capable of taking care of himself or herself in daily life and assumes an independent and responsible role in society. Finally, adolescents cannot be lumped together in terms of diagnosis, therapy, and need for psychological support with any of the other ages of life and, therefore, constitute a specific management difficulty. It is inferred, moreover, precisely because of the completion of pubertal development and, therefore, of sexual differentiation, that the approach to gender medicine begins in adolescence. Associated with this is the phenomenon, already described, of experimentation and identification with new figures, a phenomenon that can complicate the management of a cure where a chronic condition is present. All these aspects are further complicated by the process of acceptance of one's body image and the exercise of sexuality, with possible concerns about future fertility. Adolescence, therefore, carries within itself the germ of physical and psychological change, with the search for new lifestyles in keeping with one's identity. If we consider that lifestyle is the cornerstone of future health and impacts on treatments in the presence of pathologies already established, we understand how, even in terms of prevention, this phase of life is associated with important health issues. Although there is the idea that the adolescent is a healthy individual, some studies have observed that about 20–25% of subjects may have medical problems, suggesting that this age of life needs a path and/or dedicated and specific knowledge (**Adolescent medicine**) [5].

Adolescents with a long-term illness generally experienced well-being like everyone else. Three themes were found to be important for feeling well: "a feeling of acceptance of illness/disability as a natural part of life," "a feeling of support," and "a feeling of personal growth." Adolescents with long-term illnesses or disabilities experience well-being when they are allowed to prepare to live a normal life with respect to their new value system that allows for their integration into society. In other words, even the normal canons of quality of life assessment must be re-evaluated specifically for different diseases and age groups. Health care providers, however, need to focus on the care of the young person rather than the illness.

Present-day society has produced changes in family living patterns and conditions, and this has resulted in new stressors and health problems. Most children and adolescents with chronic diseases and disabilities, who were previously cared for at hospitals and institutions for long periods, are now integrated into society and they are expected to live a normal life in the conditions that currently prevail.

18.3 Health Care Transition

The issue of HCT is of absolute importance and topicality, because of its repercussions on the care plan. For this reason, it must be the object of careful reflection by paediatricians, who represent a fundamental component of the transition process. Paediatricians must deal with transition in a more conscious and effective way because some studies have shown that an inadequate transition process for adolescents affected by chronic diseases is associated with a worsening of their health status.

The goal of HCT is twofold, namely: (1) to ensure an organized process in paediatric and adult health care practices to facilitate transition preparation, transfer of care, and integration into adult-centred health care; and (2) to improve the ability of youth and young adults with and without special health care needs to manage their health care and effectively use health services.

It is clear, as explained in the second objective, that even a healthy child would have the right to transition to adult medicine in a gradual and planned way, but this aspect is beyond the scope of this volume dedicated to frailty and therefore to HCT in the strict sense.

The number of young people with long-term illnesses/disabilities has increased worldwide during the last decades. There is a lack of studies relating to the way young people regard their daily lives and factors that are important for their well-being. Improvements in chronic disease management have led to increasing numbers of fragile youth transitioning to adult healthcare. Poor transition can lead to high risks of morbidity and mortality for these citizens. For the child with a chronic or rare disease, who needs continuous care for his frailty, it is particularly delicate, the transition from paediatric care to those of the general practitioner and the specialist of the hospital centre of reference for adults, in a period of life already affected by risk behaviours typical of adolescence. Some international studies document that in this phase is higher the risk that children "get lost", abandon treatments, and do not undergo periodic check-ups, with the real danger of facing long-term complications and increased mortality [6–8]. Hence the growing attention of the medical and scientific community to the so-called "transition" of adolescents suffering from chronic diseases from a child-centred care system to an adult-oriented one. Transition is intended to prevent the loss of these patients to follow-up, which is frequently reported during this period, as well as ensure the autonomy of care. Unfortunately, in the current state of the art, the process is usually not well coordinated and is still too little widespread and standardized. Typically, a formalized transition programme is often associated with significantly lower pre-transition anxiety and greater post-transition satisfaction.

The process of health care transition (HCT) includes initial planning, the transfer itself, and the support provided during adulthood. The crucial steps to be taken for this type of medical practice are shown in Table 18.1. The steps shown in Table 18.1 are in part those proposed by The American Academy of Pediatrics and American Society of Internal Medicine consensus [9] modified according to the author's experience and

Table 18.1 Steps in the transition from child-oriented to adult-oriented healthcare

Step		Comment
1.	Identify a healthcare professional who attends to the care coordination and future healthcare planning	Small group work is preferable
2.	Identify the foundational knowledge and skills required to provide developmentally appropriate health transition services to the chronically ill patient with a specific disease	Disease-specific knowledge acquisition in transition curriculum does not necessarily correlate to task-completion skills
3.	Prepare a medical summary that provides the common knowledge base for collaboration among health care professionals engaged on both the paediatric and adult fronts	A formalized transition programme is often associated with significantly lower pre-transition anxiety and higher post-transition satisfaction
4.	Establish a written health transition plan by age 14–16 involving the youth and their caregivers and family in its development	Teams should partner with young adults to choose the right transition time considering that age at transfer initiation is not associated with satisfaction or perceived readiness to transfer
5.	Try as much as possible to move along the same guidelines adopted by the primary and preventive care service for all adolescents and young adults	Evidence-based medicine is key to optimizing resource allocation
6.	Plan periodic checks on the application of the agreed programmes, intervening on critical issues with appropriate corrective actions, with particular attention in the peri-transitional period	It is essential not to take for granted the success of the transition at the time of handover and appropriate to periodically monitor the cases entrusted to the adult specialist with whom a periodic epicritic evaluation is appropriate, especially concerning the resources dedicated

supplemented with specific comments deduced from the literature in the field.

To facilitate the implementation of HCT Programmes, Got Transition's Six Core Elements of Health Care Transition™ 3.0 is the widely adopted approach called for in the 2018 Clinical Report on Health Care Transition from the American Academy of Pediatrics, the American Academy of Family Physicians, and the American College of Physicians. The Six Core Elements considered define the basic components of a structured transition process and include customizable sample tools for each core element. The Six Core Elements are tailored to the type of practice facilitating the health care transition and are presented in three distinct packages [10].

A recent review strengthens the evidence that a structured HCT process for youth with special health care needs can show improvements in adherence to care, disease-specific measures, quality of life, self-care skills, satisfaction with care, health care utilization, and HCT process of care [11].

Currently, most countries have no guidelines on health care transition based on systematic evidence research and the process is primarily organized in local settings, partly based on disease-specific guidelines.

The existing guidelines have important limitations. Most of the actual recommendations for the HCT of young people are disease-specific, but not evidence-based, and are conducted on many chronic diseases, conditions, and intellectual and developmental disabilities, including HIV/AIDS [12, 13], type 1 diabetes [14], sickle cell disease [15], chronic kidney disease [16], autism spectrum disorder [17], and cancer [18], among others less relevant.

Only a few high-quality studies, i.e. RCTs, are available on HCT [19, 20], so evidence-based statements are possible for some, but not all, areas. Moreover, only three adult patient representatives and no adolescents/young adults themselves were involved in the Delphi consensus process. This could have strengthened the quality of the guidelines, especially in terms of their applicability and transferability.

Recently a National Institutes of Health Workshop titled Navigating Paediatric to Adult Health Care Transition has been published. The terms, criteria, standards, and actions to be taken for the planning of HCT are set in a kind of milestone for the future [21].

Transition is too often treated as an event, instead of being viewed as a gradual process of empowerment of all parties, including the patient and his or her caregivers, involved in the various care settings. Regarding this point, it is clear that during and also following the transfer, therapeutic education for the parents, as well as the young adults, requires reinforcement [22].

Risk and vulnerability encompass many dimensions of the transition from adolescence to adulthood, and the transition from paediatric, parent-supervised health care to more independent, patient-centred adult health care is no exception. There is evidence for increases in emergency hospital visits when young people with life-limiting conditions transition to adult health care. These changes are not observed for comparator groups—young people with diabetes and young people with no known long-term conditions, suggesting they are not due to other transitions happening at similar ages [23]. Special attention must therefore be paid to the most fragile cases at risk of life-threatening critical episodes.

Recently, HCT has evolved from a focus on paediatric care responsibility to a shared responsibility of paediatric and adult clinicians (physicians, nurses, social workers, and other health care providers working together to provide patient care). The crucial role of adult care clinicians in accepting and collaborating with young adults is still not only an issue of dedicated resources, but rather a challenge of education and professional training. Indeed, young adults are increasingly recognized as a vulnerable population not only in terms of their high rates of behavioural health risks but also their susceptibility to the emergence or worsening of chronic health conditions and traditionally low health care utilization.

In addition, many young adults view health care as a low priority compared to other dimensions of their adult transition (education, employment, housing, relationships, and recreation). Coordinated and dedicated HCT efforts are therefore needed to increase awareness among youth, young adults, and their families that health maintenance and continuity of care are central to achieving broader adult goals [24].

In conclusion, the transition from paediatric to adult health care represents a critical time in an adolescent's developmental trajectory, regardless of background. For youth with chronic conditions and/or developmental disabilities, this changeover can be even more critical with significant and lifelong implications. Future efforts to improve available resources and provider preparedness are and will be increasingly essential to meeting the unmet needs of frail patients.

References

1. Carrizosa J, An I, Appleton R, Camfield P, Von Moers A. Models for transition clinics. Epilepsia. 2014;55(Suppl 3):46–51. https://doi.org/10.1111/epi.12716.
2. Mohammed A, Nadeem M, Yousif T. Towards safe and effective transition from adolescence to adult care. Sudan J Paediatr. 2017;17(1):10–3.
3. Bertelloni S. Adolescentologia. Percorsi medici e socio-educativi. Milan: Tecniche Nuove Ed; 2010.
4. Sawyer SM, Azzopardi PS, Wickremarathne D, Patton GC. The age of adolescence. Lancet Child Adolesc Health. 2018;2(3):223–8. https://doi.org/10.1016/S2352-4642(18)30022-1.
5. Mackenzie RG. Adolescent medicine: a model for the millennium. Adolesc Med. 2000;11(1):13–8.
6. Macher MA, Novo R, Baudouin V. Transition de soins de l'enfance et de l'adolescence à l'âge adulte en néphrologie [Transition of care from childhood and adolescence to adulthood in nephrology]. Med Sci (Paris). 2022;38(2):182–90.
7. Mollah T, Lee D, Giles E. Impact of a new young adult inflammatory bowel disease transition clinic on patient satisfaction and clinical outcomes. J Paediatr Child Health. 2022;58(6):15907. https://doi.org/10.1111/jpc.15907.
8. Narang I, Kendzerska T, Heffernan A, Malik U, Carvalho CG, Ryan CM. Positive airway pressure usage in youth with obstructive sleep apnea following transition to adult health care. Nat Sci Sleep.

2022;2(14):153–63. https://doi.org/10.2147/NSS.S345143.
9. American Academy of Pediatrics, American Academy of Family Physicians; American College of Physicians-American Society of Internal Medicine. A consensus statement on health care transitions for young adults with special health care needs. Pediatrics. 2002;110:1304–6.
10. https://www.gottransition.org/six-core-elements/.
11. Schmidt A, Ilango SM, McManus MA, Rogers KK, White PH. Outcomes of pediatric to adult health care transition interventions: an updated systematic review. J Pediatr Nurs. 2020;51:92–107. https://doi.org/10.1016/j.pedn.2020.01.002.
12. Tanner AE, Philbin MM, Chambers BD, Ma A, Hussen S, Ware S, Lee S, Fortenberry JD. Healthcare transition for youth living with HIV: outcomes from a prospective multi-site study. J Adolesc Health. 2018;63(2):157–65. https://doi.org/10.1016/j.jadohealth.2018.02.004.
13. Yusuf H, Agwu A. Adolescents and young adults with early acquired HIV infection in the United States: unique challenges in treatment and secondary prevention. Expert Rev Anti-Infect Ther. 2020;19:457–71.
14. Monaghan M, Baumann K. Type 1 diabetes: addressing the transition from pediatric to adult-oriented health care. Res Rep Endocr Disord. 2016;6:31–40. https://doi.org/10.2147/RRED.S56609.
15. Kayle M, Docherty SL, Sloane R, Tanabe P, Maslow G, Pan W, Shah N. Transition to adult care in sickle cell disease: a longitudinal study of clinical characteristics and disease severity. Pediatr Blood Cancer. 2019;66(1):e27463. https://doi.org/10.1002/pbc.27463.
16. Javalkar K, Fenton N, Cohen S, Ferris M. Socioecologic factors as predictors of readiness for self-management and transition, medication adherence, and health care utilization among adolescents and young adults with chronic kidney disease. Prev Chronic Dis. 2014;11:E117.
17. Cheak-Zamora NC, Teti M, Maurer-Batjer A, Koegler E. Exploration and comparison of adolescents with autism spectrum disorder and their caregiver's perspectives on transitioning to adult health care and adulthood. J Pediatr Psychol. 2017;42(9):1028–39. https://doi.org/10.1093/jpepsy/jsx075.
18. Otth M, Denzler S, Koenig C, Koehler H, Scheinemann K. Transition from pediatric to adult follow-up care in childhood cancer survivors—a systematic review. J Cancer Surviv. 2021;15(1):151–62. https://doi.org/10.1007/s11764-020-00920-9.
19. Becker J, Ravens E, Pape L, Ernst G. Somatic outcomes of young people with chronic diseases participating in transition programs: a systematic review. J Transit Med. 2020;2(1):0003. https://doi.org/10.1515/jtm-2020-0003.
20. Ravens E, Becker J, Pape L, Ernst G. Psychosocial benefit and adherence of adolescents with chronic diseases participating in transition programs: a systematic review. J Transit Med. 2020;2(1):0009. https://doi.org/10.1515/jtm-2020-0009.
21. Calabrese S, Lee S, Mollica MA, Wiener L, Mendley S, Adams L, Blachman-Demner D. Navigating pediatric to adult health care transition: a national institutes of health workshop. J Pediatr. 2022;244:234–40. https://doi.org/10.1016/j.jpeds.2022.01.052.
22. Vion Genovese V, Perceval M, Gauchet A, Buscarlet-Jardine L, Pinsault N, Allenet B, Llerena C. Comment améliorer la transition au sein des CRCM: analyse des besoins des patients et de leurs parents lors de l'arrivée en service adulte [How can the transition of adolescents from a children's to an adult CF center be improved? Analysis of adolescents' and parents' needs during the post-transfer period]. Rev Mal Respir. 2022;39:132–9. https://doi.org/10.1016/j.rmr.2022.01.006.
23. Jarvis S, Flemming K, Richardson G, Fraser L. Adult healthcare is associated with more emergency healthcare for young people with life-limiting conditions. Pediatr Res. 2022;92:1458–69. https://doi.org/10.1038/s41390-022-01975-3.
24. White PH, Cooley WC. Supporting the health care transition from adolescence to adulthood in the medical home. Pediatrics. 2018;142(5):e20182587.

GPSR Compliance

The European Union's (EU) General Product Safety Regulation (GPSR) is a set of rules that requires consumer products to be safe and our obligations to ensure this.

If you have any concerns about our products, you can contact us on ProductSafety@springernature.com

In case Publisher is established outside the EU, the EU authorized representative is:

Springer Nature Customer Service Center GmbH
Europaplatz 3
69115 Heidelberg, Germany

Batch number: 09224018

Printed by Printforce, the Netherlands